JOB READINESS
for HEALTH PROFESSIONALS
SOFT SKILLS STRATEGIES FOR SUCCESS

SECOND EDITION

EVOLVE STUDY RESOURCES **FREE WITH TEXTBOOK PURCHASE**
EVOLVE.ELSEVIER.COM

ELSEVIER

ELSEVIER
SAUNDERS

3251 Riverport Lane
St. Louis, Missouri 63043

JOB READINESS for HEALTH PROFESSIONALS:
SOFT SKILLS STRATEGIES for SUCCESS, Second Edition

ISBN: 9780323430265

Notices

Knowledge and best practice in this field are constantly changing. As new research and experience broaden our understanding, changes in research methods, professional practices, or medical treatment may become necessary.

Practitioners and researchers must always rely on their own experience and knowledge in evaluating and using any information, methods, compounds, or experiments described herein. In using such information or methods they should be mindful of their own safety and the safety of others, including parties for whom they have a professional responsibility.

With respect to any drug or pharmaceutical products identified, readers are advised to check the most current information provided (i) on procedures featured or (ii) by the manufacturer of each product to be administered, to verify the recommended dose or formula, the method and duration of administration, and contraindications. It is the responsibility of practitioners, relying on their own experience and knowledge of their patients, to make diagnoses, to determine dosages and the best treatment for each individual patient, and to take all appropriate safety precautions.

To the fullest extent of the law, neither the Publisher nor the authors, contributors, or editors, assume any liability for any injury and/or damage to persons or property as a matter of products liability, negligence or otherwise, or from any use or operation of any methods, products, instructions, or ideas contained in the material herein.

Library of Congress Cataloging-in-Publication Data
Job readiness for health professionals : soft skills strategies for success.—Second edition.
    p. ; cm.
Includes bibliographical references and index.
ISBN 978-0-323-43026-5 (pbk. : alk. paper)
[DNLM: 1. Health Occupations.   2. Vocational Guidance.   W 21]
R690
610.73'7069—dc23

                                                2015032344

Senior Vice President and Director: Loren Wilson
Content Strategist: Jennifer Janson
Content Development Manager: Ellen Wurm-Cutter
Content Development Specialist: Brandi Graham, Erin Garner
Publishing Services Manager: Jeffrey Patterson
Project Manager: Sara Alsup
Designer: Ryan Cook

Printed in China

Last digit is the print number: 9 8 7 6 5 4 3 2 1

WILLIAM G. BROTTMILLER, Project Manager
Chairman, Institute for Management Studies (IMS)
Mattapoisett, Massachusetts

LEE HAROUN, MA (Education), MBA, EdD
Health Care Writer
Former Director of Maric College, San Diego
Former Regional Director of Education, Quest Education Corporation
Sunriver, Oregon

MICHELE JAWAD, CDA, RDA, BS, M.Ed
Dental Clinic Supervisor, Buchanan Dental Clinic
University of California San Francisco
San Francisco, California

JENNIFER KELLY, MA, CDA
Associate Director, Professional and Continuing Education
Chaminade University
Honolulu, Hawaii

KELLY A. ROSE, D.M.D.,CDA
Dental Assisting Instructor
Greater Lawrence Technical School
Andover, Massachusetts

REVIEWERS

GLENDA ALGAZE, CPhT, CDA, MEd
Dental Assisting Instructor, Pharmacy Technician
NAF Health Science Academy Leader
Miami Lakes Educational Center and Technical College
Miami, Florida

DEBRA BLAIS, LPN
Career Services Coordinator, Medical Assistant/
 Medical Office Specialist Instructional Lead
Nevada Career Institute
Las Vegas, Nevada

L. TAYLOR DEATHERAGE, CPC
Medical Coding Instructor
Tulsa Technology Center
Tulsa, Oklahoma

JENNIFER L. DILLARD, RMA (AMT)
Former Medical Program Chair
Everest College
Thornton, Colorado

TAMELA FREEMAN, BS, CMAA, CEHRS, CBCS
Medical Office Support Instructor
Sierra Nevada Job Corps Center
Reno, Nevada

LISA HUEHNS, M.A. Ed
Allied Health Instructor (AMT)
Lakeshore Technical College
Cleveland, Wisconsin

**BETH M. LAURENZ, MBA, BS Healthcare
 Management, AAS, CMA, Health IT certifications**
Clinician Practitioner Consultant, Implementation
 Manager, Project Management
Director of Healthcare Education
National College
Columbus, Ohio

AMY DIANE LAWRENCE, MBA/HR, CPC, CCA
Online Program Chair for Medical Administrative
 Assistant and Medical Office Billing Specialist
Ultimate Medical Academy
Tampa, Florida

BRIGITTE NIEDZWIECKI
Medical Assistant Program Director
Chippewa Valley Technical College
Eau Claire, Wisconsin

JUDITH PERELLA-ZIRKLE, MEd
Certified and Registered Dental Assistant, Director of
 Dental Assisting
Cumberland County Technical Education Center
Bridgeton, New Jersey

ELIZABETH ANN PETRELLA, MSN, RN
President and CEO
Genesee Health Careers
Flint, Michigan

**JULIE POPE, CMA(AAMA), CPMA, CPC,
 CPC-H, CPC-I**
Program Director
ATA College
Louisville, Kentucky

CYNTHIA LEWIS PORTER, CDA, EFDA, PhD
Dental Coordinator
Centura College
Norfolk, Virginia

TRACY TOMKO SCHLIEP, RN
Allied Health Instructor, Healthcare Consultant
Laurel Technical Institute
Sharon, Pennsylvania

JAIME TRACKTENBERG, BS
Program Manager, Assessment and Training
Goodwill of Southwestern Pennsylvania
Pittsburgh, Pennsylvania

**BARBARA A. WILSON, MHA, BSEd, CPC, CCS-P,
 RHIT, CRC, CIMC, CPC-P, CPMA**
Director of Coding Operations/Medical Billing and
 Coding Education Consultant
I-Code-For-You
Charlotte, North Carolina

AUDREY A. WOZNIAK, BS, AHI, RMA, EMT
MTTI/Women and Infant's Hospital
Seekonk, Massachusetts

MINDY WRAY, MA, BS, CMA(AAMA), RMA
Program Director, Medical Assisting
ECPI University
Greensboro, North Carolina

Health professionals get jobs because of their hard skills—their clinical skills and their knowledge of their profession. They *keep* jobs because of their soft skills.

Experts often possess more data than judgment.
                                                    –Colin Powell

Soft skills are about judgment and are influenced by your personality and thinking processes. They help you get along with your supervisor and your co-workers, and they enable you to be empathetic toward your patients, clients, and customers. In the long run, your soft skills may be even more important than your hard skills. Health professionals want to work with other health professionals who are kind, friendly, helpful, hard-working, punctual, team players, and flexible. Employers will not tolerate employees with toxic attitudes.

This book is about the soft skills you will need to keep and prosper in your job. Soft skills will help you earn friends, accomplishments, and promotions in your career as a health professional.

Background

Too often, the lack of soft skills holds people back in their careers and causes them to fall short of their hopes and potential. We designed this book to give you the tools necessary in fulfilling your career goals.

How We Made Sure the Content of This Book Will Help You Succeed

There are thousands of soft skills. We identified the ones that will contribute the most to the success of health professionals. We received extensive surveys from 135 health professions instructors, who know students well and possess a deep understanding of what it takes to excel on the job. Feedback came from Vo-Techs, Career Colleges, Community Colleges, and Colleges and Universities. These health professionals all work with local employers, place students in externships, and write recommendations for prospective employees.

We also asked our survey participants about how to format and teach these skills, and they generously contributed ideas and learning strategies that have worked well in their professional experience. We are grateful for the expertise they provided. The format and features they suggested are explained further in *Distinctive Features of this Text.*

Opportunities for Employment

Many young health professionals are getting jobs, but losing them. Although many health professionals are well qualified, many lack the experience necessary to know how to act on the job. Losing a job can be devastating. The soft skills discussed in this book will help you become a valuable addition to the healthcare field.

As a healthcare professional, you must possess empathy and offer meaningful care to your patients. You have worked hard to learn the skills and knowledge of your profession, as well as prepared yourself for required licensures, certifications, and entry qualifications. New therapies for diseases, disorders, and conditions are discovered and implemented every day. More elderly and disabled people are seeking complex care, living in assisted care facilities, and trying to discover ways to preserve their health as they seek more active lives and live longer than ever before. As a health professional, you have made a great choice. Your career opportunities are astounding! Make the most out of all of the opportunities available to you by thriving in your new job.

Who will benefit from this book?

Whether you are a student, a recent graduate, or a new employee in the health professions, this book is for you. Every new employee in any field needs soft skills to succeed. We have focused on the health professions because they present special challenges.

Jobs in the health professions can be stressful. People seeking health care can be difficult because they are often sick, in pain, or anxious. They are often surrounded by their concerned family members. Much of this anxiety is projected onto the health professionals. You must master the soft skills needed to handle stress. Healthcare workers endure long hours and unique pressures as they uphold standards of care and follow procedures. Even co-workers and supervisors can present additional challenges. Healthcare careers are rewarding, but they are not easy.

Approach

This book takes a storytelling approach, making knowledge vivid and memorable. Every patient has a story, and every shift at work tells a story.

Stories presented in Case Studies and "Down a Dark Road" vignettes are designed to illustrate what can happen to people who possess soft skills, and people who lack them.

Each skill is presented conversationally, summarizing the research and reasoning that supports it. The style is meant to be informal and engaging as well as authoritative. All the features explained below in *Distinctive Features of This Book* are designed to make your learning personal and engaging in order to relate this knowledge to your own life, background, abilities, and situation.

Organization

People learn to relate to the world using an "inside-out" process. Our personal experiences emerge in our self-talk which reflects our beliefs about ourselves and govern our behaviors.

This book is organized to reflect this process using six key focus points:
* Self-Management Skills
* Interpersonal Skills
* Communication Skills
* Career Building Skills
* Emotional Skills
* Go Forth and Prosper

The book is divided into 14 chapters. Within those 14 chapters, 48 soft skills are presented to promote your interactive learning.

Distinctive Features of this Textbook

Mastering soft skills is a highly engaged, hands-on process. We make every effort to involve you in this learning process through a series of activities and thought processes designed to help you relate and integrate these skills to your own life and circumstances.

Learning Objectives

We make extensive use of learning objectives because soft skills are all about the mental processes that contribute to behavior. You can always assess your learning by asking yourself if you are able to incorporate these objectives into your behavior.

Quotes

Quotes are fun and thought-provoking. They serve as touchstones for our changing thinking. The iconic actress Marlene Dietrich put it well:

I love quotations because it is a joy to find thoughts one might have, beautifully expressed with much authority by someone recognized wiser than oneself.
–Marlene Dietrich

Journal Boxes

We hope you will keep a journal as you read this book. Journals help you process and personalize this material. We suggest journal topics throughout the book, but we also hope you will add your own topics as you think of them. By the time you have read this book, you will have uniquely digested the material inside your journal. Your journal will serve as a personal version of this book. An example of a journal box is below.

> **◉← JOURNALING 2-1**
>
> Recall the last time you sought health care, whether at a walk-in clinic, a dentist's office, or a physical therapy appointment. Describe your impression of the facility. Recall the workers you interacted with. How were you treated? How did these interactions contribute to the overall impression you have of the facility?

What If? Boxes

We all know how challenging it can be to work as a health professional. Challenges occur at unexpected times in unexpected ways. Your success as a health professional depends on your ability to handle unexpected challenges. We include "What If?" boxes throughout the book to challenge your thinking with theoretical scenarios you might encounter. What If? boxes appear as follows:

> **? WHAT IF?**
>
> *What if you saw a fellow employee remove a $20 bill from a cash drawer that was open?*

Boxed Material

Content in boxes—lists and steps of a process—make information concise and memorable. It is easy to look up material that is boxed. Whenever we can summarize content or challenge your thinking, we try to box the material for you, as shown.

> **BOX 3-4**
>
> ### Diseases Caused by Stress
>
> - Diabetes
> - Hypertension
> - Metabolic syndrome
> - Atherosclerosis (hardening of the arteries)
> - Gastrointestinal disorders
> - Memory deficits
> - Ulcers
> - Sleep disorders
> - Depression

Case Studies

Much of the content of this book is presented in the form of Case Studies, one for each of the forty eight skills presented in this book. They are meant to bring each skill to life in a way that allows you to imagine how you would act when facing similar circumstances. We offer "Questions for Thought and Reflection" after each case study to promote comprehension.

"Down a Dark Road" Vignettes

There are also "Down a Dark Road" features for every skill discussed in the book. These stories illustrate what can go wrong when a new health professional fails to master a soft skill or take its importance seriously. These stories are meant to open your eyes to the real reasons why soft skills are absolutely essential to your success in your health care career.

Experiential Exercises

After each skill, we offer some experiential exercises you can practice outside of the classroom or off the job. You might even look at them before you read the skill material to gain advance insights. These exercises will help you learn more about yourself as well as the skill itself.

Cross Currents with Other Soft Skills

One of the most difficult aspects of writing a book about soft skills has been the effort to isolate one skill at a time, as if these skills are not interrelated. Therefore, "Cross Currents with Other Soft Skills" identify related skills and describe how they are related.

New Features in the Second Edition

Two All-New Chapters

Two all-new chapters have been added to the new edition, making *Job Readiness for Health Professionals* a comprehensive resource for introductory soft skills. **Being a Student** teaches skills that transcend to the workforce, including taking meaningful notes, tips for being successful when assessed, and preparing for a practicum. **Finding Your First Job** covers competencies that students need to consider and prepare for when they begin searching for their first job, including writing successful resumes and the art of interviewing.

Video Case Vignettes

Eight innovative video case studies are now available on Evolve. These vignettes provide real-life workplace scenarios for classroom discussion and student review. Video topics include:
1. Empathy: The Foundation of Caring
2. Active Listening: Connecting With Others
3. Communicating Effectively On the Job
4. Dealing with Conflict
5. Solving Problems and Making Decisions
6. Enhancing Your Promotability
7. Presenting Yourself to the Workplace
8. Interview Skills

For the Instructor

TEACH for *Job Readiness for the Health Professional* is designed to help health profession instructors prepare for class by reducing preparation time, providing new and innovative ideas to promote student learning, and helping to make full use of the rich array of resources available. Available on Evolve, TEACH includes:

* Detailed lesson plans
* Chapter-specific PowerPoint presentations

Additional instructor resources include:

* Examview Test Bank
* Video Case Assessments and Implementation Tools

A Note to the Reader

Everyone is pulling for your success. You have already done the hard part of your profession by learning the technical skills associated with your role. To complete your preparation and make you become successful and a well-rounded professional, challenge yourself to master these soft skills as well.

If you already possess some of these soft skills, share your gift and serve as a mentor to your colleagues.

Soft skills are all about personal growth. We will challenge you to step outside of your comfort zone and adopt an open mind. As the Supreme Court Judge Oliver Wendell Holmes explained it, "The imagination, once stretched by a new idea, never regains its original dimensions." Work is your canvas for achieving meaning, significance, accomplishments, and legacy. Use it to paint your masterpiece.

CONTENTS

SELF-MANAGEMENT SKILLS

CHAPTER 1

Who Are You?

- Understand your current attitude, and the reasons for your attitude.
- Explain the benefits of being organized.
- Develop a plan for managing your time.
- Differentiate between honesty and integrity.
- Define adaptability as an effective change strategy.
- Recognize that flexibility can lead to positive results.
- Identify the impact of dependability.

Adopting a Positive Mental Attitude

What the mind can conceive and believe, it can achieve.
—Napoleon Hill

LEARNING OBJECTIVE 1: ADOPTING A POSITIVE MENTAL ATTITUDE

- Analyze the origins of your attitude.
- Explain why people get and defend negative attitudes.
- Know the mechanics of changing your attitude.
- Choose the attitude you want to take to work.
- Define *self-talk* and how it affects you.
- List five strategies you can implement to make your attitude more positive.
- Adopt a strategy for personally managing change.
- Keep a journal and decide how you are going to use this tool.

Whether you've ever had a job or not, you already have an attitude toward work, and it is likely the one that you have toward life in general. Your attitude began forming when you were very young. It was created by the messages you got first from your parents and later from your teachers and friends and other influential people in your life. Now that you have an attitude, you constantly reinforce it with your self-talk—what you tell yourself every minute of every day. Your attitude expresses, both inwardly and outwardly, who you think you are.

The only question is whether your attitude is positive, negative, or somewhere in between—and whether or not you would like to change that.

Mental Attitudes

Abraham Lincoln once said, "In the end a man is more or less as happy as he makes up his mind to be." You might think that your attitude is a result of your experiences, and there is some truth to that. But mostly, your attitude is the result of your *interpretation* of your experiences.

Certainly, experiences that cause mental trauma or are accompanied by strong emotions, especially fear, can have a lasting effect. Victims of child abuse or neglect, for instance, have a lot to overcome on their way to personal achievements and satisfying relationships. Trust, once lost, is hard to recover, and without trust in others, we lack a basic tool in our quest for a satisfying life.

Fortunately, despite the fact that everyone has negative experiences in their past, most people can find ways to rise above their circumstances and live a happy, positive life if they really want to.

Negative Mental Attitudes

How many people would you predict face each day with a negative mental attitude?

Surveys suggest that at least 60% of people have a negative attitude toward their job (Figure 1-1). These people, of course, justify negative attitudes. Their supervisor doesn't like them. The work is demeaning. The pay is low. Various situations are unfair. The list goes on and on.

Still, some people in the exact same situation have positive attitudes. You may have noticed that unhappy

FIGURE 1-1 A frustrated health professional (Copyright © istock.com).

people always have explanations for why other people are happy and they are not. For instance, happy people don't have the stresses that unhappy people have. In reality, happy people experience the same challenges as everyone else, including job losses, problems with their children, money troubles, and disagreements with their loved ones. The main difference between happy people and unhappy people is attitude.

WHAT IF?

How would you respond to someone at work who is extremely negative?

One thing is for sure: Whether you are a happy person or an unhappy person, you see the world from your very own unique perspective, conditioned by your deep-set beliefs, experiences, and attitudes. These attitudes belong to you. Whether you know it or not, you act very aggressively to protect your attitudes because they are a big part of who you are. Everybody naturally rationalizes all of their experiences and circumstances in life, coloring them to fit in with their view of the world, their attitudes.

It is easy for people with negative attitudes to achieve their expectations, because they are so low. Failure has already been "pre-rationalized." Usually the blame for this supposed inevitability of failure is laid at the feet of other people and circumstances: *My parents liked my sister better. My brother was mean to me. My teacher put me in the lower class. I came from a bad neighborhood. I didn't go to college. The system is rigged.*

Surprisingly, many people with negative attitudes fear success. They may be afraid they will fail, or make things worse through their efforts. They may fear that opening doors to new opportunities may mean closing doors to comfortable options they have become used to; they focus on possible negative consequences rather than probable improvements. This can stop them from taking a few easy steps that would make their life better. Failure inevitably happens to everyone once in a while, but for people with negative attitudes, each failure serves to reinforce their fears: *I shouldn't have tried. Of course I failed; things always backfire when I step outside of my comfort zone. There is something wrong with me.* This negative self-talk reinforces their feeling that they have some imagined deficit or are undeserving. If something good happens, people with negative mental attitudes often attribute it to luck, rather than something they earned and deserved.

Positive Mental Attitudes

Just as we've seen with negative attitudes, a positive mental attitude is also a self-fulfilling prophecy. As the quote from Napoleon Hill at the beginning of this chapter says, "What the mind can conceive and believe, it can achieve." This thought isn't naïve or magical: successful people do have to work for their success. What Hill was suggesting, though, is that you have to fervently believe that success is possible before you can work for it. In other words, for hard word to lead to success, your attitude must be expectant, hopeful, resilient, persistent—in a word, positive. Of course, this is easier said than done. But the first step is to decide that you want to be positive, successful, and happy. Then, believe that these things are possible for you.

A pessimist sees the difficulty in every opportunity; an optimist sees the opportunity in every difficulty.

—Winston Churchill

To change the messages you may be sending yourself, stop and ask yourself this: "What are you thinking?" Everyone has chatter going on in their heads, conversations with yourself, personal observations, judgments, opinions, commentaries. This is your self-talk. Self-talk can reinforce negative attitudes or positive attitudes. So begin by becoming aware of your own self-talk. What are you saying to yourself? In general, is your self-talk critical, mean-spirited or judgmental? Or, in general, is it tolerant, generous or forgiving? Are you suspicious of people and their motives, or do you trust in people and believe their intentions are largely good? People with positive attitudes are not burdened by self-limiting beliefs; instead, they focus on giving and receiving positive messages; they seek out contact with other positive people. Typical positive messages can be seen in Box 1-1.

If you've been exposed to a negative environment, it's not too late to shake things up. When there is a choice to be made about the people, circumstances, and opportunities in your life, you don't have to be a prisoner of your upbringing. You can choose to be positive.

You see things; and you say, "Why?" But I dream things that never were; and I say, "Why not?"

—George Bernard Shaw

 WHAT IF?

How would you respond to someone at work who is extremely positive?

BOX 1-1

Positive Messages

- You can do it.
- Give it a try.
- I believe in you.
- Live up to your ability.
- You are one of a kind.
- You can figure it out.
- You are important to me.
- Let's do it together.
- Nothing can stop you.

If this feels new to you, start small. Sometimes it is incredibly easy to get what you want with a positive mental attitude. For instance, if you smile and greet someone, chances are good that you will get a smile and a greeting in response. If you make a habit of smiling at others, you'll begin to build your own positive reinforcements. Then, in general, you'll begin to notice that people with a sunny disposition attract other positive people. The positivity that goes with a great mental attitude brings many things into your life, including friends, opportunities, promotions, and happiness.

Negative Realities at Work

Certainly, there will always be aspects of your work that you dislike. You will have to perform tasks that are not your favorites, and you may not agree with every managerial initiative, or everything your supervisor says. You might have co-workers you don't care for. In this imperfect work world, you will have to accept some things you don't like. Let's examine these negative realities of work a little more closely.

Lack of Control

Life is full of things you cannot control, including many aspects of your job. You may be able to exert a minimal amount of influence upon, but cannot control, the leadership above you, the physical facilities, or the mix of patients seeking treatment. What do you do about the things you have little or no control over? First, recognize which elements are out of your control and accept them. Finally, seek elements you *can* control, and concentrate on them.

So what *can* you control? Virtually everything that pertains to yourself. You have already chosen your education, your friends, your aspirations. Options are liberating. When you recognize you have a choice and make a choice, you regain control. One choice you *always* have is how you choose to see and interpret your circumstances. You can be understanding or surrender to your emotions. You can be tolerant or prejudiced. You can be happy or you can be unhappy. You can forgive or hold a grudge. It's really up to you. As Castaneda said, it takes the same effort either way.

> We either make ourselves miserable, or we make
> ourselves happy. The amount of work is the same.
> —Carlos Castaneda

Constant Change

Change is a fact of life. Workplace change in particular is driven by technology, research, and innovation. For example, current high-tech security procedures at hospitals and other health care settings would have seemed foreign just a few years ago. Change is especially rampant in the practice and delivery of medicine and health care, and it's not likely to slow down during your lifetime. The sooner you accept change as an ongoing and unstoppable facet of your life (and much of it positive), the happier you will be.

Personality Clashes

Very few of us get to choose our co-workers, and nobody gets along with *everyone*. However, you do have to *work* effectively with everyone, regardless of your personal likes or dislikes. To deal better with co-workers you don't like, or who don't like you, try to analyze the situation. What is it about a particular person that you don't like? Then ask yourself whether there is anything you can do about the annoyance. Even if the annoyance is within your control, is focusing on it worth your attention, energy, and time? Alternatively, you could reframe the situation in the context of your generally positive attitude. Your responsibility is to work effectively with this individual. Can you acknowledge, then minimize their annoying qualities, and move on with the business ahead, reminding yourself that you only have to tolerate them at work?

If you are concerned that a co-worker seems to dislike you, try to find out why. Approach the person and explore the issue with him or her directly. "We don't seem to click," you might say. "Is there something I do that annoys you?" You are being straightforward, but not confrontational, seeking to understand your own behavior and how it may be creating unnecessary problems between the two of you. You may be surprised about how this exchange can open up the basis for a more positive relationship. Frequently, you may even be surprised to learn that the other person doesn't dislike you at all. If the other person identifies an issue, however, you will have to decide whether you can change that aspect of yourself. Again, the choice is yours to make.

Certainly, if there is a truly serious problem with a co-worker that interferes with your ability to work in a productive and positive manner, you have resources at work. For example, if a co-worker acts unethically, uses drugs, or tries to humiliate and intimidate you, then you need to present the problem to your supervisor and, if necessary, the Human Resources Department.

Changing Negative Realities to Positive Realities at Work

Fortunately, you will find many aspects of your work to be quite positive and enjoyable. As a health care professional, with distinctive knowledge and unique skills, you will enjoy much of what you do at work every day. You are likely to find meaning in your everyday duties of helping others with health problems. You will also probably look forward to seeing your co-workers at work every day. There will be fun events, morale-building activities, celebrations, and team meetings to look forward to (Figure 1-2).

Your positive approach, your willingness to work hard, be friendly, offer solutions to problems, and accept others will cause your co-workers to enjoy

FIGURE 1-2 A group of health professionals celebrate successful results at a team meeting.

your company and will vastly improve the quality of your own day-to-day work experience. The big take-away here is that you can *choose* the attitude you adopt and use to face the world's challenges and your personal problems.

You are in total charge of your attitude. That reality is very liberating!

 JOURNALING 1-1

Since you can choose the attitude you want to adopt, write in your journal a statement that describes the attitude you want to choose.

Create Positive Expectations

Many people miss out on opportunities because they walk into work or into meetings with no particular expectations, positive or negative. Whatever happens, happens. This passive approach to the events of your day leaves you out of control of the results and, amazingly, there *are* things you can do to exert some control over the outcomes of future events.

For one thing, you can expect things to turn out positively. More important, you can *plan* for positive outcomes. Ask yourself what you know about, for example, an upcoming meeting. You know the topic and the agenda. You know the people who will be attending, the purpose of the meeting, how long it will last, and what the results could possibly be. Then, based on this advance knowledge, do the following two things:

* **First, plan for the meeting.** Make sure you get the agenda and look it over. Is there any research you can do ahead of time, to be better prepared or actually contribute to the meeting? Consider who is coming. Ask yourself, who will lead this meeting, and who will be influential there? Are there some people who always think alike, or others who usually disagree? Who are the positive people, and who are the negative people? Is there anyone who is likely to try to sabotage the meeting? You are a health professional partly because you value relationships and have insight into others.
* **Second, plan your own actions, involvement, comments, and role.** This process is called visualization (Figure 1-3). Use your perceptual senses to imagine how the meeting will go, and how you will behave there. Smell the coffee, see the overhead lighting, hear the

FIGURE 1-3 The process of visualization.

murmurs and chatting as people arrive, see the leader's body language and meeting materials. Then plan for your own role and what outcomes you would like to see. The meeting will not go exactly as you visualized it, but you will be amazed at how much it turned out to be similar to your visualization, if you have done the preparation based on what you should know and understand your role in making desirable outcomes reality.

The future belongs to those who prepare for it today.
—Malcolm X

This process of planning and visualizing future events applies to every aspect of your day, such as sending your children off to school, encountering patients, dealing with a difficult co-worker, getting to know the new employee over lunch, working through the after-lunch slump, and mapping your commute home. Having positive expectations and a carefully visualized plan will improve the quality of your life and eliminate the negativity of passively letting things happen without your involvement.

Embrace Change

Many times, impending change generates a swirl of rumors. If you hear a rumor that concerns you, it is perfectly appropriate to discuss this rumor with your manager. This not only puts your mind at ease but also helps your manager be more effective in managing the change; either by debunking the rumor or providing information about the rumor that will make the change easier for everyone to accept. Box 1-2 explains the stages people typically go through in the process of accepting change. You may notice that, since change involves loss, the stages are not unlike the stages of grieving.

Based on your understanding of the change, you may decide to seek some training or personal development to help you grapple with the change and make yourself a more effective, versatile, and valued employee. For instance, you might decide to become an expert with the new software or medical equipment, so you can serve as a resource to others; or

Six Stages of Change Acceptance

1. Recognize that change causes anxiety, disruption, and other negative emotions. You are losing something you liked or felt used to.
2. Whenever you experience a loss, you are likely to feel anger. Choose to withhold judgment rather than lash out and say or do something you will regret later.
3. Recognize that the new way will take practice, learning, reinforcement, and habit change. Some people will stall, refuse to cooperate, or try to sabotage the change, but this will only make a difficult process worse.
4. Determine the positive aspects of the change.
5. Don't look back. Experience the benefits of the change, and start to see the change as the "new normal."
6. Integrate the change into your life. Look at how you have changed yourself, and become more versatile and resilient, as a result of accepting the change.

you may decide that you need to develop some better soft skills in the area of resilience or change management.

JOURNALING 1-2

Reflect on some unplanned changes you have experienced in your life. Maybe you had to change schools frequently and leave friends behind. Pick a change you disliked at the time. Now, ask yourself what positive outcomes occurred for you as a result of that change.

Whenever you undergo a major role change at work, you may experience a sensation called the "Imposter Complex." This is especially true when you start a new job, get promoted, or undertake new responsibilities. It takes time to make these adjustments internally. You may fear that you are not fully competent in the new role, and that everybody knows it. Actually, other people don't feel the insecurity you feel unless you project it by expressing it, appearing nervous, being reluctant to make decisions, and so on. Your best move is to "fake it till you make it," acting *as if* you are completely confident in your new role. Soon, your initial feeling of being an "imposter" will fade away.

Convert Negative Self-Talk Into Positive Self-Talk

Monitor negative feedback in your self-talk. For example, suppose you often say to yourself, "I don't deserve to be treated so nicely." Next, put these words in the mouth of someone you know really cares about you—your supervisor, your mother, your best friend. Imagine your friend saying to you, "Heidi, you don't deserve to be treated so nicely." How would that sound? That would really hurt! Why is it all right for you to say that to yourself?

Next, think of someone you don't particularly like. Imagine that this person said, "Heidi, you don't deserve to be treated so nicely." If this happened in real life, you would likely argue with this person. You would defend yourself. You deserve every good thing that happens to you. You would not tolerate this person saying something negative to you. Why would you tolerate saying it to yourself? What if somebody said such a thing to someone you love? You would be outraged. So, again, why would you say such a thing to yourself?

You don't bask in negative self-talk because you think it's a good idea. You do it because it is a habit, a bad habit. Most of the time, you are not even aware you are doing it. These are old, deeply ingrained messages that were driven into you a long time ago and which you now repeat to yourself almost unconsciously. These messages are not even true! So dare to argue with yourself. Whenever you notice negative self-talk, reject it. Tell yourself that you will *not* be accepting these messages unchallenged anymore. Instead, every time you catch yourself thinking negative thoughts, replace them with affirmations about the best parts of yourself.

> *Tell yourself that you're not pretty. Look at you, you're beautiful.*
>
> —Natalie Merchant

JOURNALING 1-3

Write a list of the ten most positive things about yourself.

Finally, tell yourself not to take everything personally. If someone cuts you off in traffic, were they targeting you, specifically? Probably not. It's much more likely that they had something on their mind or got distracted and made a mistake. Maybe they're just a lousy driver. In any case, if you carry around anger and resentment all day long, then you have made yourself the victim. Even if someone was rude to you, ignored you, or made a mean comment, it was about them, not you.

Keep a Journal

Self-talk is one way to have a conversation with yourself. Your journal is another way, and it has the advantage of being written down, which reinforces your thoughts and determination. Throughout this book, we challenge you to keep a journal, to preserve your thoughts. By keeping a journal, you can map your journey of change and then revisit significant moments along the way, remind yourself of your aspirations and your strengths, and build on your earlier insights.

At the end of this term, your journal will serve as a living change document to guide you in your future development. As a start, 10 steps to a positive mental attitude appear in Box 1-3.

BOX 1-3

10 Steps to a Positive Attitude at Work

1. Visualize and plan for success.
2. Focus on the fun, positive aspects of your work.
3. Associate with other positive people.
4. Look at the bright side of things.
5. Don't give up easily.
6. Attack problems when they first arise.
7. Engage in positive self-talk.
8. Seek balance in your life.
9. Embrace change, which is inevitable.
10. Have a support system in place at all times.

CASE STUDY 1-1
Shifting Gears

Claudette Wilson was born with a lot of disadvantages in her life. Her father disappeared shortly after her birth, and she doesn't know who he is. She has six half-brothers and half-sisters, all with different fathers, long gone. When she was fifteen, she dropped out of high school to help her mother take care of her younger brothers and sisters. As Claudette says with a laugh today, "I came from humble beginnings."

A year later, her mother decided that, more than anything else, they needed money, so she asked Claudette to get a job. She began working evenings at a nearby nursing home. She didn't have any education or training or certification, but she did have a natural ability to work with the elderly. She liked them and tried to make them laugh. She was concerned about their comfort, and she worked hard to help them bathe, change their clothes and linens, and make sure they got plenty to eat. Claudette had the patience for this kind of work. She had a big personality and loved to talk to people. She tried to get the patients to talk about their early days, and she loved it when the stories came tumbling out.

Eventually, Claudette and her boyfriend Bob moved to Rock Island, IL, where Bob got a job at John Deere as a welder in a tractor factory.

"There are some things I want in this life of ours together," Claudette told Bob one night after work.

"A house with a white picket fence?"

"Well, yes, for starters, although I don't care about the fence."

"For starters?"

"And I want to get married in a church, with a white dress."

"And a ring?"

"I don't care about the ring. But I care about what the ring stands for."

"Baby," he said, softly into her ear, "the ring stands for a circle that goes round and round and never ends, starting every day together and ending every day together, and starting over the next day and the next day, no matter what happens, no matter if the days are easy or hard, for all the days of our life."

"That's it," she said. "Here's a way in, but there's no way out. If we have children, they will know their father, and if they have children, they will know their grandfather, and that's the way it's going to be."

In Rock Island, Claudette found out about a Job Corps Center across the river in Clinton, Iowa, and she completed her high school education there and got some more training in the area of nursing assisting. Over the next five years, she worked on and off at a nursing home and she and Bob got married and had three children together, two boys and a girl. Congress passed a law that required nursing assistants working in Medicare- and Medicaid-funded facilities to be certified, so Claudette got herself certified. Bob had become a foreman at John Deere, and the young family bought a small house in a nice neighborhood with good schools.

One evening at work, Claudette heard some shouting coming from Mr. Fischer's room. As she ran to the room, she burst in just as Harry, one of the nurses, threw Mr. Fischer onto a commode and sent him speeding on the commode into a wall. Harry started at Mr. Fischer, swearing a blue streak, when Claudette shouted, "Harry, stop it!"

"I've just about had it with this stubborn old coot," said Harry, and pushed past Claudette on his way out of the room. Claudette went over to Mr. Fischer. He was shaking and crying, asking for his glasses. She got him cleaned up and dressed and brought him to the TV room where his friends congregated after dinner. She got him involved with his friends, and she was pretty sure he had forgotten all about the incident with Harry. Nevertheless, Claudette reported Harry to the Nursing Director the next day.

"That's hard to believe, that Harry would do that," the Nursing Director told her.

"I couldn't believe it either," Claudette said.

Later that day, Claudette was called back into the Nursing Director's office. "Harry denies your charge," the Director said. "Mr. Fischer doesn't remember it."

"Mr. Fischer has Alzheimer's disease. Harry is lying."

"Well, I don't know. It's one person's word against another. I don't doubt your word, Claudette. But it's not easy to get RNs. I'm just going to have to take Harry's word for it and keep a close eye on him." She paused, waiting for an argument from Claudette, but Claudette said nothing. "Under the circumstances, it doesn't seem that you and Harry are going to be able to work together."

"No, it doesn't," said Claudette.

"So I think it would be best for everybody if you just quietly resigned. Give us two weeks' notice, but leave today, and we'll pay you for the two weeks and any vacation time you have coming. I'll give you a good recommendation."

"Then, I resign," said Claudette quietly. "I'll take the money, but I don't want your recommendation. It would be meaningless to me."

When Bob got home from work that afternoon, she told him what had happened. "We don't need the money," he told her. "The kids are young. Why don't you just stay home?"

"Yes," she said. "I'm going to take a break from work."

They sat in silence for several minutes. Claudette thought back to her childhood in Lexington, where she had sometimes been a victim of discrimination, and where she saw a lot of prejudice and injustice. It had been many years since she had had that feeling, being discriminated against. She felt that the Nursing Director had fired her because that was the easiest thing for her to do, the simplest solution to the problem that Claudette had brought to her attention. She had to tell herself not to let those old feelings intrude into the day she was having today.

Finally, Bob broke the silence. "Today was a bad day," he said. "What did you learn from it?"

Claudette sat up ramrod straight. "I'll tell you what I learned, Bobby. I'm going to become a nurse."

And she did.

QUESTIONS FOR THOUGHT AND REFLECTION

1. Why was Claudette able to change her life when she moved with her husband Bob?
2. What was Claudette's idea of a better life?
3. What role did education play in Claudette's life?
4. Did Claudette exhibit second thoughts about helping Mr. Fischer or reporting Harry?
5. Do you think the Nursing Director fired Claudette because she was prejudiced against Claudette?
6. Why did Claudette decide to become a nurse? Think of three reasons.
7. Do you think a positive mental attitude had anything to do with the strong relationship between Claudette and Bob?

Down a Dark Road

Frank Kinsey was just about fed up. Ever since the physical therapy practice was bought by one of those giant for-profit hospital corporations, there had been one change after another. "I've been through a lot of these changes already," he would say, "and I've been against every one of them." Now, it had just been announced that the physical therapy practice was going to be moved to a location closer to the hospital, next to the Rehab Center. This would mean a longer commute for Frank and probably a lot of other changes that nobody even knew about yet.

In their staff meetings, Frank raised a lot of legitimate concerns. He asked how many people would have a longer commute, and about half the hands went up. "What about the move itself?" he asked. "How many days is that going to take? How many of our clients are going to have to miss sessions? The medical records will probably get screwed up. The company wants to make money, but they'll lose money. Think about the cost of the new building, and just the move itself. The phones, the computers—what a mess! We're going to lose some good people, for sure."

The practice manager, Elliott Berg, listened to Frank carefully, noting that nobody else was as vocal as Frank about the problems the move was going to cause. Still, he hadn't thought of some of the issues that Frank was giving voice to. He asked the Human Resources assistant, Melissa, to create a map that showed where all the employees lived and the old and the new locations, so he could see how the move would affect commutes. He saw that the commute would be longer for about half of the people and shorter for the other half. But he shared Frank's concern that they could lose some good people, so he made sure he knew which people had longer commutes, and he spoke with each one, even Frank, to make sure the burden would not be unreasonable, or a reason to quit.

Elliott arranged for a tour of the new building when it neared completion. Frank raised more concerns. "I don't know if our equipment is going to fit here," he said. "The waiting room is too big. Our clients are going to feel like faceless people being treated by a big faceless corporation." He went on, "These tall ceilings are going to make the place noisy. The elevator is slow—it's going to take forever to get around here. I'll bet they're going to charge us for parking here. Elliott, are they going to charge us for parking?"

"I'm not sure yet," said Elliott, "but I know that's being discussed and considered."

"Well, there's another downside," Frank said to everyone.

Elliott scheduled a meeting with Frank. "You know, Frank, I'm not the one who decided to make this move."

"I know, Elliott," Frank said sympathetically. "It's a corporate move."

"Even still," Elliott said, "I'm responsible for the success of this move, and you're not helping by bringing up every possible problem and getting everybody more concerned than they already are about the move."

"I get it, Elliott. I'll keep my big mouth shut," he said with a laugh.

The move actually went more smoothly than anyone thought. Even Frank was impressed. "It's a good thing I brought up that issue about the billing. I actually think they didn't lose too much money."

It wasn't too long before the corporation decided to merge all their systems together, which was going to mean big changes for the physical therapy group.

"What a mess," said Frank. "Can't these people leave anything alone? This whole operation is going to crash."

Elliott decided to call a staff meeting. He said, "We're going to go around the table, and everybody is going to raise one issue that concerns them about the systems integration. If you don't have an issue, you can pass. Pam, will you take notes? And Frank, just one concern per person please," and everybody laughed.

Although everyone worked hard to identify and anticipate potential problems, the systems integration had a lot of problems. It was just a hard thing, the IT Director kept saying. Problems are inevitable. You can't think of everything. Finally, Frank's bad feeling about the new corporation paid off. "See?" he said. "I told you so." He was right. When some layoffs became necessary, Frank was the first to go.

QUESTIONS FOR THOUGHT AND REFLECTION

1. What was Frank's likely effect on morale?
2. How did Frank help Elliott? How did he make Elliot's job harder?
3. What could Frank have done differently to get his concerns across?
4. Why did Elliott change the process for identifying concerns? Was this a good move? Why or why not?
5. Do you think that Frank's skills as a clinician played into the decision to lay him off?

1. To experience the discomfort of change, go to a part of your city or town that you are unfamiliar with. Walk around the streets. Go into the stores. Visit any attractions, like parks or museums. At the end of your experience, ask yourself if you are glad you went. Think about the positive experiences and feelings your excursion left you with.
2. Visualize your experience of some upcoming event you will attend. Imagine details that come from the five senses—sight, sound, taste, smell, and touch— if possible. When you attend the event, see how well you visualized it.
3. Forgive someone today.
4. Buy a journal to create your personal change journey for this course.

CROSS CURRENTS WITH OTHER SKILLS

SETTING GOALS AND PLANNING ACTIONS: Now that you are equipped with a positive mental attitude, give yourself some direction. Set goals and make plans to achieve them. Your attitude means you can achieve anything, if you can conceive and believe it. (pp. 286-291)

AIMING TO BE ADAPTABLE AND FLEXIBLE: Your attitude enables you to adopt adaptability as an effective change strategy. (pp. 25-29)

MODELING BUSINESS ETIQUETTE: Your attitude affects the way you treat patients and co-workers. (pp. 170-178)

DEALING WITH DIFFICULT PEOPLE: You will learn some tactics for this skill, but you have to bring a constructive attitude to the table. (pp. 231-238)

EXUDING OPTIMISM, ENTHUSIASM, AND POSITIVITY: Now that you have oriented your attitude in the first part of this book, work toward the last part, so you can fully realize the benefits of all your hard work. (pp. 380-384)

Managing Your Time and Organizing Your Life

The key is in not spending time, but in investing it.
—Stephen R. Covey

LEARNING OBJECTIVE 2: MANAGING YOUR TIME AND ORGANIZING YOUR LIFE

- Visualize the day ahead of time.
- Identify daily priorities with an appropriate sense of what is most important and a realistic sense of the time demand involved.

- Organize plans in a holistic and detailed manner.
- Choose and use some form of manual or electronic time management system that includes daily goals and a daily "to-do" list that puts priorities in order.
- Anticipate your next move to remain ahead of the game.
- Act proactively instead of reactively throughout the work day.
- Maintain an organized work environment.

WHAT IF?

What if everything happened "all at once?" It's 11:00, and you have three important tasks to complete: ordering insulin syringes, setting up a room for a minor in-office procedure at 11:30, and preparing blood and urinalysis lab work for an afternoon pickup. At the same time, the pharmacy is on the line confirming the amount of amoxicillin to dispense for a patient.

1. What are the criteria you would use for selecting what gets completed first?
2. What if you had a reception room full of patients and one was having trouble breathing? Where would you fit this in the scheme of your task organization?

Organizing from the Inside Out

If someone were to ask you to rate your organizational skills and your time management skills, would you say, "What's the difference?" Lots of people would. However, organization and time management are two different, but complementary, skills. While organization is tied to efficiency and how smoothly a job gets completed, time management is more about prioritizing and managing tasks, thereby using time effectively. Some people can complete a task in half the time it takes for another simply because of the effective use of their time and their ability to remain organized.

Organization begins on the inside: learning to think in an organized fashion about a goal. When you organize internally first, the rest of your outer world will line up, including your work space, tasks, and objectives. This involves thinking ahead before starting a task or project, perhaps creating lists, prioritizing tasks, and pre-thinking the activity.

Tips for Remaining Organized and Managing Your Day

- Start your work day with the big picture in mind.
- Divide your work day into hours and schedule your goals and tasks according to the time allotted.
- Be aware of those times when you are taken off task by interruptions.
- Use the systems that are in place for organizing papers; avoid allowing piles of papers to manifest in your area.
- Focus on working on one thing at a time. Be present with what you are working on or who you are working with.
- Practice anticipating the next move of the dentist, physician, nurse, or pharmacist by having things prepared ahead of time and ready to be administered according to the circumstance.

Organization is thought to be a function of the left side of the brain, while creativity is believed to be a function of the right side of the brain. Depending on your particular brain dominance, you may be naturally organized or struggle with managing tasks, projects, and meeting deadlines. Box 1-4 offers some tips for organizing and managing your day.

Being Productive Versus Being Busy

Can a person really manage time? When you think about it, in the deepest sense, time is not what you are managing, but rather, you are managing your behavior within a specific timeframe. Self-management is the best time manager. Let's say you assist a dentist with patient care from 9:00 to 5:00. How you choose to start your day will determine whether you see patients on time and whether you have enough instruments for every procedure throughout the day. If you are not prepared well in advance, you will run around all day. In the end, you will feel busy, but unproductive—and there's a big difference between the two. Being busy means you ran around all day and completed some tasks, but you did not accomplish a major objective like providing effective patient

care or producing an outcome like developing all the patient radiographs. Being productive means all your actions resulted in the completion of the major objectives for the day.

JOURNALING 1-4

Write about a time you visited a health care facility that was completely disorganized. What was the main issue and how did you feel as a patient?

Either you run the day or the day runs you.

—Jim Rohn

Being Well Rested Every Day

Nothing can make your day go better than a good night's sleep. Your brain needs downtime to release the chemicals it needs to repair cells, build synapses, and organize the day's experience in your short- and long-term memories. Sleep or rest deprivation contributes to poor decision making that can interfere with your work, your relationships, and your reputation. It adds to your stress and anxiety. It can distort your personality and it gets in the way of your ability to maintain a positive mental attitude.

WHAT IF?

What if you were a doctor and your assistant had outside personal issues that were affecting the daily routine and your assistant's ability to be organized, efficient, and focused at work? How would you handle this?

Visualizing Your Perfect Day

How would your workday look if it were perfect? When you visualize your perfect day, you see in your "mind's eye" the outcome of your day before you reach it in reality. You won't necessarily see the specifics of your day, but you will see it holistically, and how it will play out. Michael Jordan was known for visualizing himself making the play before he executed it. He saw the end from the beginning. This is a result of visualization. It's about seeing where your day will go before the day happens. When you start your day with visualization, it helps you prioritize your goals and responsibilities so that conditions point more favorably toward your end goal.

Anticipation: A Highly Valued Soft Skill in Health Care

Similar to visualization, *anticipation* is the ability to foresee the next step before it occurs to help you be properly prepared in the event something is needed. The skill of anticipation develops over time, drawing from experience and observations of similar procedures and events so that you develop a sense of what comes next before it happens, eliminating the need to scramble around at the last minute for what is needed *now*.

In dentistry, for instance, a dental assistant's ability to anticipate the dentist's next move and need allows the dentist to focus on keeping a dry field and to focus on the tooth that is being treated (Figure 1-4).

FIGURE 1-4 A dental assistant helps a dentist perform a procedure (Copyright © istock.com).

Strategies for Working Efficiently

You can prepare ahead to eliminate many of the time-wasting hassles that you know crop up each day by (1) organizing your work space and (2) developing your visualization and anticipation skills to help you accommodate the inevitable interruptions.

Organize Your Work Environment

Working in an organized and efficient manner requires a work space and environment that is neat and organized so that everything has a logical place and is easily accessible. For example, patient records in a private practice should be located in cabinets that are secure and accessible to the front office staff so they can be retrieved when patients call. These records should also be in order either by patient account or last name. Similarly, medical supplies should also be stored according to a logical and consistent system so that items can be retrieved quickly and accurately from the same cabinet or shelf every time. To maintain this, your restocking and reordering these supplies should be systematic so that you never run out. Avoid constantly moving items so the rest of your team can't find them. If you share a work station, be sure you put things exactly where you found them so that the next health care worker can access them.

Whether you work in a cubicle, a hospital work station, or an office of your own, strive to keep your in-box empty, either on your desk or in your email. Once you read mail, either take action immediately or categorize it for follow-up action. If you allow mail or email to pile up, you will feel overwhelmed trying to get on top of correspondence. You will spend more time sorting tasks instead of using that time to move forward with more pertinent goals.

Be sure to label your files appropriately. For example, label your email folders so they correspond to the email that is in the folder. Finally, keep only current projects on your desk. This will prevent you from being distracted and starting several projects at once.

Avoid Unnecessary Interruptions

Health care professionals are frequently interrupted during the day. Therefore, it is critical to learn to prioritize tasks and know when to say, "I will get back to you within 24 hours." In other words, you need to discern what is a "now" priority and what is a "later" priority. Know when you should stop what you're doing in the face of an interruption and when you should not. This usually becomes clear fairly quickly. For example, imagine drawing blood from a patient, and then leaving that patient with the needle in her arm so that you could answer the phone or tend to a patient waiting at the counter. You've left the "now" priority to tend to a "later" priority. Not only is this dangerous, but you run the risk of forgetting the first patient altogether once you've left her to become caught up in a new task. There are always plenty of distractions and demands in the health care setting.

Prioritizing tasks is not to be confused with procrastination. Procrastination is about putting off what needs to be done today and waiting until the last minute, usually because of an aversion to the task. Remain focused on the task you are handling, especially during direct patient care.

Here is the prime condition of success: concentrate your energy, thought, and capital exclusively upon the business in which you are engaged.

—Andrew Carnegie

Choose a Planner

The longest memory is shorter than the shortest pencil. That is why you need a planner to record all your appointments, commitments, notes, ideas, and aspirations. Paper and electronic choices abound. The advantage of a paper planner is that you can take it with you at all times and update it easily, whenever you need to, without having to turn it on or off or relying on battery power. They come in different formats, but most allow you to record your daily appointments, manage a to-do list, and make notes about the day's events, along with future appointment planning. The variety is so great that you can find one to fit your needs and budget. On the other hand, electronic planners are highly portable as well but make it easier to switch appointments, order and reorder priorities, and do some brainstorming. Data can be transferred to a computer or another mobile electronic device.

For health care professionals with varying work schedules, a daily planner is essential. Choose a planner that fits your lifestyle, and choose one that you will *use*!

A Time Management Strategy

Time management schemes go back to the early 1900s when efficiency expert Frederick Taylor conducted time management studies in factories to boost worker productivity and output, later publishing *Principles of Scientific Management* in 1911. The classic book on personal time management is *The Time Trap* by Alec McKenzie, published in 1972. It identified common time wasters at work, suggested ways that over-committed people can say "no," and stressed the importance of setting daily goals. Alan Lakein published his book *How to Get Control of Your Time and Your Life* in 1989, which helped people prioritize their daily to-do lists and "work smarter, not harder."

The new classic on time management is David Allen's *Getting Things Done* (GTD), published in 2001. Building on the insights of his predecessors, Allen devised a methodology, now followed by millions.

The first step in getting things done is to collect all your incomplete tasks in one central place for further processing. Whether you record everything awaiting your attention in a notebook, on sticky notes, on your computer, or even in a voice recording, the point is to get everything you have to do *off your mind* and into a central collection device. You might spend a few hours collecting all these "to-do's" initially, and then get in the habit of recording them whenever they come up or occur to you. Whether it's your sister's birthday card, the documentation you have to revise at work, or that Sunday School class you have to prepare for and teach, the idea is to get all these tasks off your mind and into a device you can trust. This practice can be a very liberating part of managing your time and your tasks!

Next, you will need to process all these undone tasks and obligations. You do this by asking yourself, "What is the next thing I have to do to move this undone task toward getting done?" Once you know the answer to this question, then you have something concrete and specific that you can insert into your time flow.

Now you are ready to place your "next actions" into your calendar and organize your life and your time. If something has to happen at a specific time, like an appointment, schedule it for that time. If something has to happen on a particular day, like paying a bill, enter it into that day. If you are waiting on something before you can take the action, like filing a lab test result in a patient's chart, enter into your calendar when you can expect to receive what you are waiting for, so you won't forget about it and you can check on it if it's late. If a next action is not time-critical, put it on your to-do list.

Schedule review periods daily and weekly to keep your schedule up to date. Every day, review and prioritize the day's events, scheduling time to prepare for them as well. Every week, collect your incomplete tasks, identify their next actions, and schedule these tasks.

Finally, the most important part of your time management system is to *do* your tasks. Anything that takes less than two minutes to do, such as emailing some lab results, should be done immediately. You don't want to wonder if you took care of a minor detail which could cause problems for you later if it is not taken care of. Anything that is scheduled should be prepared for and done at the time allotted. Have your to-do list on hand at all times, so you know what the next thing to work on is as soon as you have a break.

The steps involved in a time management system are presented in Box 1-5.

If everything you need to do is off your mind and transferred instead to your calendar or a list you constantly refer to, your time will be much less stressful, and things will get done, with little risk of falling through the cracks.

BOX 1-5

Summary of Time Management System Steps

- Collect all your undone and incomplete tasks in one central place, so they are written down rather than being a distraction in the back of your mind.
- Determine and write the "next action" for each one of your tasks, to make it crystal clear what it will take to complete each task.
- Schedule these "next actions" into your life. Appointments and other time-sensitive "next actions" go into your calendar at specific times or days. Everything else goes on your to-do list.
- Spend a few minutes organizing every day, using your calendar, your to-do lists, and your anticipation and visualization skills.
- Always have your next appointment or highest priority task teed up, so you will automatically know what to work on next to keep your life effectively managed.

CASE STUDY 1-2
The Balancing Act

Robert was having a hard time adjusting to his new position as an occupational therapist. He had gotten married just a few months before he began his career in occupational therapy. In retrospect, he thought he may have tried to do too much at once, but truly, how could he have not married the woman he loved, Matilda, whatever his career challenges night be?

But while he thought that his new marriage might be in danger of interfering with his work, it turned out to be the opposite. His upstate New York employer was delighted with Robert's Boston University credentials and immediately loaded him up with appointments. He always thought he would be home by 6:00, but he never seemed to get there before 7:00. He had so many notes and documentations to compile at the end of the day that it always took him longer than he thought. He had planned to do the documentation in the fifteen minutes between his appointments, but he also wanted to connect with the other members of the clinic staff, since he was the new person there. And once he met his new co-workers, he found he enjoyed the time he spent with them.

Regardless, Matilda, who had initially tried to be patient with Robert as he started his new job and career, was now becoming impatient. She had resolved to develop her cooking skills as a newlywed, even though her position as an operations manager at Great Lakes Shipping had its own demands. Now, her creative dishes got cold in front of her as she awaited Robert's arrival, which seemed to get later every day. Clearly, she thought—and Robert agreed—he needed to manage his time better.

Robert didn't quite know how to accomplish his new mandate, but he thought the first step might be a little healing with Matilda. He planned for some relaxation and spa treatments at the Mirror Lake Inn in nearby Lake Placid, New York, over the Labor Day weekend. They walked around the village, had lunch at the Black Bear Café, and poked around a little bookstore they found. Robert had been giving a lot of thought to what he might do to manage his time better at work and had already come up with some strategies. For instance, he was going to speak to the clinic director, Marsha, about limiting his appointments to seven a day. He resolved that he wouldn't leave his office between sessions without the documentation done, even if he didn't get a break between his sessions. To keep connected with his co-workers, he planned to bring his lunch, and planned to eat lunch every day with the gang. Still, these seemed like feeble efforts, and he lacked confidence that they would really work.

Then, in the bookstore, he came across a copy of David Allen's book, *Getting Things Done*. "That's exactly what I need to do," he thought to himself. Get things done. That afternoon, as they enjoyed some beverages while sprawling in the Adirondack chairs at the edge of the lake, he read the book. He knew he would have to reread it later, but his mind was teeming with ideas he could apply to his situation.

After they arrived home on Labor Day, Robert set aside two hours to collect all his uncompleted tasks, from trivial things like getting his oil changed to major things like planning their first Christmas holiday together as a married couple. He also included work-related tasks like reviewing the new assessment tools and ordering toys for his child clients. He also added, "Speak to Marsha about work load." Soon he had a pile of 3 × 5 cards in front of him on his desk, each with an open loop written on it.

Then he added a "next action" to every one of the uncompleted tasks he had identified, even adding a few more as they occurred to him. He took out his Day-Timer and scheduled every next action he could, and put the rest on a list. He made a special list for projects, tasks that were more complicated and would take multiple steps to achieve, like lining up internships with local employers for his clients. Finally, he grouped his tasks by location. There were things he could do only at work or only at home. Things he needed to do with his computer and things that could be batched and completed in less than two minutes each. He also batched his Saturday errands.

On Tuesday, he met with Marsha about his appointment load. Instead of just dumping the problem in her lap, he had a number of ideas and proposals. The Occupational Therapy Assistant, Ernie, could take some of the load. Some of the appointments could be reduced from 45 minutes to 25 minutes, because they were just check-ins, so Robert could see two clients in the time he would normally see one. He and Marsha discussed the possibility of recruiting an O.T. with a specialty in pediatrics, since children were becoming a larger part of the practice. In the end, they agreed on some short-term solutions and some longer-term solutions. "I'm married with three kids," she told him. "I understand the situation, and I appreciate your being proactive."

That evening, Robert was home by 5:15, even before Matilda. He wished he knew how to cook, so he could really make her evening. But he wasn't totally inept in the kitchen. Cheese and crackers was one of his signature dishes, and he possessed corkscrew skills.

QUESTIONS FOR THOUGHT AND REFLECTION

1. Why was Robert unable to anticipate how long his work would take him?
2. What other priorities emerged at work that Robert might not have considered?
3. Describe the importance of work/life balance in Robert's situation.
4. How did Robert manage the meeting with Marsha?
5. What will Robert have to do to make these time management improvements stick in his life?

Down a Dark Road

Natalie, a dental assistant with a few years of experience, worked for a busy private dental practice. She had good dental skills, but she was distractible and inconsistent. One day, she rolled in late to work to find her boss, Dr. Cho, frantically setting up the room for the first patient, the one

Natalie passed in the reception room on her way in. Natalie put her purse and lunch away and then seated the patient. The day was a bit frantic, since Natalie did not come in 30 minutes before the start of the day to set up all the procedure trays and run the sterilizer full of needed instruments.

As the day progressed, the team ran behind 30 to 45 minutes on each patient. They did not have enough hand pieces for drilling because they were not sterilized, nor were they ready for each patient. The dentist had to assist Natalie the whole day in order to catch up. The team was not afforded a lunch because they still had patients who were scheduled on time but could not be seen on time.

As the day progressed, the 3:00 patient was in the chair waiting for his gold crown to be permanently cemented, but the crown was not back from the lab. Natalie went to the receptionist, Karen, to inquire about the lab case, and the receptionist said she confirmed the patient's appointment without knowing whether the crown was returned from the lab.

Natalie informed the dentist that the case was not returned. The dentist was upset. He didn't know what to do about the patient because he was leaving on a trip. When he informed the patient that the crown wasn't done yet, the patient was upset. "Why did you confirm my appointment if you didn't have the crown back?" "What a disorganized place!" he murmured as he departed to reschedule his appointment.

The dentist let the patient know that he would give him a discount for the inconvenience, and while the patient was grateful, he was still upset that he had to fight traffic and arrive on time, only to have no treatment done.

The next patient was seated while the previous one rescheduled his appointment and got his parking validated. This patient was in a wheelchair and required nitrous oxide (N_2O_2) sedation. It took some time, and the assistance of the patient's wife, to transfer the patient into the treatment chair. Once they were successful in transferring the patient, the patient's wife left for an hour to shop and said she would return in an hour or so to pick him up. They leaned the patient back and rolled in the nitrous oxide tanks, only to realize that the oxygen tank was empty, and there was no backup tank. Natalie said she forgot to order another one. She said she didn't have a system for ordering just before the tanks were empty. As a result, the dentist had to seat the patient up and explain that he couldn't treat him because they only had the nitrous but not the oxygen tank. The patient had to sit there for an hour until his wife returned to assist him back into the wheelchair, untreated.

Everyone was off key and couldn't wait until this day ended. A day that was supposed to end at 5:00 ended at 6:00 because the clinical area was such a mess from the pile-up of used instruments and equipment to be sterilized. Everyone felt unproductive and reactive to everything going on around them. At 6:00, everyone ran off to try to beat traffic home.

The next day, Natalie came in on time in the morning but returned from lunch 30 minutes late. The afternoon was a repeat of the previous day.

Natalie's boss, Dr. Cho, decided to discuss Natalie's performance with her and explain how it affected his business this past week. He decided to wait until the end of the day, so that all the patients were treated and their conversation didn't affect the outcome of the day. It was a difficult conversation for several reasons. He procrastinated in having this conversation. He risked her being upset and quitting, or worse yet, continuing the same behavior. Finally, he just didn't like negative communication and conflict. Dr. Cho was frustrated by the amount of time he has invested in how he is going to handle this, costing him stress and company time.

At the end of the day, he met with Natalie to discuss how her behavior and irresponsibility was affecting his practice. She apologized and explained that she was partying one of the nights and was hungover, which led her to be unfocused at work. The other night she had a problem with her boyfriend. Although Dr. Cho was concerned about his assistant's life, he was more concerned about his practice and the care of his patients. He gave her a verbal warning about her behavior and told her in no uncertain terms that it had to improve, or she would be fired.

QUESTIONS FOR THOUGHT AND REFLECTION

1. What are two main issues in this case study?
2. How did Natalie's lack of self-management affect the team?
3. How would you resolve the two situations where the patient arrived but nothing was ready?
4. How could the events of this day have been avoided?
5. What is the relationship between arriving on time and running on time?

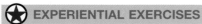

1. Identify and write on the board as many things that you believe are issues outside of work that could possibly affect your work and the outcome of your day at work. Separate on the board those things you believe are within your control and those you believe are not.

2. Role-play in pairs (one doctor and one assistant) how you as a doctor would address the disorganization of an assistant and how this affects patient care.

3. Define the following terms and provide a personal example for each:
   a. Procrastination
   b. Distraction
   c. Interruption

4. Select one thing to do today and do only that for the majority of your day. If you are in sterilization, focus only on sterilizing and doing this well. If you are prepping rooms, do only that today. The goal is to teach you how to be laser focused on one thing until completion.

5. Contact a nursing facility and ask for a tour of the facility. At the end of your tour, indicate whether you would have a relative stay there. Determine the level of organization of the place and whether systems are in place for patient care. Would you recommend this facility for care? Why or why not?

6. Think about a time when something in your personal life affected your work at a job or at school. At what point do you believe the event or situation interfered with your professional life?

⊘ CROSS CURRENTS WITH OTHER SOFT SKILLS

SETTING GOALS AND PLANNING ACTIONS: Knowing how much time and energy you have as it applies to your day and how you allocate your time and energy to achieve target goals. (pp. 286-291)

GAINING ENERGY, PERSISTENCE, AND PERSEVERANCE: Being able to manage your time and organize your life will make room for attacking your work with renewed vigor. (pp. 190-197)

MANAGING STRESS: Nothing eases stress like being organized and knowing what to do next. (pp. 203-210)

SEPARATING YOUR WORK AND PERSONAL PROBLEMS: An integrated time management system will improve balance in your life. It will make it clear that you can only take care of work-related problems when you are at work and home-related problems when you are not at work. (pp. 370-375)

Achieving Honesty and Integrity

In looking for people to hire, you look for three qualities: integrity, intelligence, and energy. And if they don't have the first, the other two will kill you.

—Warren Buffett

LEARNING OBJECTIVE 3: ACHIEVING HONESTY AND INTEGRITY

- Define the relationship between honesty and integrity.
- Recognize why people are tempted to lie or be dishonest.
- Develop a plan for maintaining your integrity.
- Identify ethical dilemmas in the workplace and how to deal with them.

The world presents itself in shades of gray. It's not always clear what the right thing to do is. Nowhere is this more evident than in the world of health care.

Honesty and integrity are two key ships against this storm. *Honesty* is defined in the dictionary as "adherence to the truth." *Integrity* is defined as "adherence to moral values," of which honesty is core. Both words include the concepts of being fair and incorruptible. As health care professionals, we can cling to honesty and integrity to help us navigate the ethical rough waters we sometimes find ourselves in at work.

Your Integrity at Stake

Consider the kinds of challenges to honesty and integrity that can arise in a health care setting:

* You could be recruited to participate in a Medicare fraud scheme by falsifying records.
* You could learn confidential medical information about someone you know personally.
* Someone could lie about their religion to get time off.
* You might observe a patient being mistreated by a co-worker.
* A colleague might have falsified her resume to get her job.
* You might have an infectious disease but consider going to work anyway.
* Your certification might have lapsed, but nobody would know.

* Your co-worker signed up for a conference but just took the day off.
* You observe a co-worker pocket some cash he found in a pair of jeans cut off a patient in the emergency room.

As you can see, there are innumerable opportunities to be dishonest at work in health care settings. In many cases, the dishonest person might never be caught, although chances of getting caught increase with every additional instance of dishonesty.

Real integrity is doing the right thing, knowing that nobody's going to know whether you did it or not.

—Oprah Winfrey

As a health professional, you are well equipped to resist temptations and always strive to do the right thing in all circumstances. Usually, being honest will be fairly easy for you. Although remaining honest will require courage in a few extreme circumstances, the habit of speaking truthfully should come easily to you. It is said that lying is a habit, but so is telling the truth, one so much easier to form.

No legacy is so rich as honesty.

—William Shakespeare

Challenges to Integrity

The benefits of telling the truth and acting with integrity are so obvious that no one needs to be convinced of their wisdom. Yet, people lie all the time. To understand why, review the reasons in Box 1-6.

BOX 1-6

Why People Lie

- People are ashamed of what they did.
- People fear retribution or revenge.
- People fear being punished.
- People fear losing support.
- People fear change.
- People fear they will become unpopular.
- People want to be seen in a positive light.
- People hate being wrong.
- People don't want to lose face or be shown up.
- People don't want to take responsibility when they make bad decisions.

You can see that the challenge in being truthful comes when you have something to lose by acting with integrity: a co-worker could become hostile toward you; your employer could lose some money; a patient might be angry to learn that he has been treated unethically. Then, there are the really serious consequences that go with acting with integrity: you could lose your job; other people could lose their jobs; your employer could be sued; someone could be in legal trouble. Even highly ethical people might have to take a deep breath before taking actions consistent with their personal integrity when these serious consequences are the likely result.

Finally, the person of integrity stands to lose something even more important: if they make an unethical decision rather than accept the consequences, they lose their integrity, and that is the greatest loss of all. The consequences of acting with integrity could be serious, but they will be manageable. The consequences of acting without integrity could be disastrous and unmanageable.

You usually can't control the timing of the need to make an important ethical decision. More often than not, you will be suddenly confronted with circumstances you did not anticipate, so it is important to imagine the dilemmas that can arise now, near the beginning of your career, so you will be well prepared and know what to do when the big ethical decisions come along.

 WHAT IF?

What if you saw a fellow employee remove a $20 bill from a cash drawer that was open?

Armed for Integrity

You can strengthen your integrity muscles by developing traits and strategies to serve you in times of crisis. For example, as a health care professional, you probably already have a highly developed sense of empathy, the ability to deeply understand the feelings of others. When you can put yourself in other people's situations, you are in a good position to make an ethical decision you can be proud of.

Our emotions contribute to our humanity. But if you develop the ability to check your emotions so you can deliver a more crafted response, you are not as likely to make a situation worse by just responding emotionally. Even if the circumstances you find yourself in make you feel angry, disappointed, frustrated,

FIGURE 1-5 Empathetic hospital workers interact with an elderly patient (Copyright © istock.com).

or regretful, you should learn to take a deep breath so you can ask yourself, "How should I respond rationally to this situation?" Learn how to disagree in a constructive, respectful, civil manner.

Humility is another quality to develop (Figure 1-5). It puts your ego in the background, because ego injuries often lead to ill-considered and defensive responses. You know who you are; you don't need to put your hurt ego ahead of a well-considered response.

Blaming accomplishes very little. It usually makes a situation worse by making everyone defensive, and it creates hard feelings. Worse, it tends to generate excuses, not solutions. As a person of integrity, you want to focus on solutions to the morally ambiguous situations that challenge your integrity. Plus, each time you take accountability for your actions, it makes you stronger and makes it easier to do the right thing the next time. For example, the person who double-bills Medicare may think they are just doing what they are told. But if you take personal accountability for your role in any fraudulent activity, you will know what to do.

As noted before, the bigger the consequences of your honest behavior, the more courage it takes to be honest. At times like this, your self-confidence comes into play. If you are confident in your behavior, you will be able to exhibit the courage you are occasionally called upon to display. You can bolster your confidence by thinking about what other highly ethical people would do in the situation; pick your role models in advance and use your vision of their moral courage to support yourself in a challenging situation. Or imagine that someday your children, or someone else whose opinion of you matters, will find out what you have done, whether for better or worse.

Finally, remember the big picture, keeping in mind the overriding benefits of being honest, which are briefly summarized in Box 1-7.

Lies and the Body Language of Lying

Lies, Half-Lies, and Lies of Silence

There are many kinds of lies, including lies of kindness. For instance, you may decide not to tell an Alzheimer's patient looking for his wife that she is dead. You may feel it is unkind to plunge the poor man into renewed grief every single day. Nor would you go out of your way to hurt someone's feelings by telling them the truth about inconsequential things, like their new hair style.

Many people avoid telling the truth by remaining silent when they should not. If you have information that is needed to make a good decision, correct a mistake, or prevent bad behavior, and you make the choice not to disclose it, you have essentially lied by omission. Another serious lie is the half-truth: disclosing information selectively to give the wrong impression or misdirect someone's attention away from a serious matter.

A half-truth is a whole lie.

—Yiddish Proverb

Finally, gossip and speculation have no place in the health care community. They serve no purpose; they raise anxiety and lower morale. The truth is plenty for most people to digest, without having to sort out facts from rumors. Gossip that is false can have hurtful consequences.

A lie gets halfway around the world before the truth has a chance to put its pants on.

—Winston Churchill

The Body Language of Lying

If you're telling the truth, your body language will confirm it. If someone is lying, their body language will very likely reveal it. However, we have to be careful about interpreting body language: it is not a foolproof guide to lying. A person who is telling the truth, but is under a great deal of stress, may exhibit body language consistent with lying. By contrast, people who are great actors or who have the psychiatric character disorder of antisocial behavior or sociopathic disorder can lie without being betrayed by their body language. But the vast majority of people give nonverbal signs of lying.

What Can You Do to Influence the High Integrity of Your Workplace?

Your first line of defense against being asked to do something dishonest is to be the kind of person who exhibits integrity. You do this in small ways; you don't have to wear a shirt that says "Person of Integrity." For instance, you stand in for someone who is busy doing something else. You clean up an examination room so it is ready for the next person. You defend someone who is being teased. You focus in on an individual patient when chaos is all around you. You discreetly correct a colleague who has made a mistake. Soon, you will be respected for your integrity, and no one is likely to ask you to violate it.

In the same way, you can hold your colleagues to high levels of integrity. For example, you can praise someone who displays integrity. If someone is acting dishonestly, you can quietly question them about it. If they are rude or unkind, you can even say something like "I was disappointed to see you treat that patient rudely. That's not usually like you." Make sure that you have a code of conduct that you live and work by, and you expect the same from others. Your actions speak louder than your words.

People with strong characters have a high sense of what psychologists call "self-efficacy." Such people believe that, by their behavior and high standards, they positively affect others and, indeed, improve the entire organization. After all, when a patient encounters you, they judge the entire facility on the quality of their interaction with you. You enhance your self-efficacy when you perform your job competently and confidently, when you back up a friend or co-worker, and when your supervisor can count on you to do the right thing every time.

 JOURNALING 1-7

Do you act the same when you're by yourself as you would in front of other people? Think of an instance where you made a difficult but ethical decision, even though nobody else knew about it. Record this incident in your journal and reflect on how your actions made you feel.

Confronting Ethical Dilemmas

When you are confronted with an ethical dilemma at work, you have been placed in a delicate situation. You have to have an uncomfortable conversation; you may have to disclose information you wish you did not have; you may have to put something you value, like your job or friendships, on the line. It is important to think about how to handle these rare situations with skill.

As a general rule, you want to focus on the problem and its solutions, and less on the people involved. Of course, problems and people are difficult to separate, but you might think about how you would most effectively address a child who had misbehaved. If you were handling it right, you might say "I don't like your behavior" instead of "I don't like you."

When your integrity is challenged in some way, check your emotions and get all the facts you can. Let's take a simple example. A co-worker is very busy and asks you to document that she gave a patient a bed bath when you are pretty sure she didn't. You have been placed in an ethical dilemma. You have the patient's chart, and your co-worker asks you to do this in an offhand way, since you are already doing your own documentation in the chart anyway. Your first reaction might be to be offended. This person is asking you to lie, and take legal responsibility for it. Everybody should do their own documentation anyway. Before you react and say the first thing on your mind, though, you should get the facts. "Did you really give her a bath?" If the co-worker insists that she did, you will want to ask the patient, or someone else who knows, or at least go to the patient's room and see if there is any evidence of the patient having been given a bath. If, and only if, you can confirm that the patient was given a bath, can you ethically document the facts, such as "Mary states she gave Mrs. Parsons a bath, and Mrs. Parsons confirmed it." Before you confront this dilemma, you want as many of the facts as you can gather.

If you cannot confirm what your co-worker has claimed, then you have to take the action that preserves your integrity. "It doesn't seem that this patient received a bed bath this evening, Mary, so I can't document that in her chart." You have chosen language that doesn't directly accuse your co-worker but states your ethical response clearly.

You may know that this co-worker frequently asks other people to do her documentation for her. But do not get into this discussion. Past behavior is off the point and could lead to a different and unproductive discussion. Maybe the co-worker is a poor speller or has poor handwriting and doesn't like to do documentation. Stick with the current problem.

If your co-worker argues with you, you will just have to repeat your position and make it clear you are sticking to your principles. "I can't document what I can't verify." At this point, your co-worker may be angry or annoyed with you, but that is a small price to pay for your integrity.

In any case, you have not accused or blamed her. You have stated what you can or cannot do, and you have given your co-worker a chance to respond. Suppose she says, "I'm sorry I put you in that position. I've been so busy, and I just didn't have time to give her a bath, although I know she needs one."

At that point, you have to be happy that your co-worker at least has the honesty to admit her mistake. Because of the approach you have taken, you can help resolve the situation by focusing on the solution, and not your co-worker's bad behavior. "I'll help

you give her a bath right now," you might say. Or, "Let's ask Alicia to give her a bath when she gets in." It's great if you can preserve your relationship with your co-worker. But the important thing is that you preserved your integrity and reinforced to everyone the nature of your character.

Guidelines for Acting with Integrity in the Health Care Workplace

* Be on time. Health care facilities depend on promptness and punctuality.
* Treat every patient's private medical information with discretion. Do not talk about patients with other people not directly involved with their care. Act to protect their privacy.
* Do not gossip. If you get information you cannot trust, verify it rather than spread it.
* Complete your work and clean up afterwards.
* If you say you are going to do something, follow through and do it, so others know they can depend on you.
* Document patient care accurately and in a timely, professional manner.

*Honesty is the best policy. If I lose mine honor,
I lose myself.*

—William Shakespeare

CASE STUDY **1-3**
The Courage of Her Convictions

Isobel had seen signs of it before, but she had pushed it to the back of her mind, not quite sure that she had seen what she had seen. The last thing she ever expected to see from Mario was Medicare fraud.

It started last August when Mr. Hemminger asked Isobel Sotelo, the senior medical assistant at the medical practice, about a Medicare claim that had been filed that he didn't know anything about. Isobel copied the paperwork Mr. Hemminger brought in and later asked Mario about it. She and Mario had started together at North Central Orthopedic Associates many years ago. Mario had started out as a Medical Insurance Coder, but he had been

promoted over the years and now functioned as the business manager.

She showed Mario the documentation and said, "Do you know what this is about?"

"Hmmm, no. Let me see that. Hmmm, I wonder if this was supposed to be for someone else. Hmmm, and you're sure he didn't have these services performed?"

"He said no," said Isobel.

"Hmmm, well, I'll straighten it out," he told her, and she never gave it a second thought.

Until it seemed to happen again. Only this time, the person with the complaint was Dr. Fessenden, a professor emeritus at the University. Unlike Mr. Hemminger, who could be forgetful, Dr. Fessenden was pretty sure he was not mistaken about what was going on here. He was going to discuss it personally with Dr. Griffiths, and Isobel encouraged him. Later, she saw Mario and Dr. Griffiths in Mario's office, scrutinizing the paperwork and having a hushed conversation.

A few months passed, and then it came up again. This time, it was the daughter of Mrs. Hanson, one of Dr. Griffiths' patients at the nursing home. There seemed to be some bills for durable medical equipment that Mrs. Hanson never got, and a bill for "foot surgery," when Dr. Griffiths had only trimmed her toenails.

Isobel took this documentation to Mario. "I can't ignore this anymore," she said.

"Ignore what?"

"These fraudulent Medicare charges."

"What? Whoa! That's a very serious allegation Isobel. Very, very serious. People go to jail for that. I'm very surprised to hear you say this, Isobel, an old friend like you."

"I can't ignore it anymore."

Mario buried his nose in the latest documentation and motioned for Isobel to sit down.

"I just think these must be mistakes. Maybe I billed the services to the wrong people. I'll have to research this."

He looked up and made eye contact with his old friend Isobel. He could see she wasn't buying it. "Look, Isobel, we're just trying to maximize our Medicare reimbursement. You know we provide all kinds of free services here, and not everybody even takes Medicare patients anymore."

"Free services, Mario?"

Mario laughed abruptly and covered his mouth with his hand. "Well, I just don't know…what to say." He laughed again and brushed his hair back vigorously. "I guess I'm in a bit of a fix here."

"You needed the money?"

Mario said nothing, staring at the documentation.

"I'm just," he said after a moment, "sort of in the middle. It's really Mark," he said, referring to Dr. Griffiths. "He asked me, uh. I'm going to tell him to stop. This is just a mistake." He looked up at Isobel. And his gaze bore into her gaze, as if pleading with her to understand and overlook. "Let's keep this between you and me, and I'll put a stop to it."

Isobel said nothing. She rose and left the room.

Back at the front desk, Isobel was in a daze. A patient approached her, and it took her a moment to notice. She helped the patient and decided to throw herself back into her work and think about what she should do when she had a chance to give the matter her full attention. Before the end of the day, though, Mario asked her to come to his office. He ushered her in and closed the door. There, sitting in the chair behind the door, was Dr. Griffiths.

"Hello, Isobel," he said with a wan smile. "Mario tells me you have some concerns about some errant medical bills."

"Errant? Yes, they were for equipment and services that weren't provided." Isobel took a very slow deep breath. This was not a situation she ever wanted to find herself in. She liked Dr. Griffiths. He had been good to her. He was a good doctor. And Mario, he was a friend.

"Well, that's a very serious statement, Isobel, 'not provided,'" said the doctor. "I'm very sorry this all was brought to your attention. It should not have been. When Dr. Fessenden came in, you rightly referred him to me, and it was all straightened out. I think this is all just a big misunderstanding, don't you?"

"Very big," she said with a forced smile, looking into her lap. She knew that Dr. Griffiths would not be having this conversation with her if this wasn't Medicare fraud she had stumbled across.

"Good, good," he said. "If anything of this nature ever concerns you again, you come and see me, all right?"

She nodded and stood, asking permission with her eyes to be dismissed. Dr. Griffiths opened the door for her. "I'm glad we got this all straightened out," he told her.

That evening, Isobel went on the Medicare site on the Internet, the Office of the Inspector General. She copied down the number, and the next morning she called it. As instructed, she assembled all the documentation she had copied and saved and wrote a statement of her concerns, and she sent it to Washington by Postal Express. By then, she was a few minutes late for work. She felt afraid. She didn't know where this would lead. She worried about Mario, and even Dr. Griffiths. When she got to work, she quietly resigned.

QUESTIONS FOR THOUGHT AND REFLECTION

1. Did Isobel ask to be placed in this situation?
2. Do you think that Isobel was correct, that Medicare fraud was taking place?
3. What did it cost Isobel to preserve her integrity?
4. Could Isobel have taken an easier path?
5. Would you have the courage of your integrity that Isobel has?

Down a Dark Road

Even though it was only his fourth day on the job, Carl was late again. "Traffic," he muttered.

"Why don't you leave earlier?" asked Susan. "You're always late."

"If I left earlier," he said, "I'd get here even later." He started laying out his theory of timing and the Kennedy Expressway, but everybody dispersed. They had work to do.

When Alyssa took her midmorning coffee break, Carl was already in the breakroom, paging through a magazine. "Hi. Hey," he said, "have you seen these new Smart Phones? I was the first one to get an Android, and now they have a new generation. I want to get FaceTime so I can talk to my brother live. He's a big shot at the Chinese Embassy in Beijing. I'd be waking him up in the middle of the night. How about you, who would you call?"

"I don't know, Carl. I have a lot on my mind."

"Me too."

At 11:30, Carl asked his supervisor, Mike, if he could leave 15 minutes early for lunch. "I'm meeting a friend for a little handball, and I'll never get there on time if I don't leave early."

Mike said, "No. And try to get here on time in the future." In a little while, Mike noticed that Carl was hanging around the lobby, apparently waiting until the stroke of noon, so he could be out the door.

Later that afternoon, Susan approached Mike and said, "You're not going to believe this. I just saw the new guy Carl take a twenty dollar bill from a patient and put it in his pocket."

"Susan," said Mike, with a grave look on his face. "Are you absolutely sure?"

"I wouldn't say anything if I weren't," she said.

Mike took a few moments to compose himself and plan the words he would use with Carl.

Approaching Carl, Mike said, "I understand you received a $20 bill from a patient."

Carl smiled broadly. "What, somebody squealed on me?"

Mike ignored him. "You took cash from a patient."

"Not really," said Carl. "It was a tip."

Mike just looked at him, not breaking eye contact, not blinking.

"The guy just wanted to make sure his lab results would get to his doctor before his next appointment."

"We don't charge for the prompt delivery of lab results, Carl. What was the patient's name?"

"Well, I could probably look it up, why?"

"Because I'm going to return it to him as soon as you're out of the building."

QUESTIONS FOR THOUGHT AND REFLECTION

1. Does Carl have any credibility with his co-workers?

2. Why do you think Carl lies so much?

3. What do you think Carl told the patient to get the $20 bill?

4. How would you rate Mike as a supervisor?

★ EXPERIENTIAL EXERCISES

1. Give someone some straight talk. Plan the conversation in advance, and select the words and phrases you will use, including the ones you plan to come back to in the face of argument, emotions, or disagreement.

2. Arrange a debate, assigning ethically indefensible positions in advance to yourself, so you can hear what it sounds like to argue for something you find morally repugnant.

3. Go see a movie that features a character you think you will admire. Think about this character the next time you face an ethical dilemma. What would *she* have done?

4. The next time you think that someone is telling you something that isn't truthful, observe the person's body language to see if there are any clues that betray him or her.

CROSS CURRENTS WITH OTHER SOFT SKILLS

BUILDING TRUST: Without honesty and integrity, there can be no trust. (pp. 212-218)

DEALING WITH DIFFICULT PEOPLE: Honesty and integrity are the foundations for all relationships, especially difficult ones, where your character can be challenged. (pp. 231-238)

BUILDING SELF-ESTEEM: Once you choose honesty and integrity as the hallmarks of your character, self-esteem will take care of itself. (pp. 350-356)

TAKING ACCOUNTABILITY: This is how you demonstrate your integrity. (pp. 333-336)

Aiming to Be Adaptable and Flexible

To adapt, is to move ahead.

—Byron Pulsifer

LEARNING OBJECTIVE 4: AIMING TO BE ADAPTABLE AND FLEXIBLE

- Apply an adaptive behavior to a new situation.
- Be prepared to be flexible in the face of an emergency or unplanned event.
- Adapt to new technology and products introduced into your facility.
- Develop a methodology for accepting and implementing disruptive changes.
- Understand how to use teams and colleagues to manage change.

A young mental health worker tells his friends that what he likes about his job is that he never knows what to expect from day to day. "It could be quiet, or it could be crazy, you never know. But it's never quiet or crazy in the same way twice. You have to think on your feet." Although psychiatric facilities may be a little less predictable than others, the fact is that, in all health care facilities, unexpected changes and surprises are only minutes from walking in the door at all times.

The difference between adaptability and flexibility is in their permanence. When we adapt, we make a permanent change, from the old way to the new way, such as from x-ray film to digital x-rays. Flexibility is a quality that enables you to make adjustments on the fly, like filling in for someone or taking an emergency. The difference between being adaptable and being flexible is that being adaptable focuses on the skills one needs to respond to disruptive change, whereas being flexible is a personality trait that reflects your willingness to make last-minute changes to support the broader goals of an organization.

To succeed as a health care professional, you must use your critical thinking skills to help you embrace the unexpected. You don't want to merely tolerate change; you want to embrace it if possible. A group of Allied Health students were asked what they thought being adaptable and flexible meant to future health care workers, and a few of their responses are included in Box 1-8.

JOURNALING 1-8

Think about a situation at work or in your life in which you had to adapt to a problem. How did you handle it? Were you able to adapt without discomfort? Could you understand how your ability to adapt in a positive manner influenced the situation in a good way?

All is flux.

—Heraclitus

Drivers of the Need to Adapt and Be Flexible

Change drives the need to adapt, and change is rampant. Chief among these is technology. We know these changes will come. But there will also be changes in policies, laws, regulations, and management. Then, there are the changes more difficult to anticipate, like schedules and emergencies, which require flexibility.

BOX 1-8

Definitions of *Adaptability* and *Flexibility* from Allied Health Students

- "Being adaptable means doing something when asked, even if you aren't prepared for it."
- "I think being adaptable means being able to work with a patient if they are having difficulties or are difficult to work on, sometimes you might have to adapt your approach to them."
- "Being flexible means being willing to change hours or days if asked, maybe not have as long a lunch as you would like because you are needed."
- "I have had to be flexible with my time as an intern when someone did not make it in that day and they threw me into a new area of assisting the doctor."
- "It means being part of the team, taking pride in doing well, and providing the best care for your patients, no matter what."

Changes in Technology

These changes are reflected in medical equipment, imaging techniques, dental materials, better or more accurate instruments, and new treatments and surgical procedures. Once a new innovation hits the market, there is some pressure for all hospitals and health care facilities to adopt the latest procedure as soon as possible, to remain competitive. Many cost factors drive the acquisition of new technologies. Patients, insurance companies, and Medicare and Medicaid can be billed more for tests and procedures involving newer equipment. In some cases, new equipment could drive reductions in cost. For instance, the current push to install electronic medical records will save money by eliminating duplicate tests, eliminating physical storage areas, and requiring less manual maintenance.

Obviously technological advances drive better diagnostics, care, and treatment. Even the electronic medical records systems mentioned above will enable a patient's medical records to be collected in one place, giving practitioners better information to improve diagnostics and treatment.

Health Care–Related Laws and Regulations

Thousands of laws and tens of thousands of regulations govern the delivery of health care. Federal laws like the Patient Protection and Affordable Care Act of 2010, for example, will drive changes in the delivery of health care for years to come. Court challenges and decisions will continually alter its effect, and it will no doubt be amended and refined in the coming years. The Health Insurance Portability and Accountability Act of 1996 (HIPAA) drove huge changes in the way protected medical information (PMI) was handled by health care professionals, but these changes have now been broadly accepted and integrated. Federal laws are enforced by various federal agencies, which must write the regulations that determine how the law will manifest itself at the local hospital or clinic. In addition, each state has its own laws and regulations that affect how health care is managed in your particular state. For instance, the licensing of virtually all health professionals is handled at the state level. Even local ordinances and regulations affect factors like traffic and parking, noise levels, fire codes, and safety. All these rules can have an effect on you as an individual health care provider, and changes in them require you to adapt. Some changes can be significant.

New Policies, New Management, and Managerial Initiatives

Although laws affect like facilities alike, each facility has its own governance, that is, its own owners, boards, directors, executives, and managers. These people make decisions about how the facility will be organized and managed and ensure that all applicable laws and regulations are being complied with. They will act to make their organization more competitive and attractive to its customers. They will make capital expenditures and establish checks and balances to control costs.

Beyond the basics, business leaders are always working to improve things. You will see revamped performance review procedures, new ways to measure productivity, new and better security procedures, new construction, new medical records systems, new strategic initiatives—the list is endless. As a health care professional, you will have to find ways to deal with these changes.

Unanticipated Changes

Finally, all kinds of unexpected events occur in the field of health care. Emergencies crop up. Schedules often change. Employees are late or behind schedule. They are out sick or away from their station. Patients get worse suddenly, or arrive in groups. Family members can be harder to manage than the patients themselves. Clients may make unusual or unreasonable requests. The phones will go down, the computers will blow up, and chaos can reign all around.

Effects of Disruptive and Unexpected Changes

It's not surprising that all this complexity and rapid and pervasive change causes problems for health professionals. Without strategies and interventions, health care professionals can experience significant distress. In severe cases, the effects can lead to illness and burnout.

Stress is a physiological response to changes in the environment requiring the need to adapt. It is an involuntary response involving the autonomic nervous systems and hormonal changes. Managing stress is discussed in detail in Chapter 5. In addition, we have all experienced anxiety, but anxiety at work is particularly uncomfortable and, in fact, dangerous. Anxiety impairs critical thinking and decision-making abilities and can actually stop you in your tracks, not knowing what to do next. Controlling anxiety will be discussed in detail in Chapter 12.

Strategies to Being Adaptable

Adaptability will determine successful performance in a changing health care environment. Focus, problem solving, critical thinking skills, and being a team player are all important aspects of being both adaptable and flexible.

Pace and Focus

All changes are by definition unfamiliar at first. Go slow. You need to understand the need for the change and what it will mean for you, your workflow, your patients, and your facility. You will need to build new skills, which takes time and patience. If possible, work from a plan; this can be particularly helpful if you are asked to make a significant change: planning enables you to impose conditions on your acceptance of additional responsibilities to ensure your success. For example, you may want a quick tutorial on the use of new equipment, or an orientation on the preferences of a doctor you may be assisting. Every outcome will improve if you adequately prepare for the change.

Once you have made a microanalysis of what it will take for you to successfully manage a change, focus on the big picture too, the relationship between the change and the organization's mission and goals. It is much easier to embrace and implement a change if you see its purpose and desirability.

> *Enjoying success requires the ability to adapt. Only by being open to change will you have a true opportunity to get the most from your talent.*
>
> —Nolan Ryan

Finally, focus on how you can help your supervisor achieve her goals. She will obviously be responsible for seeing that the change is implemented successfully, and you can support her in that endeavor. There is no greater feeling than getting heartfelt thanks from a supervisor who recognizes what a great job you did of pitching in during an emergency or a time of unexpected need.

Finally, look ahead, not back. In times of rapid or unexpected changes, safety is ahead of you, not behind you. Box 1-9 summarizes a change methodology you can live with and embrace.

BOX 1-9

Five-Point Process for Remaining Adaptable and Flexible in the Face of Change

1. When it is necessary to make a change, put out of your mind your preconception of what you *were* going to do, and concentrate on what you *now* have to do.
2. Although you may feel apprehensive about the change in plans, try to embrace it, as if it were a learning opportunity, a challenge, a unique opportunity to contribute, or a chance to help your supervisor.
3. Throw yourself into the new activity. Make the best of the situation by seeing it as a necessary development.
4. Recognize that you were able to take on these unexpected changes. See yourself as resilient.
5. Incorporate your new abilities into the person you bring to work every day, adding value for your employer and esteem to your self-concept.

CASE STUDY 1-4
Two Faces of Lisa

Lisa, Dr. Wu's RDA, shows up to work her regular shift. As she's preparing her day and reading through the various procedures and patient charts, the front office manager comes in and tells her that Dr. Janklowicz's assistant will not be in that morning. "You will have to assist for both dentists today, Lisa."

Dr. Janklowicz is a fairly new dentist, and one that Lisa has not worked for or been trained for yet. Lisa is at the office 40 minutes early and has already set up for her regular dentist and the first patient. Lisa gets her morning coffee and goes down to the other end of the building and begins to prepare for Dr. Janklowicz's first patient. Even though the equipment is not the same and is new to her, Lisa is ready to problem solve and make it work. She reads through the day's schedule and does as much as she can to be ready for Dr. Janklowicz's first patient.

When Dr. Wu gets to the office, Lisa explains the morning to him and how she will now have to run between the two of them for the next four hours. But Lisa assures both doctors, as she has looked over the schedule for both of them. She knows the procedures, and when they need her help the most, she will be working with them by coordinating the procedures and times between them. Even though Lisa will be doing double the work load and running around a lot, she knows that problems can arise and will do her best to make the situation as "normal" as possible for everyone, in order to keep everyone as comfortable as possible.

QUESTIONS FOR THOUGHT AND REFLECTION

1. How was Lisa's response to this problem an adaptive behavior?
2. How was Lisa flexible during this unexpected situation?
3. How did Lisa's behavior help the dentist, the office manager, and the patients involved?
4. What would you have done?
5. Do you think her willingness to help made everyone's day better? How?

Down a Dark Road

Let's examine Case Study 1-4 again and consider what could have happened without the adaptive and flexible behavior that Lisa used.

Lisa, Dr. Wu's RDA, shows up to work her regular shift. As she's preparing her day and reading through the various procedures and patient charts, the front office manager comes and tells her that Dr. Janklowicz's assistant will not be in that morning. "You will have to assist for both dentists today, Lisa."

Lisa immediately panics and tells the front office manager, "There is no way I can do both jobs." She and the office manager get into a brief argument about the reasons why she should be willing to do so.

Grudgingly, with a sour look, Lisa agrees. Lisa has not worked for or been trained to assist Dr. Janklowicz, but she figures, "Oh well, not my problem." Lisa gets her morning coffee and the latest *People Magazine* and relaxes until her first patient for Dr. Wu arrives. Dr. Wu gets to the office, Lisa seats the patient, and then goes back to her desk to check her Facebook page. Meanwhile, Dr. Janklowicz arrives and goes into his office to wait for his assistant to come get him for his first patient.

Dr. Wu is ready to start on his patient, and he uses the "call bell" to alert Lisa that he is ready. While Lisa and Dr. Wu are in the middle of their first patient, the office manager comes to get Lisa, and wants to know why the room is not set up or the patient seated for Dr. Janklowicz. The patient has been in the waiting room for at least 10 minutes. Lisa tells Dr. Wu, "Oops. I have to go help the other dentist." Lisa is frantically running around, setting up the room for Dr. Janklowicz and the first patient, as well as figuring out what the first procedure is, and where everything is kept. The patient has now been out in the waiting room for 20 minutes and is at the front desk, angry and causing an unpleasant scene. Dr. Janklowicz comes out of his office to find out what is going on, only to discover that his assistant won't be there for the morning and that Lisa has not prepared the room or the patient for the procedure. Not only is the patient angry, but now they are 20 minutes behind.

QUESTIONS FOR THOUGHT AND REFLECTION

1. How does this second scenario differ from the first? What part of Lisa's behavior in this story is adaptable or flexible?

2. How did Lisa's response affect the doctors, the office manager, and the patients?

3. Compare and contrast the two scenarios and list some things that made a negative impact during the second version of the scenario.

4. Has this changed how you would handle or think about the situation if it was you?

5. Do you think the way a person handles unexpected problems can make a difference in the feel of the practice as a whole, the day, the patient's experience, and your co-workers' mood?

⭐ EXPERIENTIAL EXERCISES

1. This week while in class, see if you can identify a time when you, your classmates, or your instructor had to adapt to a situation. What was the problem? How was it adapted? How did this help the class? Yourself?

2. See if you can adapt a situation to improve it for yourself, your classmates, or someone in your family. What was the problem? How did you adapt it? What were the results? How did you feel when applying this solution or adaptive behavior?

3. Can you think of a time or times when you had to be flexible in a situation? What was it? Why did you have to be flexible? What might have happened if you were not flexible? Who might have suffered?

4. Over the next couple of days, see if you can find a situation in which you might be flexible. Write down each of these times and how you were flexible, how this helped in the situation, and who benefited from it.

◎ CROSS CURRENTS WITH OTHER SOFT SKILLS

LISTENING ACTIVELY: These skills will help you assess what is needed that will require your flexibility. (pp. 263-269)

MANAGING YOUR TIME AND ORGANIZING YOUR LIFE: If you are organized and in control of your time, you will be able to adapt and respond when circumstances demand it. (pp. 11-18)

THINKING CRITICALLY: Every day you will be called upon to make rapid decisions that call for prioritizing in the face of changing information. (pp. 320-325)

Striving for Tolerance

Anger and intolerance are the enemies of correct understanding.

—Mohandas Gandhi

LEARNING OBJECTIVE 5: STRIVING FOR TOLERANCE

- Identify why you must confront any biases you may have to succeed as a health care professional.
- Define how prejudices are formed and reinforced.
- Understand the importance of being aware of any biases you may have.
- Articulate the concept of secondary gains of biases.
- Describe how biases can be eliminated.

Suspicion, misunderstanding, prejudice, and hatred come about by overemphasizing the differences among people and groups of people. Tolerance is built on appreciating what we have in common—and learning to *celebrate* those differences that can enhance our lives.

The Need for Tolerance

The United States is a diverse country. We are a country of immigrants, with people from literally every country. Moreover, we base our national values on equal opportunity, equality before the law, and universal suffrage.

This is not a nation but a teeming nation of nations.

—Walt Whitman

FIGURE 1-6 Two health care professionals discuss patient information (Copyright © istock.com).

Health care organizations value diversity in their own workforce. Your co-workers were hired in part because of the unique perspectives they bring to the workforce in the form of their racial, ethnic, economic, social, educational, language, and religious backgrounds. Moreover, employers want to present a mirror image to their diverse patients, so they feel welcome and accepted the minute they walk in the door. You bring your own unique perspective to the job. You expect tolerance, and so does everyone else. As a health care professional, you don't get to choose which patients come to your facility for care and treatment. Everyone is entitled to equal treatment. Furthermore, you must be willing to work in teams with all kinds of people from diverse backgrounds (Figure 1-6). Tolerance is an important part of the skill set you bring to your work.

The Roots of Intolerance

To ensure that, as a health care professional, you are truly tolerant of your co-workers and clientele of all different races, cultures, and convictions, it is important to understand how intolerance develops.

Bias

Bias is an attitude of preferring one thing over another—which is fine when you are rooting for your favorite sports team. But bias against a specific category can cause conflict in the workplace. Rigid biases against those who are different can be difficult to overcome because it is a conditioned response, usually learned from childhood, by being exposed to unrelenting negative reinforcement about the objects of their bias. Then, later in life, biased people are unconsciously selective of the information received, noticing information that reinforces their bias and failing to notice or accept information that runs counter to their biases. Common biases are listed in Box 1-10.

Stereotyping

All of us are susceptible to bias; it isn't just a feature of other people who may be more ignorant than we are. This is because our brains are constantly categorizing information we encounter, so we don't have to follow the same thinking process every time we encounter something new. This process, called stereotyping, enables us to quickly pigeonhole new people and experiences, allowing us to say that "this new thing is just like some old thing that I'm already familiar with." It's a mental shortcut that enables us to move along rapidly as we encounter new things in our daily experience. There is nothing inherently wrong with stereotyping, and we all do it because of the way our brain is structured. In fact, without stereotyping, the world would be a much tougher place to navigate, particularly in these times of rapid change and rampant innovation and novelty.

Nevertheless, stereotypes are by definition generalizations, but there are all kinds of exceptions to generalizations. Even the most intelligent, thoughtful, and discerning people fall into the trap of letting their stereotypes do their thinking for them. In health care, this can lead to bad decisions. For instance, it has been documented that attractive patients receive less pain medication than unattractive patients with the same disease and pain level. This has been attributed to the stereotype that says attractive people are healthier than unattractive people.

Heuristics, or Rules of Thumb

Heuristics are general rules of thumb that guide our thinking and decision making. Generally, they are good guides and so serve as mental shortcuts in our thinking. For example, a lost child might trust a man in a police uniform, but few others. Through a mechanism called social proof, a young man may look to his girlfriend's mother for guidance on manners in a restaurant. People depend on rules of thumb because we resort to them when we feel unsure, and these rules do, in fact, work most of the time. Followed automatically without further thought, rules can lead to and reinforce biases.

"Groupthink" and Conforming

A tightly knit group tends to adopt common thinking, leading to biases. Also, once you are deeply committed to one group, there is a tendency to think that your group is better than other groups and to see people as members of groups, with all the broad characteristics you ascribe to that group, and not as individuals with unique characteristics. Similarly, if you are overly concerned about what others think, you may adopt biases you think they hold, so you will be in conformity with people whose opinions matter to you.

 WHAT IF?

What if you felt pressure from a group you identify with to share the group's bias against another group? What could you do?

Remedies for Intolerance

Since biases are attitudes, they can be challenged by thinking about them and refusing to let them function automatically—that is, stopping them from being expressed in actions. Interrupt this process, so that, when you see a person you are biased against, you insert active thinking before you take the preprogrammed action of shunning or acting in a hostile manner toward the person. However, an even better solution is to overcome your biases. Let's look now at steps toward ending a bias.

Awareness

The first step toward overcoming a bias is to notice that you have one. Then, pledge to be aware of it when confronted by the object of your bias. By examining the individual instead of his or her "type," you might find that the trait you are biased against is only a small part of the person—or does not even exist.

In health care facilities, biases cannot prevail. Because of the high stakes involved in health care, it is natural to want to rethink any biases. Rethinking is the beginning of the end of biases.

JOURNALING 1-10

Think about a friend you were originally biased against until you got to know the person. What was your bias and how did your friend overcome your bias to emerge as an individual?

Know the Secondary Gains of Your Biases

Most biases have secondary gains—something you are getting out of your bias. It is important to recognize these secondary gains and understand what little purpose they serve. For example, ex-smokers can be very intolerant of smokers. They can feel superior to others who have not been able to do the hard work of overcoming a cigarette addiction. This feeling of superiority is a secondary gain. Secondary gains, whether real or imagined, can come in astonishing varieties and can be hard to overcome. Box 1-11 offers a short list to get you thinking.

Examine Your Biases

Use the scientist inside of you to really look at any biases you may become aware of in yourself. How did this bias develop? Where did you get it? Who reinforced it? What were the characteristics of this group that reinforced your bias? Why did it once seem valid, and why are you not so sure now? Is it necessary for everyone to share your views, values, and

BOX 1-11

Secondary Gains from Biases

- Sense of superiority
- Blame can be assigned
- Predictions come true
- Status quo is defended
- Protection from loss of status
- Protection from emotional pain
- Convenience: biases are mental shortcuts
- No guilt

WHAT IF?

What if you felt compassion for somebody from a minority group different from yours? How would you show empathy?

Act As If You Are Not Biased

Now that you are aware of any biases you may have and understand the importance of eliminating the worst of them, you can examine your biases to determine if any of them result in secondary gains, such as feeling superior or belonging to a group. Once you identify these gains, you can eliminate the biases that interfere with your work and your personal life. Being aware of and learning about biases helps to eliminate them. To take things a step further, act *as if* you are not biased. Seek interactions and understanding with people you may hold a bias toward. Go out of your way. Be patient. Your attitude and your bias will not change right away, but it will begin to crumble. Why? Because you discover that stereotypes don't hold up. Instead, people are much more complicated, interesting, and surprising than you might expect. Even your friends who are different than you add richness and understanding to your life. You will also find that they bring unique talents, skills, and perspectives to the job, and contribute to your team in ways that only they can.

goals? Is a difference of opinion enough to justify a bias? You want to be a social scientist studying your attitudes that qualify as biases.

I used to think anyone doing anything weird was weird. Now I know that it is the people that call others weird that are weird.

—Paul McCartney

Who are your heroes and role models? Are they all similar to you? Can you think of reasons to admire people in groups different from your own? Thoroughly examining your biases helps to expose erroneous thinking, in turn demonstrating more clearly that they are really not valid.

Use Empathy

As a health care professional, your empathy should be strong. Use your empathy to put yourself in the place of people you are prejudiced against. See things

I don't like that man. I must get to know him better.

—Abraham Lincoln

CASE STUDY 1-5
Ex-Con

Bill Wilson warned the hospital that his CORI—his criminal background check—would come back with negative news. He had served eight years in state prison for drug trafficking. He had checked the box on the application that said "Have you ever been convicted of a felony?" He had written in, "May I explain?"

"I did a stupid thing when I was a teenager," he told the Human Resources Director. "The strict Rockefeller drug

laws were in effect then. I got caught with too much marijuana, but I never sold any. I have not taken any drugs now for over ten years. I go to Narcotics Anonymous meetings, and I have a sponsor. I also sponsor others, and I volunteer in drug treatment centers. Still, I pay for what I did every day. Most people won't hire me because I'm an ex-con. I always wanted to be a lawyer, but my conviction made it unlikely that I would ever be allowed to sit for the bar exam.

When I was in prison, I learned how to be a medic, and when I got out, I got my degree in Respiratory Therapy. I understand how people feel, but I'm a good person. Will you give me a chance?"

The HR Director was noncommittal. "Let's see what the CORI says, and then we'll decide."

Bill nodded, rose, and shook her hand. "Thank you for your consideration."

Outside, he sighed. This has been the story of his life. The only jobs he could get were laboring jobs. Maybe he should have learned one of the construction trades, or how to drive a rig or heavy equipment, or just tried to get into the military.

Inside, the HR Director, Georgia James, arranged a meeting with the hiring manager, Philip Acosta, the Head of Respiratory Therapy, and Jim Mandeville, Chief of Pulmonary Medicine. The feedback they gave on their interviews with Bill Wilson was positive, and she needed to facilitate a hiring decision made with the full disclosure of Wilson's background.

At the meeting, Georgia explained that the CORI report was negative. Wilson had been convicted of a felony, trafficking drugs, and served eight years in Attica State Prison in upstate New York.

"Wow," said Philip.

"What's a CORI Report?" asked Dr. Mandeville.

"Criminal Offender Record Information. It's a criminal background check."

"Huh. Well, I guess that's it. Too bad. I kind of liked him."

"Actually, although we are required to get a CORI before we make an offer to new employees, there is nothing that says we can't hire the person, if we feel the circumstances warrant it."

"No, no. We can't have a drug trafficker working in a hospital. I think we all understand that."

Georgia proceeded carefully. She didn't want anyone to think she was biased in favor of ex-offenders. "Let's just take a quick look at the CORI report and the facts before we move on," she said. "He had almost six ounces of marijuana in his possession. By law, that amount was automatically considered trafficking at the time. Mr. Wilson claims he never sold any drugs, but he has accepted his punishment and paid his debt to society."

"Well, that's most unfortunate for poor Mr. Wilson," said Dr. Mandeville, with a smile and wink at Philip. "But I don't think we should hire a marijuana smoker as a Respiratory Therapist. Do you, Philip?"

"That wouldn't seem to make a lot of sense, Jim. Is there anything else we should know, though, Georgia?"

Georgia then explained the circumstances as Bill Wilson related them. Georgia had also called the drug treatment center where Bill volunteered, and they offered a glowing recommendation for him.

"Look, Georgia," said Dr. Mandeville. "I'm sure we would all like to help Mr. Wilson. He seemed like a fine man before all this came up. But really, Georgia, a drug user? Have you ever known a *former* drug user? I mean, come on."

"Actually, there are millions."

Dr. Mandeville rolled his eyes.

"Like your friend, Dr. Barton."

"Let's not get personal," said Dr. Mandeville, losing whatever good humor he was still trying to show. "Dr. Barton was under a lot of stress. His wife divorced him. He's an extraordinary man, one in a million. Do you know what he had to go through to get off the stuff? It cost him over $200,000 out of his own pocket." His voice was rising now. Georgia did not want to be the target of his famous temper. But then Philip spoke up. "I'm willing to give Wilson a chance, but under only one condition," he said.

"What, drug testing around the clock?" exclaimed Dr. Mandeville.

"No. I'll hire him if you agree to give him a chance to show that he can change like Dave Barton did."

That silenced Dr. Mandeville for a moment. "Barton didn't go to prison," he muttered, but he said nothing more, because he knew that not everyone had David Barton's resources. Dr. Mandeville rose and went over to the window overlooking the river below. He said nothing for long enough that everyone was experiencing some discomfort. Georgia knew that the decision would now be based on the next words out of Dr. Mandeville's mouth. Philip collected all his papers and exchanged a glance at Georgia, who smiled weakly.

"Yes," said Dr. Mandeville. "We need to hire this man." He turned toward Philip. "He has my support."

"I'll let Mr. Wilson know that," Georgia said quietly.

QUESTIONS FOR THOUGHT AND REFLECTION

1. Was there any reason not to hire Bill Wilson, other than his CORI report?
2. Do you think ex-offenders should be allowed to work in hospitals?
3. What made Dr. Mandeville turn against Bill Wilson?
4. Can you find any instances of personal courage in this story?
5. Do you believe that Dr. Mandeville will support Bill Wilson on the job? Why or why not?
6. Do you think that the HR department, Philip Acosta, or Bill Wilson himself should disclose his past felony conviction to the staff members in the Respiratory Therapy Department? Why or why not?

Down a Dark Road

Mike had been a Lab Tech for a few years before he got a new job at the state university's student health center. The first thing that surprised Mike was the diversity of students who sought health care at his new job. He had worked in a suburban lab previously, and he had never been exposed to the clientele he was now meeting.

He went to school with a few African American and Hispanic people in the past, so he had some exposure to different cultures. However, the staff members at the Student Health Center represented different racial and ethnic backgrounds, people who represented groups he had never encountered before, like John Yee, one of the doctors, and Jayakumar, the pharmacist. To be sure, Mike wasn't sure if that was his first or his last or his only name. But Jayakumar seemed like a nice guy, and Mike actually felt pretty positive about being exposed to a wider world of people, although it was hard for him to think of all of these people as Americans, even though he knew they were citizens.

Dealing with the student patients was harder for Mike, though. As a phlebotomist, he had to touch them, find the arteries, invade each other's personal space. He didn't know what to say by way of conversation while he was in the rather intimate and uncomfortable act of drawing blood, so he developed a kind of professional script that he used to get him through these difficult moments. He would introduce himself formally and ask them a few pre-prepared questions. Had they had blood drawn before? Did they prefer their right or left arm? He would mutter what he was doing as he worked to fill the silence and, perhaps, to prevent any real conversation.

Some patients were particularly difficult for Mike. Africans and African Americans with very dark skin were hard. He often had trouble finding the arteries, but he learned to take some deep breaths and determine to be as patient as possible. He found large African American men physically intimidating, and he prayed he could find their vessels quickly and get them out of a lab room that always seemed way too small when they were in there. He felt strangely compassionate toward small Asian women. They seemed so delicate. Mike didn't want to hurt them, and he handled them very gently.

One day a Muslim woman in a hijab arrived to have her blood drawn. Mike really had no idea what to do. To him, it was like taking blood from a nun. Should he really be touching this woman, and asking her to reveal the lower half of her arm? While he was thinking all this, she said, "Is it possible to have my blood drawn by a woman?"

"Nope," said Mike. "I'm the only tech here. You can come back on Monday, but I think your doctor wants these results before then."

"Yes, he does. It's all right. I have my husband's permission."

"Permission?" said Mike. That didn't sit well with him. "Well, I never had anybody in a burka before. What do you want to do?"

"It's not a burka," she said. "It's a hijab. A burka covers everything but the eyes."

"Whatever," said Mike.

"I can pull back the sleeve on my abaya," she said, "but I would like you to sterilize the site with one of these," she said, pulling a jar of damp pads from somewhere within her gown. "They don't have alcohol."

Mike rolled his eyes but used the non-alcoholic pad she offered, and he quickly drew two tubes of blood.

Later that afternoon, Mike had a young Middle Eastern man, and just the appearance of this patient put Mike in a surly mood.

"You Muslim?" said Mike, startling the man, who nodded. "Any special procedures or rituals?" said Mike.

"No," said the man, confused, not sure if Mike was being hostile or sarcastic. Soon he knew.

"Do you have your wife's permission?" said Mike.

"I'm not married. Is there anyone else who can do this?"

"Nope, you're stuck with me." He grabbed the man's wrist harshly and started rubbing the site with an alcohol pad. "Don't worry about the alcohol." he said. He jabbed the man's arm coarsely with the needle, not really seeking an artery. He wiggled the needle around, making the man wince in pain. "Don't worry," said Mike. "I'll find one eventually."

"What are you doing!" Mike whirled around to see that Dr. Yee had been at the door. He had no idea what Dr. Yee had heard or seen. "Remove that needle and meet me in my office." As Mike left the room, he could hear Dr. Yee apologizing and taking over the blood draw himself.

Mike didn't spend much time in Dr. Yee's office. He was on his way home within a half hour, his personal items in the trunk of his car.

QUESTIONS FOR THOUGHT AND REFLECTION

1. Mike tried to act professional in the face of uncomfortable situations. Was he successful?
2. In your opinion, was Mike a "good man who did a bad thing," or are there deeper flaws in his character?
3. In your opinion, did Mike have good clinical skills?
4. What could Mike have done to deal better with his cultural biases?

1. Adopt a role model or personal hero from a race, culture, or background that is totally different from yours. Find out enough about this individual that you could articulate why this person is a role model to you.
2. Think about the wars that the United States has been involved with over its history. Think about the enemy people we have fought—the British, Mexicans, Northerners and Southerners, the Germans, Italians, and Japanese, the Vietnamese. How did we treat these groups when we were biased against them, and how do we see them today? Today, in the War against Terror, we are fighting Muslim extremists. Yet Islam, like Christianity, is a religion of peace. Are you biased against Muslims, or are you able to evaluate them individually?
3. Read *Black Like Me* by John Howard Griffin, the true story of a white journalist from Mansfield, Texas, who, in 1953, darkened the color of his skin under medical supervision and posed as an unemployed black man riding Greyhound buses across the deep south when the Civil Rights era was just beginning. The bias you see through Griffin's eyes will open yours.
4. Approach someone you may be biased against. Learn all you can by using your active listening skills.

CROSS CURRENTS WITH OTHER SOFT SKILLS

MODELING BUSINESS ETIQUETTE: Business etiquette mandates that you at least mask your prejudices with pleasant behavior, the first step toward overcoming your biases. (pp. 170-178)

SHOWING EMPATHY, SENSITIVITY, AND CARING: Seeing issues from the point of view of others is an effective way to overcome prejudices. (pp. 218-222)

VALUING MULTICULTURAL COMPETENCE: This will help you see people of different backgrounds as an asset rather than a chore. (pp. 238-242)

LISTENING ACTIVELY: The way to crush a bias is to get to know the person behind the label. Questioning and listening are the ways to do that. (pp. 263-269)

PRACTICING PATIENCE: Patience is a virtue you will need to overcome biases that are rigid and took years to form. (pp. 361-364)

Being Dependable

The while we keep a man waiting, he reflects on our shortcomings.

—**French Proverb**

LEARNING OBJECTIVE 6: BEING DEPENDABLE

- Provide examples of being dependable.
- Determine the dependability skills you have and those that you want to work on.
- Establish how your personal ethics, habits, or beliefs affect your personal dependability.
- Display dependable behavior with your co-workers.

Dependability is especially needed in health care because you are in charge of someone else's well-being. Ask yourself, "What does being dependable mean to me?" You might also ask yourself how you would rate your current level of dependability while on the job, in school, or during your interactions with others. Is it at the level you would want others to be? Do you need to work on it? How can you become more dependable? How does dependability affect your ability to do well on the job?

◀ JOURNALING 1-11

Think about a situation in which you depended on someone and they let you down. Or, can you think of an instance when you disappointed someone by being undependable? How did you feel? How did that affect your day and your feelings? What would you have liked to happen?

Allied Health students were asked what they thought being dependable meant, and some of their responses are presented in Box 1-12. Generally, being dependable can be viewed in terms of how much an employee can be counted on to do the job. Can the employee work as a valued team member, following rules and laws that govern the health care worker's job? Is he or she self-motivated and a problem solver and able to step up and lead when needed? Developing a reputation for being dependable can raise your income, your personal status, and your importance to the organization, all very important goals in today's unstable job market and economy.

> *Diamonds are only chunks of coal that stuck to their jobs.*
>
> —Minnie Richard Smith

Behaviors of People Who Are Dependable

You only get to claim the character trait of being dependable if you can be depended upon every single time, no exceptions. In fact, dependability is a quality bestowed upon you by others who experience you as a dependable person. What are the behaviors associated with dependability? Several steps for building trust are summarized in Box 1-13, and others are discussed in greater detail below.

Punctuality

No one enjoys being late (Figure 1-7). You get anxious and stressed. You rehearse excuses in your mind, knowing that none of them are acceptable. You inch closer to the car in front of you. You run across wet parking lots. You pace in front of elevators. In the world of health care, punctuality is essential. The whole operation depends on everything starting on time, from shifts to treatments to meetings to patient

FIGURE 1-7 A health professional practices good time management skills through punctuality.

appointments. Some people see punctuality as a time management issue, but it is actually a respect issue. If you respect the time of your patients and co-workers, as well as your own time, you will arrive on time if not early.

Here are two easy tricks you can use to develop this essential habit: Always assume that getting there will take longer than you think and set your alarm early. Viewing yourself as punctual can make you more driven to be on time.

Do What You Say You Will Do

It sounds simple: Do what you say you will do. But why doesn't everyone follow this simple rule?

For one thing, many people can't say "no." They want to be seen as cooperative, but their failure to deliver brands them as the opposite. Other people have good intentions, but fail to estimate how long things will take or what other obligations they have committed to. Before you say "yes," think things through carefully to be sure you can actually deliver, and say "no" when you have to. It can be far wiser to under-promise and then over-deliver.

Set a Positive Example for Others to Follow

Stop to identify the positive role models in your own life, and try to look for at least one good role model you might look to at work for guidance in a tough situation. When you are modeling your own behavior on someone you respect and admire, you become a positive example—and role model—for others.

CASE STUDY 1-6
Mr. Smith Goes to the Dentist

Monday is a very busy day, and Sonia has a special patient coming in, Mr. Smith. Mr. Smith is a 90-year-old man who does not have a personal care giver and walks to his appointment on his own. He is a sweet, elderly man who requires a lot of attention when he comes to the office. But he brings the staff flowers from his yard, and sometimes cookies or candy. Because she knows Mr. Smith is on the schedule, Sonia plans her morning to allow her the time to give Mr. Smith the extra care and guidance he will require for his appointment. Mr. Smith often needs help reading his forms, understanding the procedure, and getting to the operatory and in and out of the chair. Because of his age, he often gets confused and out of sorts, but he recognizes Sonia, and she keeps him calm and comfortable. He trusts her.

Today, Mr. Smith arrives a bit out of breath from his morning walk. He has a big grin on his face and a bunch of large pink flowers in his hand from his yard. Sonia greets him with a smile. She takes the flowers and gets a vase while she has him take a seat in the waiting room. The other women in the office, and a couple of the doctors, marvel at Sonia's ability to handle Mr. Smith and make him so comfortable. He is so much work. When the doctor is ready, Sonia takes time from her regular duties to go get Mr. Smith and help seat him for his appointment. Mr. Smith vaguely forgets why he is at the office, and Sonia spends some time reminding him. She parts after handing him a magazine and receiving a compliment that she is a "fine young lady."

QUESTIONS FOR THOUGHT AND REFLECTION

1. Can you pick out Sonia's dependable behaviors?
2. How were these behaviors being dependable?
3. Did Sonia's actions help the patient?
4. Would you be able to handle such a patient? Why or why not?

Down a Dark Road

Let's revisit Case Study 1-6, now with a few changes:

Monday is a very busy day. Sonia wakes up with a major headache. She knows she probably should not have gone out last night and partied. Oh well, she thought. The office will just have to manage without her. The office opens at 8:00. But Sonia doesn't call or text anyone until 8:30 because she has rolled back into bed and fallen asleep. Meanwhile, at the office, Mr. Smith has arrived. He is a very nice 90-year-old man who has walked to his appointment with his usual flowers in hand. When he arrives there 15 minutes early, the office is locked, and the building dark. Mr. Smith begins to second-guess himself. "Was I supposed to be here today?" he wonders. But he is tired from his walk, so he figures he will rest a bit and see if anyone shows up. One of the back office employees shows up, a bit late and in a hurry to get her own preparation done before her patient arrives. She greets Mr. Smith briefly, opens the door, and allows him to seat himself. She tells him to "hold onto" the flowers.

Mr. Smith is becoming a bit worried and slightly agitated. "Where is Sonia? Who is that girl?" The other receptionist comes in about this time. She usually doesn't have to get there until 9:00, but by now she got a text from Sonia, and she has had to find someone else to take her two kids to school. Because she is flustered and off key due to the last-minute rushing, she doesn't really have the time to "deal" with Mr. Smith. She grudgingly takes the flowers and tells him to "sit tight." "Someone will be with you as soon as possible." By now, Mr. Smith is getting pretty agitated and he is starting not to feel so well.

Mr. Smith's doctor arrives and tells one of the assistants to put him in his room so he can get started. Mr. Smith asks the assistant why he is there, and she tells him she doesn't know. Now Mr. Smith starts to panic and get agitated. His blood pressure is going up. It takes the doctor a while to calm him down and reassure him. Now, the doctor will be behind all morning, and the front desk will be short staffed. Mr. Smith will be disoriented all day because all this confusion has upset him.

QUESTIONS FOR THOUGHT AND REFLECTION

1. What are some of the obvious differences between the two scenarios? How about the less obvious differences?
2. How did Sonia's lack of dependability change this scenario?
3. How did her behavior affect the patient in particular and the office as a whole?
4. What does Sonia's behavior say about her personal values? How about her work ethic?
5. Can you see in these examples how dependability ties into other soft skills? How?

⭐ EXPERIENTIAL EXERCISES

1. During the next few weeks, while working, at school, or even in your personal life, see if you can identify others who display dependability. In what way? How did this make a positive impact on those around you?
2. For one week, go out of your way to display the ability to be dependable. Look for ways in which you can practice this skill. Write down what the situation was, what you did, and the reaction it caused. Did it help others? Did others take notice and remark on it? How did you feel? Was this easy or hard? Why?
3. Make a list of role models you hope to emulate in your life.

🔄 CROSS CURRENTS WITH OTHER SOFT SKILLS

MODELING BUSINESS ETIQUETTE: Dependability is an excellent segue to business etiquette. (pp. 170-178)
BUILDING TRUST: Trust is the essence of dependability. (pp. 212-218)
TAKING ACCOUNTABILITY: Only you can create the track record that others will mark as dependable. (pp. 333-336)

Bibliography

Griffin RA, Polit DF, Byrne MW. Stereotyping and nurses' recommendations for treating pain in hospitalized children. Res Nurs Health 30(6):655-666, December 2007. DOI: 10.1002/nur.20209. Copyright © 2007 Wiley Periodicals, Inc.

CHAPTER 2

Being a Student

THEMES TO CONSIDER

- Understand the importance of developing good note-taking skills.
- Use effective listening techniques to take advantage of learning opportunities.
- Choose a note-taking format and develop review techniques that work for you.
- Explain how tests are part of the daily life of a health care professional.
- Use tests as incentives to learn.
- Apply effective techniques and strategies to improve your performance on classroom tests and professional exams.
- Choose positive actions to help you succeed in your externship.
- Describe what you hope to accomplish in your externship.
- Describe the qualifications that will increase your value at your externship site.
- Apply your study skills to maximize your externship.
- Describe the characteristics and behaviors of a competent intern.
- Explain how to apply your externship experience to your job search.

Taking Notes for School Success

He listens well who takes notes.

—Dante Alighieri

LEARNING OBJECTIVE 1: TAKING NOTES FOR SCHOOL SUCCESS

- Explain why it is important to take good notes in class.
- List ways you can improve your listening skills and then put them into practice.
- Understand how your learning style affects your ability to take and review class notes.
- Describe how you should prepare before class in order to listen actively and take good notes.
- List ways that instructors help you know what to record during their lectures.
- Describe the three main note-taking methods.
- Explain how students can learn from the notes they take in class.

Taking good notes combines the art of listening and the act of selective writing—choosing what to write down. Many students report having trouble taking good notes, but it is a skill you can master. You actually have a big advantage in class because you can hear and take in words much faster than your instructors can speak!

Taking notes in class is just the first step in creating a personalized learning tool. Your notes are not complete when the instructor finishes the lecture. To make them useful, you still need to edit them and review them regularly. You will see how to do this later in this chapter.

JOURNALING 2-1

Think about your note-taking skills. Have the class notes you've taken in the past helped you to learn, master skills, and prepare for tests?

★ EXPERIENTIAL EXERCISE

Review the notes you have taken in one of your classes. How complete are they? How useful do you think they will be for reviewing and learning?

Listen Actively in Class

Most of the successful people I've known are the ones who do more listening than talking.

—Bernard M. Baruch

You cannot record what you do not hear, so good listening skills are necessary for taking good notes. Being a good listener is an important professional skill, so the classroom is the perfect opportunity to learn information and to acquire a life skill at the same time. See Box 2-1 for ways to develop good listening skills in the classroom.

Learning Styles and Listening

More than half of all people are visual learners. This explains why it is difficult for many students to pay continual attention during lectures. If you are a visual learner, here are some techniques to help you get the most from lectures:

* Complete any reading assignments before class.
* Avoid sitting near visual distractions.
* Keep your eyes on the instructor.
* Pay special attention to visual prompts such as writing on the board, PowerPoint slides, or other visual aids.
* Ask the instructor to write down any words or phrases you don't understand.
* During lectures, refer to your textbook or handouts that relate to the material.

If you are a kinesthetic (hands-on) learner, you can benefit from the physical activity of writing when you take notes. Here are some other ideas to help you improve your listening skills in class:

* Think about how you will use the information you hear during lectures.

BOX 2-1

Developing Good Listening Skills in Class

- Have a positive attitude about learning to listen.
- Leave your mental baggage at the classroom door.
- Sit where you can both see and hear well.
- Concentrate on the content of the lecture.
- Reel in your mind when it wanders and focus on the lecture.
- Keep an open mind about what you hear.

* Imagine yourself interacting physically with the topic, such as performing procedures or operating a machine.
* Make slight movements that do not disrupt others but keep you somewhat physically active. For example, count off the steps of a procedure with your fingers, stretch your legs, or take occasional deep breaths.

◀ JOURNALING 2-2

What kind of learner are you? How might this affect how you take notes?

★ EXPERIENTIAL EXERCISES

1. Choose a class in which to pay special attention to your listening skills. Are you able to continually focus on what the instructor is saying? Do you tend to get distracted? Do you comprehend what the instructor is saying?
2. Practice active listening when communicating with friends and family members.

Prepare Before Class

By failing to prepare, you are preparing to fail.
—Benjamin Franklin

Preparing for classes is an important part of taking good notes. If you simply forget about class between meetings and just show up each time as the instructor begins to speak, you will miss out on a good part of your educational investment.

Be sure to complete any assigned reading and other homework. There is nothing more frustrating than trying to follow a lecture in which the instructor assumes you know at least a little about the subject—and you know nothing!

Plan to arrive at class a few minutes early so you can be ready when the lecture starts. Arrive with a positive attitude, and be ready to get as much benefit from the instruction as possible.

Use a Binder

Notes are useless if you cannot find or identify them, so good organization is essential. A loose-leaf binder is a good choice because it is the easiest and most flexible way to organize. You can add new information in any order you wish, something you can't do with spiral notebooks. Binders allow you to insert revisions of your notes along with handouts, assignments, and skill check-off sheets. They also offer the best protection against weather and keep papers flat and neat.

If you use more than one binder, be sure to label them on the outside. You don't want to arrive at your anatomy class only to discover you have your pharmacology notes!

The Cornell Note-Taking System

The Cornell system is a method for laying out, editing, and studying from your notes. A key feature of the system is leaving plenty of blank space on each page so you can add information when you review and edit your notes.

To do this, set up each page on which you will take notes by drawing a line about 2½ inches from the left side. Then draw a line about 2 inches from the bottom. Figure 2-1 shows this page layout.

The large space in the center is for writing your notes during class. The left side is used after class to write key words, headings, questions, and other notes. The bottom space is for writing short summaries. There will be more information about using these spaces later in this chapter.

Decide What to Record

Instructors can say a lot during a class, and sometimes it is difficult to decide what to write down. You need to write down enough to understand your notes later. At the same time, you can't—and shouldn't—try to record every word.

Use what you have read about the topic to form a mental overview of the material. Listen for the main ideas in class, as instructors often give clues about what is most important. Here are some common instructor behaviors that say, "Write this down!"

* Saying, "This is important" or "You'll need to know this when you're working."
* Emphasizing certain words or ideas.
* Expressing extra interest or enthusiasm.
* Illustrating points with stories and examples.
* Asking questions of students during the lecture.

Box 2-2 contains a list of questions to keep in mind as you listen in class and study your notes. They can help you keep yourself on track mentally and help you focus on the main points of the lecture.

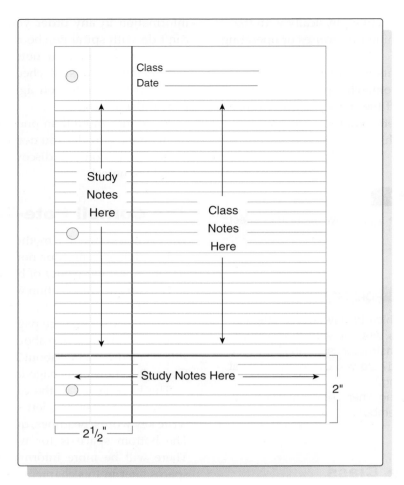

FIGURE 2-1 Example of setting up a page when using the Cornell note-taking system. After class, write additions and revisions on the reverse sides of the pages.

⭐ **EXPERIENTIAL EXERCISES**

1. During the next week, practice listening for hints from your instructors that will help you organize your notes.
2. At the same time, listen for clues your instructors give about what is most important for you to learn and remember.

BOX 2-2

Guiding Questions

- Why is this important?
- How does it work?
- What are the main parts?
- Why is it done this way?
- How is it done? How will I do this? When will I do this?

Choose a Note-Taking Method

There are several ways you can organize lecture content as you record it. When choosing how to take notes, consider your learning style, your instructor's way of lecturing, and the subject. The most important thing is to become proficient at it so you can focus on the content of the lecture.

The next three sections illustrate common note-taking methods. Each is written in the format being presented so you can see what it looks like. See Box 2-3 for note-taking tips that apply to any method. Figure 2-2 contains an example of notes written using an informal outline, the most common method.

Informal Outlines

How to use
    Indent to list and organize material
    Write phrases
    Don't label outline with numbers or letters

INFORMAL OUTLINE

Anxiety = response to perceived threat
    Cannot converse well
        Misses nonverbal cues
Helping anxious patients
    Get attention
        Slow conversation
        Help to focus
        Validate concern
Anxiety interferes with memory
    Create memory aids
            Write down appointments
        Give written instructions
Severe anxiety = panic attack = medical problem
    Physical symptoms
            Hyperventilation
        Rapid heart rate
        Unresponsive
        Numbness in fingers and toes
        Sensation of fluid in ears
        Feeling of dread
Helping with severe anxiety
    Acknowledge and accept to help patient gain control
        Decreases patient's fear
    Encourage slow deep breaths
        Do not use paper bag
                Causes decrease in blood oxygen
    Help patient validate and recognize significance
Explain symptoms
Stay with patient
Discuss handling anxiety
    Advise physician

FIGURE 2-2 Example of notes using an informal outline. This is probably the most commonly used method. (Data from Bonewit-West K, Hunt S, Applegate E: *Today's medical assistant: Clinical & administrative procedures*, ed 2, St Louis, 2013, Elsevier.)

BOX 2-3

Success Tips for Note-Taking

- Create your own abbreviations and symbols.
- Leave some blank space between major ideas.
- Write out examples, definitions, formulas, and calculations.
- Write on only one side of the page.
- Write as neatly as possible.
- Use an erasable pen.

When to use
    You are a linear thinker
    Lecture is easy to follow
Advantages
    Helps you organize material and ideas
    Keeps material in logical order
Disadvantages
    Difficult if lecture is disorganized or rambling
    May distract you from lecture content as you try
        to create the outline

Key Words and Phrases

Main ideas
Relationships between ideas
Supporting facts
Good for auditory learners
Fill details in later

Paragraphs

Writing in paragraphs can be effective when a lecture is hard to follow. Use phrases. Create a paragraph for each main idea. It is not necessary to write complete sentences. You can use abbreviations and shortened forms of words (e.g., Not nec to write compl sent. Can use abbrev, short forms/words). Mark important points during lectures. Organize and fill in details later.

This can be difficult for some students. They must write quickly and neatly enough to read later. It can be good for hands-on learners because it involves activity.

WHAT IF?

Suppose a classmate were ill and missed class and asked to borrow your notes. Would he or she find them useful?

★ EXPERIENTIAL EXERCISES

1. Choose the class note-taking method you believe would be best for you. Try it during the next few class lectures you attend and see how it works.
2. If the first method you chose doesn't work well for you, either revise it or try another method for a few days.

Make Your Notes Work for You

The average person forgets half of what was said during a typical class lecture within 24 hours of hearing it. So it's important to review your notes within a day of taking them.

Begin your review by reading over your notes and filling in any missing words or writing out the words you abbreviated. Next, fill in ideas or reorganize your notes as needed. If there are gaps or notes you don't understand, look for answers in your textbook, ask a classmate, or check with your instructor.

Consider rewriting your notes if they are very disorganized or incomplete. This revision will also serve

as a good review of the material. Use a highlighter or colored pen to mark key words and phrases. Write questions or notes in the space on the side and bottom of the page. See Figures 2-3 and 2-4 for examples.

? WHAT IF?

What if you've been taking notes in your classes but haven't had time to review them? When you finally get to it, you find that you don't understand much of what you wrote and that your notes seem incomplete. What should you do now?

Review Productively

The most important way to use your notes is to review them often, at least twice a week. The key to long-term memory is repetition over time. Keep in mind that you are not simply learning to pass the next test, but you are gathering knowledge to succeed on the job.

The best way to review is to write key words or questions in the blank space on the left. Box 2-4 has a list of sample questions. Cover your notes on the right-center of the page and answer the questions or define or explain the key words. This review method forces you to think and helps transfer the content of your notes into your long-term memory. Many experts also recommend reviewing out loud, especially when you are asking and answering your questions, as the best way to learn and retain new information. Use what you know about your learning styles when studying your notes. Here are a few ways to do this:

* Visual: Picture the words and concepts in your mind. Label drawings. Draw sketches.
* Auditory: Review out loud. Record your notes and review by listening to them.

BOX 2-4

Examples of Review Questions

- What is the definition of _____?
- What is the meaning of _____?
- What are the steps in performing _____?
- What is important to remember about _____?
- Why must you _____?
- What are the principal parts of _____?
- How does _____ function?
- What is the purpose of _____?

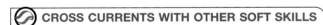

FIGURE 2-3 Notes are more useful if, when reviewing, you add details, write questions, note sources for more information, and mark key concepts. (From Haroun L, *Career development for health professionals: success in school and on the job*, ed 4, St Louis, 2016, Elsevier.)

* Kinesthetic: Stand up and move around as you review. Use movements and gestures to emphasize important points. Act out content.
* Interactive: Review with a study partner.
* Global: Write out the concepts and create a list of supporting facts.
* Linear: Look for logical patterns in the material.

CROSS CURRENTS WITH OTHER SOFT SKILLS

SHOWING EMPATHY, SENSITIVITY, AND CARING: You must be able to listen attentively to people in order to demonstrate empathy and caring. (pp. 218-222)

PROFESSIONAL PHONE TECHNIQUE: Taking accurate notes to record phone calls is an essential workplace skill. (pp. 257-261)

FIGURE 2-4 Make up questions based on your notes and write them in the left margin. Cover the main section and review by answering your "quiz" questions. This is reported to be *the* most effective way to learn from reading. (Data from Bonewit-West K, Hunt S, Applegate E: *Today's medical assistant: Clinical & administrative procedures*, ed 2, St Louis, 2013, Elsevier.)

YOUR QUIZ QUESTIONS	LECTURE NOTES
What is the definition of anxiety?	Anxiety = response to perceived threat Cannot converse well
How can anxiety affect patient behavior?	Misses nonverbal cues

What are ways the health care professional can help anxious patients?	Helping anxious patients
	Get attention
	    Slow conversation
	    Help to focus
	    Validate concern

What can the health care professional do to help anxious patients remember important information?	Anxiety interferes with memory
	    Create memory aids
	Write down appointments
	    Give written instructions

What is a panic attack?
What are the physical symptoms associated with severe anxiety?
	Severe anxiety = panic attack =
	        medical problem
	Physical symptoms
	Hyperventilation
	Rapid heart rate
	    Unresponsive
	    Numbness in fingers and toes
	    Sensation of fluid in ears
	    Feeling of dread

What actions can the health care professional take to help patients who are experiencing severe anxiety?	Helping with severe anxiety
	    Stay with patient
	Acknowledge and accept patient's
	    feelings
	Help patient validate and recognize
	    significance of anxiety
	Explain symptoms
	Discuss ways of handling anxiety
	Advise physician

Why is breathing into a paper bag no longer recommended for patients who are hyperventilating?	Do not have patients breathe into paper bag Causes decrease in blood oxygen

CASE STUDY 2-1

Jan is excited about starting her practical nursing program. She dropped out of high school to get married and was happy raising her four children. She got her GED a few years ago, but she always regretted not getting more education. Last year, her husband Frank was in a serious car accident and spent time in the hospital, followed by weeks in a rehabilitation facility.

During that time Jan saw the work performed by the nurses who attended to Frank. She could see what a positive difference the good ones made in Frank's attitude and progress. Jan noticed that it was the practical nurses who seemed to have a lot of contact with him, and the kind of career with direct patient contact and the opportunity to make a difference appealed to her. Going into health care would also give her the training she could use to continue Frank's long-term care at home and to replace the income that Frank could no longer earn.

Her first few days in school are almost a blur. There is so much to absorb: school policies and rules to remember, classes to attend, and people's names to learn. She feels a lot of pressure to do her best because she had to take out a student loan, and the last thing she wants is to have wasted the money.

Jan attends all her classes, but it's been many years since she was in school and she's beginning to panic. She never was a top student and is finding it difficult to always follow her instructors' lectures. When she gets home and looks over her notes, they don't all make sense. There are gaps, they are unorganized, and she's pretty sure many of the words aren't spelled correctly. At least she can't find them in her textbooks.

At first, Jan is afraid to say anything. She's older than many of the other students and believes that she should be able to do this at her age. After all, her children did well in school, and she would be embarrassed to admit she is having trouble. Instead, she works extra hard studying in the evenings and tries harder to concentrate in class.

Jan does not do well on her first quizzes and begins to question whether she can be successful in this program. She worries a lot about this and actually loses a few nights' sleep. Finally, she admits to Frank that she believes she has made a mistake.

"Let's take a good look at this," he tells her. "You've been out of school for more than 30 years. That's a long time."

"You're right about that," Jan admits.

"So, remember when we first got married? Did you know how to cook? How to keep a house? Why no, you had no experience being in charge of a household. But you learned—and ended up being the best cook in the neighborhood!"

"Okay, so what's that got to do with the trouble I'm having in school?" Jan asks.

"I think it means that you have to learn how to learn this new stuff. There are probably some techniques—like when you learned to cook—that you just need to know about," Frank says.

"That does make some sense," Jan responds. "Maybe I should talk with my instructors and see if I can get some help learning to learn."

The next day, Jan made appointments to meet with her instructors. They asked her a lot of questions about how she was studying, whether she read the assignments in her textbook, and finally—how good were the notes she took in class. After looking these over, her anatomy instructor smiled and said, "I think I know where we can start working on your study skills." Over time, with work and the help of her instructors, Jan learned to take notes that she could use to help her learn and succeed in her classes.

QUESTIONS FOR THOUGHT AND REFLECTION

1. How is Jan's situation a common one for older returning students?
2. What are some reasons why she waited so long to ask for help?
3. Why do you think she was having so much trouble taking notes?
4. How was Frank able to help Jan see her problems more realistically?
5. What suggestions do you think her instructors gave her?

Down a Dark Road

Dan Abrams felt he was lucky. He attended school to become a physical therapist assistant with his girlfriend, Ashley. If it weren't for her taking notes in class and helping him review for tests, he probably wouldn't have made it through graduation. Ashley took great notes in class and always gave Dan copies to study. Taking notes just wasn't his thing. He attended many of the classes, but he wasn't interested in learning to take good notes. After all, he would be working with patients, so when would he ever use note-taking again?

Dan got a job at a small physical therapy practice and really enjoyed helping patients with their exercises. He communicated well with his supervisor, Doug Anderson, and got along well with the patients.

After he had been on the job for a couple of months, the patient load declined and Doug had to let the receptionist go. He felt badly about this, but he needed to cut expenses to keep the office open. This meant there would be some cross-training among the employees. The PT assistants, for example, would have to take turns answering the phones, taking messages, scheduling appointments, and taking the histories of new patients.

When the time came for Dan to take on some of these new duties, he decided to give it his best, but after taking down a few phone messages incorrectly and recording patient data inaccurately, he began to panic. He just didn't seem to be able to focus intently on what people were saying. His mind tended to wander and he would lose track before he could get their words or information down on paper.

Doug's priority was on keeping his business going and he finally told Dan that if he couldn't get it together, he would have to let him go. Doug simply didn't have the time to correct the mistakes and take the losses they were causing.

QUESTIONS FOR THOUGHT AND REFLECTION

1. What does Dan's experience demonstrate about the relationship of study skills and job skills?
2. How did Ashley make a mistake by giving Dan her notes to study?
3. Do you think Dan will make it as a physical therapist assistant? Why or why not?

Reading to Learn

To read without reflecting is like eating without digesting.

—Edmund Burke

LEARNING OBJECTIVE 2: READING TO LEARN

- List the reasons why reading helps students benefit from their studies.
- Understand the purpose of prereading.
- Explain how to use headings to make you an active learner.
- List and describe the parts of a typical textbook.
- Explain the question-answer method as it is used when reading.

Reading, along with listening and taking notes, is one of the most important ways you will acquire information as a student. Like effective listening, reading to learn requires you to pay attention and participate actively. For example, if you were reading instructions about how to perform a medical procedure, you would ask yourself, "Do I understand this? What, exactly am I supposed to do?" And then you would read carefully to make sure you got it right.

The goal when reading your textbooks and other materials is to understand and think about what you will do with your new knowledge. Completing your reading assignments has several benefits. These are listed in Box 2-5.

JOURNALING 2-3

Do you enjoy reading? Why or why not?
Do you read to learn new things?
How would you rate your reading skills?

Getting Ready to Read

There are several prereading activities you can do to make it easier and more beneficial. The first is to clear your mind of clutter. Reading requires concentration. If you have something bothering you that can be handled quickly, take care of it before you start studying. If it will take more than a few minutes, write it down so you'll remember to deal with it later.

The next step is to find a place that encourages reading rather than sleeping or daydreaming. Many students find that a straight-backed chair at a desk works best. Also, make sure the lighting is adequate.

BOX 2-5

Benefits of Completing Reading Assignments

- The more ways you take in information, the more likely you are to remember it. Your memory paths are created and maintained by repeated use.
- Reading will give you background information for class lectures.
- Textbooks are a permanent way of saving information. You can review over and over.
- Books usually contain more supporting details, examples, graphics, and organizational aids than lectures.

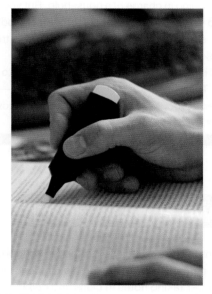

FIGURE 2-5 Highlighting important passages is a good way to actively study (Copyright © istock.com).

An uncomfortable environment can tire you and cut your reading and studying time short.

You need more than just a textbook to read actively, so gather your tools: notebook, pen or pencil, highlighter or colored pen, and dictionary (Figure 2-5). (Bonus: getting in the habit of gathering what you need is a good health care practice. You wouldn't want to interrupt a patient procedure because you forgot to bring something from the supply room.)

Previewing

Work smarter, not harder.

Many methods have been suggested for getting the most from your reading, but they all recommend that you preview the material you are about to read. This means quickly skimming the entire selection, learning any new vocabulary, paying attention to the headings, and using clues in the text to anticipate the content. Pay special attention to the lists at the beginning of chapters: vocabulary, objectives, and introduction. See Box 2-6 for a complete list of the features that textbooks include to help students.

 EXPERIENTIAL EXERCISE

Look over your current textbooks. Using the list in Box 2-6, list the features they contain.

When previewing, headings provide a logical structure to guide your reading. Try to relate them to information you already know. The following example of headings comes from a chapter entitled "Interacting with Patients" in *Today's Medical Assistant* (Bonewit-West, 2009)[1]:

Communicating with Patients
Verbal and Nonverbal Communication
Interference with Communication
Listening Skills
Nonverbal Measures to Facilitate Communication
Interviewing Techniques
    Close Questions
    Open Questions
    Keeping the Conversation Going
    Drawing Out Patients
    Avoiding Responses that Inhibit Communication

Before even reading the chapter, you can learn at least three things from these headings:

1. Interviewing techniques are used when communicating with patients.
2. There are at least two kinds of questions.
3. Some types of responses can interfere with communication.

Knowing this, you create questions in your mind and anticipate what you will be reading. You are now an active reader.

You may be thinking that previewing is a waste of time and that it would be better to just jump into the reading and get it done; however, this is not true, as many studies have shown. Previewing is actually an excellent use of your time.

 EXPERIENTIAL EXERCISES

1. From this or any other textbook, write a list of 10 chapter headings or chapter objectives.
2. Convert each heading or objective into a study question.

BOX 2-6

Anatomy of a Textbook

- **Preface**: Introductory section stating the purpose of the book and a list of its features.
- **Table of contents**: Often contains detailed outlines of chapter content.
- **Appendices**: Extra materials at the back of the book. Examples: list of professional organizations, guidelines for infection control, a metric conversion chart.
- **Index**: Alphabetical listing of all the topics in the book and the page numbers on which they appear.
- **Bibliography and/or references**: List of source materials used by the author and/or recommended readings for students who want more information.
- **Glossary**: Alphabetical list of words with their definitions.
- **Vocabulary or key terms**: Lists of words, with or without definitions, usually placed at the beginning of chapters.
- **Learning objectives**: Statements telling students what they should learn or be able to do after studying the material in the chapter.
- **Section headings**: Words or phrases that divide and identify various parts of the text. Serve as a "heads up" about what is to follow.

 WHAT IF?

What if you find that some of your textbooks contain many words you don't know and are difficult to understand?

Getting the Most from Your Reading

When you have finished your previewing and start reading, there are actions you can take to increase your learning. The first, and the one proven to be by far the most effective, is to ask and answer questions, out loud, about the material. To use this method, change each section heading into a question and look for the answer as you read. See Table 2-1 for examples of questions based on a few of the headings from "Interacting with Patients." You will get the most benefit if you say the answers out loud, even if you do so quietly.

TABLE 2-1
Examples Using the Self-Questioning Study Method

Section Headings	Study Questions
Verbal and nonverbal communication	What is the difference between verbal and nonverbal communication? How are the two types of communication used by health care professionals when working with patients?
Interference with communication	Give two examples of factors that can interfere with effective communication.
Listening skills	What are good listening skills? How can good listening skills be developed? Why are good listening skills important when working with patients?
Closed question	What is the definition of a closed question? What is an example of a closed question? When should closed questions be used when interviewing a patient?

BOX 2-7

Suggested Symbols to Use When Reading

- T = the instructor has indicated you will be tested on this
- ?? = I don't understand and need to ask about this
- * = this information is important
- ** = this information is *very* important
- circled word = this is a new word for me

BOX 2-8

Success Tips for Reading

- Look up unfamiliar words as you come to them.
- Take advantage of illustrations, charts, lists, and boxed text.
- Read through procedures carefully, paying special attention to the rationales (i.e., reasons for doing something in a certain way).
- Read in short sessions.
- Don't worry about your reading speed. Your goal is not speed; it is comprehension.

The second reading activity is marking your book in some way: underlining, highlighting, writing questions or key words in the margins, or using symbols. Do the highlighting or underlining *after* you have read a section. Otherwise, you are likely to mark too much material, thus defeating the purpose of highlighting. See Box 2-7 for a list of suggested symbols.

A tool that combines the features of a highlighter and pen is a colored pen. When it is used to underline, the color draws attention for easy review. Use the same pen to write in your book. This tool saves time because you don't have to switch back and forth between a highlighter and a pen. See Box 2-8 for more success tips for reading.

CASE STUDY 2-2
To Read or Not to Read

Emily Hasbrow didn't really know what to do with herself after graduating from high school. After reading an article in the local paper about careers in massage therapy, her mom said, "Emily, you are a perfect fit for this occupation. You've spent the last year moping around the house, not knowing what to do with yourself. You're really good with your hands, and you like people. Maybe you can get a job on one of those cruise ships. That would really be fun."

When her mother agreed to let her continue living at home rent-free and to help her with school expenses, Emily finally decided to go ahead and give the program a try. She passed the school's entrance exam, bought the necessary books and uniform, and started attending classes the following week.

Emily thought the classes were okay although not as interesting as she had hoped. And the homework—good grief! Did the instructors really expect the students to do that much reading? After a few days of slugging through her assignments, Emily decided that since she was going to class and taking decent notes, she couldn't see any reason to waste her time reading the textbook. When her mom asked about homework, Emily explained that there really "wasn't any." All the work was completed in class.

Emily was able to pass, with C's, the short weekly quizzes in her classes, but she had a surprise when the class had their mid-term exam. Where did the instructor get these questions? Emily couldn't remember having heard anything about some of this information. She had attended every class—had she fallen asleep or something?

When the tests were returned and Emily had earned a D, she went to see her instructor, Ms. Shepherd, to find out what had happened. Had Ms. Shepherd given them the exam intended for a different class?

The instructor explained, "Emily, looking over your test, it appears that the questions you missed were on the information contained in the readings I assigned. They are in your textbook and in the supplementary reading material. Didn't you ever look at these?"

Emily looked down. She didn't want to admit that she hadn't been doing the reading, as she thought it was a waste of her time. All she could say was, "Well, I guess I goofed up. I thought you were covering everything we needed to know in your lectures."

Ms. Shepherd smiled. "There's no way I have the time in class to cover everything you will need to know on the job. That's why I give the reading assignments."

"Okay," said Emily. "I get your point. I'm going to have to decide how I want to spend my time and how much my education means to me."

QUESTIONS FOR THOUGHT AND REFLECTION

1. Do you think Emily is really interested in becoming a massage therapist?
2. What mistake did she make when deciding how to spend her study time?
3. What kind of attitude does Emily have about school?
4. Do you think she will stay in school and pursue this career? Why or why not?

Down a Dark Road

Megan is glad to be finished with school—well, almost finished. She is now working at her externship site, a pharmacy located in a large grocery store where she is practicing what she learned in her pharmacy technician program. Megan is glad to be working because, as she told her friend, Amy, "I'm just so tired of reading boring books and doing homework assignments every night."

Amy, who is studying to be a nurse, agreed that studying could become tiring but seemed necessary if they were to learn all they needed to know for their careers.

Megan is not happy to learn that Ted, the pharmacist who was her supervisor, expects her read the employee procedure manual before she can start working with customers.

"Oh, great," she tells Amy one night on the phone. "Now I have to do *more* reading. I thought I was done with that."

"Well," Amy replied, "there might be important things about the pharmacy that you need to know."

"I just don't think I have it in me to go through that stupid manual," Megan said. "I think I'll just pay attention to what the employees are doing and ask questions when I need to."

Amy didn't think this was a good idea, but she had her own studying to do and didn't want to argue.

Megan followed her plan. She paid special attention to the actions of the pharmacy technicians and asked them questions about things she was unsure of. She thought she was doing just fine and told Ted that yes, she had read the manual from "cover to cover" and was ready to work with customers. The first couple of days went smoothly, but on the third day it seemed that every customer had some kind of question that Megan couldn't answer. Those that she couldn't bluff her way through, she asked the experienced technicians.

At the end of the day, Ted called her into the office behind the pharmacy. "Megan," he said. "I need the truth. There were questions today you were asking the staff that you would have known if you had read the procedure manual. Did you read the manual?"

Megan answered, "The truth? No, I didn't. I thought it might be a waste of time and that I could learn in other ways."

Ted sighed. "If you had told me this in the first place—the truth, rather than lying about having read it, I would let you have a second chance to read and study the manual and try again. But in this case, I'm afraid I'm going to have to ask the school to end your externship."

QUESTIONS FOR THOUGHT AND REFLECTION

1. What do you think of Megan's decision to learn about the pharmacy procedures by observing and asking questions instead of reading the manual?
2. Should Ted have tested Megan on the material rather than taking her word for it that she had read it?
3. Do you think Ted was fair in terminating Megan's externship?
4. What do you think Megan should do now?

Doing Research to Learn

LEARNING OBJECTIVE 3: DOING RESEARCH TO LEARN

- Become familiar with library resources in your area.
- Explain how to evaluate websites for credibility.
- Use the Internet to research topics of interest.
- List examples of reliable websites that contain health care information.

Research is not limited to finding information for a paper you have to write. We do research all the time, such as when we investigate which car to buy or how to find the best auto insurance. Research simply means finding sources of reliable information and obtaining what we need from those sources.

Libraries

You should get to know both your school library and your local public library. If there are other schools of higher education nearby, ask whether they allow the public to use their libraries. Some give checkout privileges for a yearly fee. Many hospitals and clinics have libraries for employees as well as for the public.

Today's libraries have many resources in addition to books and journals. Most offer Internet services, DVDs, and other multimedia materials. Every library is different. Walk around and explore. Look for informational brochures and how-to guides, and ask the librarian for help.

The Internet

The Internet is a rich source of all types of information. Box 2-9 contains a list of examples of what is available.

If you don't own a computer, check with your school to find out what is available. A complete discussion on how to search the Internet is outside the scope of this book; however, it is easy to use and doesn't require a lot of computer experience. You can learn more by entering the key words "Internet tutorials" or "online search tutorials."

You can find information on the Internet in several ways. The first is by using a website address. All sites have one, just like houses. If you know the address, you simply type it in. If you don't know which sites have the information you need, you can use a program called a search engine. You simply enter key words, and the search is on. You will be presented with a list of websites that contain information of various kinds about your topic. Here are the three general search engines recommended by the University of California (UC), Berkeley:

* Google: www.google.com
* Yahoo! Search: www.search.yahoo.com
* Exalead: www.exalead.com (UC Berkeley)

Some search engines are limited by subject area. The following are examples that you may find useful:

* Health: www.healthline.com
* Science: www.sciencedirect.com

General subject directories contain information categorized by topic, including health. The following two examples are recommended by UC Berkeley[2]:

* www.ipl.org
* www.about.com/health

Evaluating Websites

The Internet is not controlled by any organization or agency that checks on content or keeps it up-to-date. For serious research be sure to check the credibility of the information supplier. Here are some questions you should ask about a website:

1. Who is the sponsor? Universities, government agencies, many professional organizations, research institutes, and established publishers are usually good sources. This is not to say that commercial sites do not contain good information. Just note whether their purpose is to inform or to advertise a product. The endings of the web address indicate sponsorship:
   a. University: .edu
   b. Government: .gov
   c. Professional organization: .org
   d. Commercial enterprise: .com
2. Who is the author? He or she should have education and/or experience in the subject matter. Can you contact the author?
3. What is the purpose of the website? Many sites are designed to sell products or persuade readers to believe in a cause. The material provided may be biased.
4. How are claims supported? Check for statistics and references to original sources of information.
5. How current is the information? Are dates given? Advances and changes in health care occur continually.
6. What is the purpose of the website and its contents? To present facts? To give an opinion? To sell a product or service?

See Box 2-10 for a list of reliable websites that contain a wealth of information about health topics.

★ EXPERIENTIAL EXERCISES

1. Choose a topic in which you have an interest. Locate five sources of what you consider to be reliable information.
2. Briefly describe each source and explain why you believe it to be reliable.

Tests: Part of School, Part of Life

Think of a test as a challenge instead of a threat.

—Walter Pauk

- Explain how the daily tasks of health care professionals are actually tests of their knowledge.
- List the skills you can learn from preparing for and taking tests in school.

Taking tests is not limited to your life as a student. The truth is that life is full of tests. Employment interviews are a form of test with the purpose of assessing your ability to present yourself and your qualifications for the job. To legally work in many occupations, such as practical/vocational nurse and radiologic technologist, you must pass a professional exam. Other occupations, such as medical assistant, have voluntary tests to obtain certification that improve your chances of getting a job.

Tests on the Job

Once on the job, you are, in a sense, being tested every day. Although you may not think of your everyday tasks as tests, they are applications of what you have learned, and your ability to perform them correctly will be noted by your patients, co-workers, and supervisor. The annual employee performance evaluation is a type of test in which your supervisor writes a report about your work and then meets with you to discuss it. This document is then placed in your personnel file. Learning to perform "when it counts" is a valuable skill. For example, the mother of the infant in Figure 2-6 wants to know that the health care professional giving the injection has "passed the test" and is qualified to safely perform this task.

See Table 2-2 for examples of test-taking in school, during the job search, and on the job, and see Figure 2-7 for a sample employee performance review.

JOURNALING 2-4

What are some other similarities between classroom tests and working on the job? Think about past experiences, outside the classroom, in which you felt you were being "tested."

WHAT IF?

You are on your externship and the physician asks you to do a lab test. You learned and practiced this procedure in class, but at the moment, you just can't remember all the steps.

FIGURE 2-6 The mother of this infant wants to know that the health care professional giving the injection has "passed the test" and is qualified to safely perform this task (Copyright © istock.com).

TABLE 2-2
Applications of Test-Taking Skills

School	Job Search	On the Job
Take daily quizzes	Prepare for national and/or professional exams	Perform daily work accurately and completely
Review and take final exams	Present self successfully at job interviews	Participate in annual performance evaluation with supervisor
Demonstrate practical skills	Answer interviewer's questions effectively	It's all a test!

Wellness Plus Physicians Group
Employee Performance Review

Name:_____   Position: _____

Hire Date: _____   Date of Last
                                                         Performance
Supervisor: _____   Evaluation:_____

Rating Scale: 1 = Excellent   2 = Very Good   3 = Satisfactory   4 = Needs some improvement   5 = Needs much improvement

A. Quality of work performed   Comments:

   Rating   1   2   3   4   5

B. Use of judgment   Comments:

   Rating   1   2   3   4   5

C. Dependability   Comments:

   Rating   1   2   3   4   5

D. Cooperation with others   Comments:

   Rating   1   2   3   4   5

E. Appearance and hygiene   Comments:

   Rating   1   2   3   4   5

F. Attendance and punctuality   Comments:

   Rating   1   2   3   4   5

G. Time management   Comments:

   Rating   1   2   3   4   5

H. Proper use of equipment   Comments:
   and supplies

   Rating   1   2   3   4   5

I. Ability to work independently   Comments:

   Rating   1   2   3   4   5

(1)

FIGURE 2-7 Sample Performance Review.

**Wellness Plus Physicians Group
Employee Performance Review**

Rating Scale: 1 = Excellent   2 = Very Good   3 = Satisfactory   4 = Needs some improvement   5 = Needs much improvement

J. Communication skills   Comments:
    Rating   1   2   3   4   5

K. Willingness to take direction   Comments:
    and suggestions
    Rating   1   2   3   4   5

L. Ability to adapt to change   Comments:
    Rating   1   2   3   4   5

Employee's greatest strengths: _____
_____

Progress in meeting goals from last review: _____
_____

New goals for improvement: _____
_____

Plan for achieving goals: _____
_____

Overall evaluation of this employee: _____
_____

Reviewed by: _____

Date: _____

Employee signature _____

Date: _____
    (Signature does not necessarily
    mean agreement)

(2)

FIGURE 2-7, cont'd

Use Tests to Your Advantage

Classroom tests and work on the job both involve interpreting sets of instructions (questions and job tasks), performing within time limits (class session and appointment schedules), following given standards (instructor criteria and facility protocols), and being measured by indicators of the level of performance (grades, patient satisfaction, evaluations, and raises). In reality, performing on the job is more serious in terms of requirements and consequences than any classroom quiz or final exam. Students can repeat a test—or a class, if necessary—but correcting a medical error, winning back an unhappy patient, or reversing the poor opinion of your supervisor is more difficult. At the extreme is the possible damage done by an incorrect procedure or inaccurate medication dosage.

The intention here is not to terrorize the future health care professional but to put the subject of tests in the classroom in perspective. Tests are a fact of life, and if approached with the right attitude, classroom tests can provide you with opportunities to increase your learning. For example, tests encourage students to study. Most of us perform best when there is a consequence for our actions.

Tests also teach you to work under pressure, which is a daily reality for health care professionals. You can never take your tasks for granted, and classroom tests provide practice for working calmly and efficiently when it counts. Planning and preparing ahead, thinking about what you are doing, and performing to the best of your ability are habits that apply to both test-taking and work.

Finally, test results give you opportunities to improve and advance your learning. Review your answers to discover which material you haven't mastered. What did you not understand? What do you need to ask the instructor? What should you review again? Fill in the gaps in your knowledge now, while you are still in school.

JOURNALING 2-5

How can you approach tests with a positive attitude? What can you learn from taking tests? How can tests help you become a better health care professional?

Realities About Tests

LEARNING OBJECTIVE 5: REALITIES ABOUT TESTS

- Explain the concept of tests as a sampling of student knowledge.

- Explain how tests provide instructors with feedback about their teaching.
- Describe the best action to take if you believe a test is unfair.

Tests only ask for samples of what you are expected to know. Many students express disappointment when everything they studied does not appear on a test. They believe they have wasted their time and should have had to study only what was on the test. The truth is that health care professionals must know a lot of information. If instructors included everything on tests that students need to know, the tests would be so long that there would only be time for taking exams and no time left for teaching! Samples are reliable indicators of overall knowledge. For example, if you are expected to learn 1000 medical terms, the instructor may randomly select 50 for a test. Knowing more than what is on the test is a requirement for job success, not a waste of your time.

Classroom tests provide instructors with feedback about their teaching. Tests help them adjust their classroom strategies to ensure that their students have every opportunity to master the subject and skills. If many students do poorly on all or part of a test, it may be an indication that the information was not presented effectively and needs to be repeated.

Poorly prepared tests do exist. Test writing is a skill, and good test questions are not easy to create. Even instructors with good intentions may write some questions that are unclear and confusing. They may teach more than one class and forget exactly which material was—and was not—presented in each section. They may ask questions that are different from those they announced would be on the test. This does happen, and the best strategy is to ask the instructor politely to review the information.

⭐ EXPERIENTIAL EXERCISE

Describe five ways you can use tests to your advantage as you prepare for a career in health care.

Preparing Effectively for Tests

LEARNING OBJECTIVE 6: PREPARING EFFECTIVELY FOR TESTS

- List several techniques for preparing to do well on tests.
- Explain how to use study tools to prepare for tests.

The best way to prepare for tests is the same way you prepare yourself for career success: start preparing early, and study to learn so you master the content of your courses. Here are a few study techniques that lead to successful test-taking:

* Manage your time so studying is a priority.
* Identify and use study techniques that correspond with your preferred learning styles.
* Use learning techniques that help move information into your long-term memory, such as repetition.
* Take good notes in class, and review them often.
* Read your textbooks actively, and review them regularly.
* Seek help early if you are having trouble.

Steps for Successful Test-Taking

In addition to practicing good study habits, there are specific steps you can take to prepare for important tests.

1. Find out as much as possible about the test. Gather your notes and handouts, and ask the instructor for suggestions on how to best prepare. Suggested questions to ask your instructor: "What type of questions will be asked (such as multiple choice and true-false)?" "Will there be a time limit?" "Will it be given at the beginning or end of class?" "Will you review the material first?"

2. Quickly review your notes, textbook, handouts, and any other class materials to check your comprehension. Is there is anything you don't understand or can't remember, even after reviewing? Write a list of questions about the subject to ask in class. (This is why you start your review early, not the night before the exam!)

3. Make a schedule, and divide what you have to review over the time you have available so you won't run out of time before you have a chance to review everything.

4. Use the study tools you developed when you reviewed throughout the class. See Box 2-11 for a few ideas.

5. Identify and concentrate on the material you find most difficult and have the most trouble remembering.

6. Use the practice questions and quizzes you created from your class notes and from your reading. Try to recall the answers without looking at your notes or textbook. This may be the *single best way* to prepare for classroom tests.

BOX 2-11

Study Tools for Test Preparation

- Key words or questions to prompt recall of notes and text
- Outlines, charts, or mind maps to help you organize the material and make it meaningful for you
- Flash cards to practice recall. Put aside the ones that you know well, and concentrate on the ones you have the most difficulty remembering. Your goal is to move all of the cards into the "know-these" pile.
- Saying aloud or writing answers to your prompts and practice questions

JOURNALING 2-6

Think about your past test-taking experiences. Do you tend to get very nervous? What study techniques have you used to prepare? Do you usually feel prepared?

EXPERIENTIAL EXERCISES

1. Choose at least three study techniques to use when you prepare for your next test.
2. Create a plan for using these ideas, including the actions you will take and a study schedule.
3. After you have taken the test, write a paragraph describing how the strategies worked for you.
4. Are there other strategies you would like to try? If so, describe them.

The Anxiety Monster

LEARNING OBJECTIVE 7: THE ANXIETY MONSTER

- Describe methods for controlling test anxiety.
- Explain the purpose and process of desensitization.
- Describe how to deal with procrastination and feelings of being overwhelmed.

You have studied throughout the class, you have reviewed for the test, and you feel pretty secure about your knowledge of the material—but you are still panic-stricken by the idea of your final exam. You just know you'll freeze up and won't be able to remember a thing. You may even feel physically ill when you enter the classroom on test days. There just doesn't seem to be any way around it; you just "can't take tests." This is a real problem for many students, and solving it is an important step toward achieving your professional goals. Here are some actions you can take to help you manage test anxiety:

* Evaluate your study habits and test review methods. Can you improve them? Are you really using your study time efficiently? For example, some students spend a lot of time reading notes over and over but never actually quizzing themselves without looking at the written information. They think they know it, but without their book or notes, they can't remember very much.

* Think about your test preparation. It may seem like you are spending a lot of time reviewing because you feel worn out by it. In reality, if you engage in a marathon review session the last two days before the test, you may feel as if you studied a lot but are too tired to remember much of the material.

* Be honest with yourself. Do you have trouble understanding your classes but don't ask for help because you are embarrassed? Remember that instructors are there to help you, and asking for help is not nearly as embarrassing as failing a test or finding that you lack information needed to perform your job.

* Don't let your classmates freak you out. If you worry about competing with them, such as finishing the test first or earning a higher grade, you can get distracted from focusing on your own performance. Your education is not a race with winners and losers; the goal of a health care program is for everyone to win by graduating as a competent professional. Although the awarding of grades tends to set up a competitive environment, modern health care is delivered by teams of individuals who must work cooperatively, not competitively. Some classmates are even more anxious about tests than you. These people often express their nervousness by talking a lot and predicting total gloom and doom. Be upbeat with them rather than letting their negative talk increase your own anxiety. Avoid participating in "this is horrible" conversations around test time.

* Join forces with positive students. Organize a small group to review, share ideas, quiz one another, and cheer one another on. Have each person make up a few test questions and quiz the others. Seek out classmates who are dependable and will contribute to the group. Keep the number small (three to five) so everyone can make a contribution. Use visualizations and positive self-talk to promote learning and good test performance.

* Practice good health habits and stress-management techniques. Physical exercise releases endorphins, the body's natural tranquilizers. Do your best to get enough sleep before major tests so you're not exhausted. Take deep breaths to help quiet the mind.

? WHAT IF?

Your medical terminology class is more difficult than you expected. Your classmates constantly complain about how it is "impossible" to memorize so many terms, the instructor expects too much, and so on. Their constant talk is beginning to freak you out.

Desensitization

If you review thoroughly and try the suggestions for relieving anxiety but still find yourself freezing up during exams and feeling as if even dynamite couldn't blast facts out of your brain, you can try a technique called "desensitization." This is a treatment developed for people who have anxieties that interfere with their daily lives. It works by providing exposure to small doses of the source of the fear and then gradually increasing the size and number of exposures. Develop a plan to increase your exposure to tests. Have a friend or family member make up and give you tests, starting with short quizzes. Make them as realistic as possible. For example, set and stay within a time limit. Ask your instructor to give you practice tests. Find out if you can take these in a classroom under conditions as close to those of a real test as possible. Many sponsors of professional exams have sample tests you can take. These techniques may seem like a lot of work and even a little embarrassing, but if test anxiety is running your future career off track, desensitization is worth trying.

Don't Trip Yourself Up

Some students procrastinate in preparing for tests (and starting other projects, such as term papers) because they are afraid of failing. Their fear causes a kind of paralysis that prevents them from taking positive steps to prepare. For other students, not studying creates an excuse for failure. After all, if they try their best and still fail an exam, this might mean they lack ability. Another problem is feeling overwhelmed. Students who feel there is just too much to learn may decide to give up without really trying. If any of these behaviors sound familiar, make a deal with yourself to try something new. Study throughout the course, use the suggestions in this chapter on preparing for tests, ask for help, and work with a study group. The chances are very good you will experience success, and that can be habit-forming!

FIGURE 2-8 A multiple choice answer sheet (Copyright © istock.com).

JOURNALING 2-7

Procrastination is a common problem. Do you tend to put off studying and preparing ahead for tests? If so, can you think of ways to encourage yourself to develop better study habits?

The Day of the Test

LEARNING OBJECTIVE 8: THE DAY OF THE TEST

- Explain why you should plan to arrive early on the day of a test.
- List last-minute pretest actions that can help you perform better on tests.
- Describe ways to better understand what you are to do on a test.

It's the day of the test and you feel reasonably prepared. You certainly don't want to perform poorly just because you failed to follow some commonsense test-taking guidelines. Here are some helpful hints you can apply to any test situation:

* You deserve a good start, so plan to arrive early. Don't stress yourself out by rushing in late, scrambling to find a seat, and missing the introductory instructions.
* Bring your supplies, including books, notes, and a calculator (if these are allowed). An erasable pen (blue or black ink) works well because you can make corrections neatly and your instructor will be able to read your answers.
* Read and/or listen to all instructions. Ask the instructor to explain anything you don't

understand. This is not the time to be shy. You have a right to know exactly what is expected.
* Quickly review the *entire* test before starting. Read *all* of the directions on every page. If you have questions and the test has already begun, go to the instructor and ask them quietly.
* If there are different types of questions, note which ones will take the most time to answer and/or are worth the most points. Then quickly plan how to divide your time among the different parts of the test.
* If the test is longer and/or more difficult than you expected, do *not* panic. Take a deep breath, follow the guidelines, answer the easiest questions first, and focus on doing your best.
* When there are different types of questions, it is usually best to move from the shortest to the longest answers: true-false, multiple choice, matching, fill-in, short essay, long essay (Figure 2-8). This is like giving yourself a warm-up. Also, the questions that have the answers provided for you to choose from may give you ideas for answering questions in which you must supply the answers from recall.
* Limit the time you spend on questions you find very difficult or don't know. Mark them and return later after you complete the rest.
* Proofread your answers before you turn in your test. Did you answer all the questions? Mark the correct boxes on the answer sheet? Follow all directions correctly? Check for spelling errors, words left out, and other careless errors.
* Use all the time allowed if you need it. You don't earn extra points by finishing early, and hurrying may cost you a few correct answers.

Specific Test-Taking Techniques

- Explain the best way to do well on tests.
- Explain why knowing about various test formats can help you perform better on tests.
- List the techniques for improving your chances of correctly answering true-false, multiple-choice, matching, fill-in-the-blank, short answer, and essay questions.

The well-being of patients depends on what and how well health care professionals master the knowledge necessary for their professions. The purpose of studying is to learn for the future, not just to pass tests. And the *best* way to do well on tests is to thoroughly know your material. That said, it is also true that learning about commonly used test formats can help you to be more effective in showing what you know. Students who are unfamiliar with question formats can waste time and energy figuring them out.

It is important to keep in mind that some of the techniques suggested for answering test questions would be downright dangerous if applied to working in health care. For example, most study skills books recommend that if there is no penalty for incorrect answers, go ahead and guess. With true-false questions, you have a 50% chance of answering correctly, but with most multiple-choice questions, the chance is only 25%. But there is no room in health care for a 50% chance of correct performance. Some tasks, such as administering medications, must be 100% correct. There is no guesswork allowed!

The suggestions given in the following sections are only guidelines and *do not substitute for learning the material.*

True-False Questions

Examples

Read each of the following statements. If the statement is true, circle the T. If it is false, circle the F.

T F 1. Classroom tests are always good indicators of how well students understand a subject.

T F 2. Test performance can be improved by cramming as much as possible the day before the test is given.

T F 3. Reviewing material regularly throughout the course is the best way to do well on tests.

Suggested Techniques for Answering

- Be sure that every part of the answer is correct. If any part of it is false, the entire answer is false.
- Watch out for words like "always" and "never." Few things in life are that final, and statements with these words are often false. (There are exceptions, however. For example, there are safety rules in health care that must always be followed and legal rules, such as those concerning the release of patient records, that can never be violated.)
- Answers with middle-of-the-road words like "usually," "sometimes," and "often" tend to be true (except as previously noted).
- Do not spend a lot of time on true-false questions you really don't know, especially if they are at the beginning of a test that also contains more time-consuming questions.
- Guess only as a last resort (and only if there is no penalty).

Multiple-Choice Questions

Examples

Circle the letter to the left of the response that best answers each question.

1. Which is the best reason for learning to spell correctly?
   - **A** Patients are impressed by correct spelling.
   - **B** Patient care can be negatively affected if words are misspelled on medical documentation.
   - **C** Students who spell correctly get better grades in school.
   - **D** Good spelling skills increase the chances of receiving a promotion at work.
2. The Cornell note-taking system has proven helpful to students because it:
   - **A** prevents them from having to review notes after class.
   - **B** helps them record everything the instructor says.
   - **C** provides a format that encourages review.
   - **D** teaches specific active listening techniques.

Suggested Techniques for Answering

- Read the instructions and questions carefully. If the question asks you to identify the "best" answer, it is possible that more than one is correct. In the first sample question, all answers are good reasons for spelling correctly. So you need to think about which is the *most* important reason, and that is patient safety. Therefore, B is the correct answer.

* If the directions state to select the "correct" answer (as opposed to the "best," "most complete," etc.), consider each statement separately, and then ask yourself if it is true or false. (Many professional exams, such as the Certified Medical Assistant exam, are multiple choice.)
* Read through all the answers before selecting one.
* Immediately eliminate answers that are obviously incorrect.
* If the answer requires a math calculation, do the problem yourself before you look at the answers.
* Match each answer to the question rather than comparing the answers to one another.
* If you are guessing, choose an answer that has information you recognize.
* You can sometimes eliminate choices by using logic. For example, if two answers say basically the same thing, they must both be incorrect. As with true-false answers, if any part of a statement is wrong, the entire answer must be wrong. If the answer is silly or farfetched (instructors sometimes like to have a little fun), eliminate it immediately.
* If you are allowed to write on the test, circle or underline key words in the question to focus your attention when you read the answers.

Matching Questions

Examples

On the line to the left of each number in Column A, write the letter from Column B that explains one of its uses.

	Column A	Column B
___ 1.	Comma	A. Substitutes for letters that are dropped when contractions are formed
___ 2.	Semicolon	B. Indicates a change of thought within a sentence
___ 3.	Colon	C. Connects two sentences into one long sentence when a connective word is used
___ 4.	Apostrophe	D. Follows the greeting in a formal business letter
___ 5.	Dash	E. Connects two sentences into one long sentence without the use of a connective word
		F. Is placed at the end of a sentence

Suggested Techniques for Answering

* Read the instructions carefully. Note whether any item can be used more than once.
* Quickly count each column to see if both columns have the same number of items. Sometimes they do not. It is possible that an item may be used more than once or that one item is not used at all.
* Read through both columns before you write in any answers.
* Do the ones you know first.
* Some students find it easier to read the longer answers first (usually placed in the right-hand column) and then look for the shorter match. See which method works best for you.
* Mark or cross out each item as you use it if you are allowed to write on the test paper.

Fill-in-the-Blank Questions

Examples

Fill in each blank with a word or phrase that correctly completes the sentence.

1. The huge group of interconnecting computers located around the world is called the _____.
2. Learners who are both visual and global sometimes find that _____ is a useful note-taking technique to record information in a way that clearly shows relationships.
3. An explanation of why a procedure is performed in a certain way is called the _____.

Suggested Techniques for Answering

* Read the entire statement before attempting to fill in the blank(s).
* Write answers that fit the form and content of the words around them. For example, if the last word before the blank is "the," you know the answer is a noun.
* It sometimes helps to convert the phrase into a question in which the answer is the correct fill-in.
* The length of the space *may* be a clue to the answer, but there is a chance the person who typed the test didn't even know the answers and randomly chose the lengths. Therefore, this is not a reliable way to select an answer.

Short-Answer Questions

Examples

Write a short answer to each of the following questions, using the spaces provided. Some questions have several parts. Your answers do not need to be complete sentences.

1. List three reasons why many educators recommend using a three-ring binder to keep your notes and class materials in order.
2. Explain why previewing is a critical part of the reading process.
3. Describe four ways of starting to write a paper when you are having trouble determining exactly what to write and/or how to organize it.

Suggested Techniques for Answering

* Read the instructions to find key words that tell you exactly what is expected in the answer. Are you asked to explain? Give two examples? List five reasons? Define? Give the steps?
* If you are asked to write several sentences, answer the question as directly and completely as possible without padding with unnecessary information.
* If you don't know the entire answer, write down as much as you do know. You may receive partial credit.

Essay Questions

Example

Write a well-organized essay at least one page long explaining the meaning of this statement: "Study skills are career skills." Support your answer with examples and references to the National Health Care Skill Standards and the requirements of employers. You will be graded on how well you demonstrate understanding of the concept, as well as on spelling and grammar.

Suggested Techniques for Answering

* As with short-answer questions, read the instructions carefully to find out what you are to include in your answer. Provide evidence for your response? Give examples to illustrate? Give the sequence? Explain reasons and purposes? Defend your answer? Compare and contrast?
* Don't write answers that are too short. Even if the question does not specifically ask for examples or evidence, you should fully explain or defend your answer.
* Don't spend time with a lot of words that don't really mean anything, such as repeating the question or writing a long introduction. Answer questions directly.
* If you have trouble organizing an answer in your head, quickly jot down a few key ideas, an outline, or a mind map.
* Use the rule that journalists use when they write a newspaper article: state the most important

information first by answering the question as quickly as possible. Use the rest of the time to develop your answer, write examples, provide evidence, and so on to support your answer. This way, if you run out of time, you know you have included the most important information.
* Include the principal ideas of the course, as appropriate, especially those the instructor emphasized.
* Use the principles of good writing discussed in the chapter on writing strategies: good organization and correct grammar and spelling.

⭐ EXPERIENTIAL EXERCISES

1. Study the strategies given in this section for the various types of test questions.
2. Use the strategies when taking your next quiz or test.
3. Do you believe the strategies were helpful? Explain.
4. Discuss this statement: "Test-taking strategies are not a substitute for learning."

❓ WHAT IF?

You studied all the material you understood would be on a weekly test. However, some of the questions don't seem to be related to the week's lessons.

After the Test

LEARNING OBJECTIVE 10: AFTER THE TEST

■ List the actions that students should take if they perform poorly on a test.
■ Describe common test-taking problems students have and what they can do to resolve them.

Much as you'd like to forget about the test you just took, don't! Just like athletes who analyze each game to learn which plays worked and which didn't, you can use debriefing to your advantage. As soon as possible after finishing the test, review your notes and books to find the answers to the questions you were unsure about or just didn't know.

When the test is returned in class, try not to react emotionally. If you earned a top score, give yourself credit. Continue to review the material from time to time to reinforce and retain important facts and

TABLE 2-3
Common Test-Taking Problems

The Problem	What to Do
You didn't study at all or waited until the last minute and crammed.	You know what to do!
You studied but couldn't remember the information when you needed it for the test.	Check your understanding. Information you don't understand well can be very difficult to remember. Did you use prompts to study and review the material without looking at the answers? Or did you simply reread your notes and textbook? Passive review, or simply looking at the material, is not an effective learning technique for most people.
You were extremely anxious during the test and froze.	Review the section in this chapter on anxiety and try using the techniques. If they don't work for you, seek additional help.
You made careless errors.	Allow time to proofread your test before turning it in.
You didn't understand what the questions meant.	When you are studying, be sure to look up any words you don't know. During the test, ask the instructor for clarification. If English is your second language, see your instructor for help.
The questions were not what you expected. For example, you memorized a list of facts and definitions, but the test asked you to apply information to new situations.	Review your notes or other information about the test to see if you misunderstood. Be sure to attend all classes so you will hear announcements about test content. If you believe the instructor was unclear about the format and/or content of the test, speak to him or her privately.

information. If you did poorly, don't lose heart. Instead, try the following:

* Listen to any review the instructor gives of the test.
* If you have to return it to the instructor, take notes on a separate sheet of paper listing what you missed.
* Pay special attention to the questions you missed and write down the correct answers.
* If the instructor explains information, be sure to take notes.
* Ask questions about anything you don't understand.
* If your instructor does not discuss the test with the class and you did poorly, make an appointment to discuss it privately.

At your earliest opportunity, review your notes and the marks you made in your books. Did you miss some of the major points? Study the wrong material? Not really understand it? What can you do to improve your performance the next time? See Table 2-3 for suggestions on how to deal with test problems commonly encountered by students.

Professional Exams

LEARNING OBJECTIVE 11:
PROFESSIONAL EXAMS

- Explain the purpose of professional exams in health care.
- Describe who administers professional exams.
- List the types of credentials awarded to those who pass professional exams.
- Explain how students can prepare to perform well on professional exams.

Many health care professions have exams you must pass to work in the field. The purpose of professional exams is to ensure high standards for practitioners by testing for knowledge and competence. These exams may be administered by a governmental agency or a professional organization. Passing them allows the professional to use one of several special designations such as "licensed," "certified," or "registered."

Most exams require a fee. Your school may have included this cost in your tuition or fees. The school may also assist you in applying to take the exam. Some exams are given year round and others only on certain dates. Find out whether professional exams are required for your occupation. Learn as much as possible about the exam(s) while you are still in school.

Some professions do not require formal approval (certification, licensing, etc.) for graduates to work. At the same time, voluntary testing is available and recommended for many careers. For example, most states do not have licensing requirements for medical assistants. (States do regulate what procedures medical assistants can and cannot perform.) Many physicians, however, prefer to hire only certified or registered medical assistants, designations earned by passing professional exams administered by the American Association of Medical Assistants and the American Medical Technologists, respectively. Some health insurance companies and government programs, such as Medicare, require physicians to hire only credentialed professionals.

Success Tips for Passing Professional Exams

* Start preparing early. This suggestion is not intended to add further stress to your already busy class and study schedule. It is a reminder that if you prepare over a period of time, you will learn more and experience less stress when the time comes to actually take the test.
* Keep your notes, handouts, and textbooks organized so you can find and use them for review before the exam.
* Pay attention to any information and advice your instructor gives you about the content of professional exams.
* Some textbooks refer to specific exams and requirements of professional organizations, and the authors of the textbooks design their content and review questions to help students prepare throughout their courses. Take advantage of these features!
* Find out if there are review books available in your school library or for purchase or online materials to help you focus your studies on mastering the material likely to appear on the exam.
* Practice tests are available for many exams. Check with your professional organization.

* Find out whether review workshops are available in your area.
* Plan to take the exam as soon as possible after you become eligible. This is usually upon graduation from your program, although some occupations also require work experience. You are less likely to forget information and lose your confidence if you do not wait too long.

⭐ EXPERIENTIAL EXERCISES

1. Learn about the required or voluntary professional exams for your future occupation. (Sources of information: *Occupational Outlook Handbook* at http://www.bls.gov/ooh/ and your professional organization.)
2. Take practice exams or study review questions, if they are available.

Some Honest Talk About Cheating

LEARNING OBJECTIVE 12: SOME HONEST TALK ABOUT CHEATING

■ Explain why cheating is a serious offense for health care students.
■ Explain the potential consequences for the patients of students who cheat.

Health care professionals must follow high ethical standards. High-quality patient care and safety depend on their actions, and there is no room for cheating in any form. Furthermore, governmental regulations have increased, and audits of health care facilities are common. The consequences for fraud, taking shortcuts, and even trying to just "get by" are severe, including costly fines and closures of health care facilities.

You may believe cheating on tests in school isn't as serious as cheating on the job, but this is not true. Health care graduates who cheat to pass their classes, instead of learning what they need to know on the job, may become dangerous practitioners. You are in the process of becoming a professional, and what you do now is setting the groundwork for your future actions. Integrity (honesty, sincerity) is an essential characteristic of the health care professional, and cheating undermines that integrity.

Even if you do not cheat yourself, helping others to do so promotes incompetence in the health care system. Would you or one of your family members want to be treated by "professionals" who cheated to pass their classes? Do you want to carry the load at work for a co-worker who is used to taking the easy way out? Helping friends cheat allows them to avoid taking responsibility for themselves. This can lead to the habit of dependence and unsatisfactory performance on the job, resulting in negative consequences for everyone.

 JOURNALING 2-8

Have you ever felt tempted to cheat, or have you cheated on a test? How did you feel afterward? Why is cheating in a health care class an especially serious offense? What are some possible future effects on the job for students who passed their classes by cheating instead of studying?

? WHAT IF?

A classmate tells you she couldn't study for an exam because her ex-husband has been harassing her. She asks you to help her out by sharing your test answers during the exam. You sit together in the back row, so it is unlikely the instructor will see you.

CASE STUDY 2-3

Rosa Gonzalez is the first in her family to pursue studies beyond high school. She is enrolled in a dialysis technician program. Although she finds her classes interesting, they are also very challenging. They are much more difficult than those she took in high school. As she told her friend, Amelia, "High school classes were pretty easy. I didn't really have to study that much to get by."

Amelia, who is now working in her family's store, replied, "This is why I didn't go to college. I'm earning enough in the store and don't have the hassle of studying and tests to worry about."

Rosa told her friend that she really wanted something more out of life—that she thought health care would be really interesting and satisfying. "But," she said sadly, "maybe I've made a mistake."

After receiving a D on her first major exam, Rosa felt ready to give up. That evening, she said to her mother, "Mama, I'm so discouraged. I'm thinking about dropping out of school." "But Rosa," her mother replied, "I thought this meant so much to you."

"I know," said Rosa. "It did—or I thought it did. But I'm afraid I'm too dumb or something. I'm just not getting it." Her mother thought for a moment. "Rosa, I know that you're not dumb. Listen, you're paying good tuition money for school. Why don't you talk with your instructor and see if she can give you some help?"

Later that night, Rosa thought over what her mother had said. It did make some sense. She had taken out loans to pay for school. Maybe she should do more than just sit in class. The next day, she made an appointment with her instructor, Ms. Santori. As they talked, Ms. Santori asked about Rosa's study habits. "Well," Rosa said, "I really don't have a lot of time to study. And in high school, I just paid attention in class and did okay. I didn't have to do that much to get by."

Ms. Santori pointed out, "Getting by won't do here, Rosa. You're training for an important career that affects patient health and safety. The tasks you'll be performing must be done correctly and accurately. You've got to be prepared."

Rosa admitted that she hadn't thought about it that way. She asked Ms. Santori for suggestions about improving her time management and study habits to do better.

"Rosa," said Ms. Santori, "I like your attitude. I'd be glad to help you. We can get started today by looking at your out-of-class schedule and exactly what you do when studying for tests."

QUESTIONS FOR THOUGHT AND REFLECTION

1. Why is Rosa having difficulties handling college-level classes?
2. Is Amelia right that Rosa should think about getting a job rather than more education after high school?
3. What suggestions do you think Ms. Santori will give Rosa?
4. Do you think Rosa will complete her program and succeed as a dialysis technician? Why or why not?

Down a Dark Road

Jed Stuart's parents always expected that he would attend college. They hoped he would attend the university where they met and became engaged, thinking he would enjoy living in a fraternity, attending parties and football games, and participating in other college activities. Jed, however, really didn't consider himself to be the "college type." He was never very social, but preferred staying home and playing video games and watching sports and movies on television.

During his senior year of high school, his parents insisted that he start making plans. "Jed," his father told him, "you've got to start thinking about your future." "Dad," Jed said, "I'm really not interested in going away to school and living in a dorm with a bunch of guys I don't know."

"Well," his dad said, "you know our house rules. After high school, you either need to go to school or get a job and pay some rent if you want to live here. You'll be an adult, and you'll have to act like one."

Jed realized that the only jobs he would qualify for didn't pay much. And although he wasn't crazy about continuing his education, he knew he didn't want to be stuck in a dead-end job for the rest of his life. He knew from the career exploration class that seniors were required to attend that jobs in health care were pretty promising. And he had seen some ads for schools that were close by so he could continue living at home.

Jed talked with the admissions counsellor at a local college about the various programs offered. He decided to apply for the medical coding program. He liked the idea of mainly working alone, and the job prospects and salary sounded pretty good. He decided he would enroll in the program after graduation in June.

Once in college, Jed thought his classes were okay. The main thing he didn't like was having to work with other students when group projects were assigned. He also was reluctant to ask questions in class when there was something he didn't understand. Besides being shy, he believed it was the instructors' responsibility to explain the material well enough so that students could understand the material. This was his reasoning for not spending much time studying his textbooks. If the instructors didn't explain it in class, he figured that it must not be that important.

Jed passed the first few short quizzes in his classes, but he failed the midterm exams in two classes. As he told his parents, "The instructors in these classes really aren't that good. The students haven't worked with this stuff before. How do they expect us to learn it if they can't explain it well?"

QUESTIONS FOR THOUGHT AND REFLECTION

1. What do you think about Jed's reasons for selecting a medical coding program?
2. Do you think he will do well on future tests?
3. Do you think Jed will complete the program?
4. How is his attitude about working with others and speaking up in class affecting his academic success?
5. Is his opinion about the instructors' responsibilities correct? Why or why not?
6. What responsibilities do students have for succeeding in their programs?

Preparing for an Externship

The Importance of the Externship

LEARNING OBJECTIVE 13: THE IMPORTANCE OF THE EXTERNSHIP

- Explain the purpose and benefits of the externship.
- Consider what qualities you can offer to the site where you do your externship.
- Write out goals you want to achieve as you complete your externship.

Your externship can be one of the most valuable parts of your education. It provides the final link between your education and your future career, building a bridge between school and the world of work. Experienced professionals and/or externship instructors will guide your work in a real occupational setting. Take advantage of this exciting phase of your education to do the following:

* Apply the skills learned in class.
* Gain confidence in performing these skills.
* Learn firsthand about the expectations of employers.
* Practice working with patients.
* Think and problem-solve in real-life situations.
* Gain a clearer idea of what kind of job you would like after graduation.

* Demonstrate your abilities to a potential employer (students are sometimes hired to work at their externship site after graduation).

A successful externship requires your full attention and effort. Some students make the mistake of thinking that this part of their education is just one more assignment, especially if the externship is graded on a pass-fail basis. But nothing could be further from the truth! During your externship, you will deal with real people and real problems. At this time, you will begin to establish your professional reputation and influence your ability to get a job.

← JOURNALING 2-9

Think about your personal characteristics. Which ones do you believe will most help you have a successful externship experience? Which ones do you need to work on to increase the benefits you will receive from your experience (e.g., shyness, impatience, or difficulty being on time)?

Set Goals for Your Externship Experience

What do you hope to learn from your externship? You will increase your chances of benefiting if you write out goals that express specifically what you want to learn; what skills you hope to practice and/or acquire; and what you hope to accomplish by the end of the externship.

It is recommended that you research the facility as much as possible before beginning your externship. This will help you anticipate, prepare good questions for your supervisor, and set appropriate goals. Once at the site, share your goals with your supervisor and discuss what the site expects of you.

Ask if you can meet with your supervisor regularly, such as once a week, to discuss your progress and request feedback about your work. At the same time, conduct your own personal progress checks to see if you are meeting your own expectations and goals.

★ EXPERIENTIAL EXERCISES

1. Learn as much as you can about your future externship site. Look for a website and/or printed material. Ask your instructor for information.
2. Write three goals for your externship experience.

Getting Off to a Good Start

LEARNING OBJECTIVE 14: GETTING OFF TO A GOOD START

- Explain what is meant by "shift your focus" as you begin your externship.
- Develop the habit of practicing empathy with the people in your life.
- Explain the importance of developing and maintaining a positive attitude.
- Describe ways of making a good first impression as you begin your externship.
- Use your study skills to help you learn on your externship.

The first days of your externship can be busy and stressful. Do your best, but at the same time, be patient with yourself. It takes time to make the adjustment from school to a workplace. As an intern, you may not be 100% confident of your abilities and feel a little anxious about your performance. Keep in mind that no one expects you to know everything. There are three actions you can take to help you get a good start:
1. Shift your focus.
2. Develop and maintain a positive attitude.
3. Make a good first impression.
4. Learn all you can about the externship site and your duties.

Shift Your Focus

As a student, your main concerns are mastering new material, learning new skills, completing assignments, and performing well on tests and evaluations. Your principal responsibility is to yourself, perhaps to a family and a job, and to your personal progress. On your externship, you will need to shift your attention to the goals and needs of others: the employer, the patients, and your co-workers. You are now accountable to people who are depending on what you do and how well you do it. Keep in mind that patients and others consider you as part of the staff. You now represent the organization, as well as yourself.

Empathy

Understanding the feelings and experiences of others—patients, supervisors, and co-workers—is essential. People who have experienced an illness or injury sometimes feel as if they have lost control of their lives. The empathy expressed by caregivers and other support personnel can be a critical component of their recovery. Empathy is also important in relationships with supervisors and co-workers. Mutual understanding promotes effective working relationships.

Each of us will interpret a given set of circumstances differently. Your externship will give you opportunities to work with people with different cultural backgrounds, levels of education, religious beliefs, and life experiences. Difficulties and misunderstandings arise because most of us take our assumptions for granted and don't see them as only *one* possibility out of many.

Here are some suggestions for developing empathy:

* Listen carefully to what the other person is saying. You must know his or her view before you can begin to understand, and you can't know unless you listen.
* Don't judge what you hear. You are gathering information to help you understand the other person, not to decide if he or she is right or wrong.
* Ask questions or give feedback to ensure that you have received the other person's message as it was intended.

An important point to keep in mind is that it's not necessary to agree with the beliefs of others. You must simply be aware of them and how they influence their perceptions and actions.

❓ WHAT IF?

What if a patient who has a common cold complains to you because the physician would not prescribe antibiotics? She doesn't understand that viruses cannot be killed by antibiotics and insists that the doctor isn't willing to help her.

◀ JOURNALING 2-10

Describe a situation in which someone made you feel as if he or she understood and respected you. How was this communicated to you?

Develop and Maintain a Positive Attitude

Approach your externship with enthusiasm and a positive attitude. As explained in previous chapters, it is helpful when you create positive expectations. Look forward to putting your skills into

BOX 2-12

Focus on the Positive

- Do an inventory of the good things in your life, or start a gratitude journal in which you regularly record everything for which you are grateful.
- Keep things in perspective.
- Fix your sights on your goals.
- Distinguish between what you can and cannot change, and concentrate your efforts on what you can change.
- Find sources of help and inspiration.
- Visualize the satisfaction you can receive by overcoming a difficult situation.
- Challenge your negative beliefs.

practice, meeting and learning from interesting people, and securing a good recommendation from your supervisor.

We can choose our reactions to people and events. If you find a staff member at your externship site to be especially annoying, it is natural to become angry or frustrated. But how does this benefit *you*? Negative feelings drain energy and may interfere with your focus on your work. This person is now not only annoying, but has, in a sense, taken over your emotions. Don't give negative people that power.

Choosing to approach life with a positive attitude releases you from the control of circumstances and frees you to focus fully on what has meaning for you. See Box 2-12 for suggestions on how to develop a positive approach to life.

Make a Good First Impression

The saying "You have only one chance to make a first impression" is worth thinking about. People tend to make judgments about others very quickly and often on the basis of very little information. On your externship, others will be forming opinions about the level of your professionalism and competence. There are some key factors under your control that influence first impressions: punctuality, appearance, and courtesy (Figure 2-9).

It is critical that you arrive on time to your externship site, *especially* on your first day. Plan to arrive at least 15 minutes early on that first day. If you haven't been to the location already, do a trial run during similar traffic conditions before your start date.

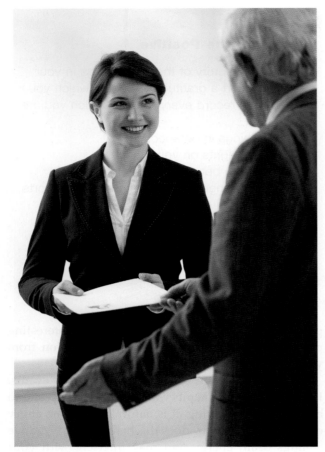

FIGURE 2-9 A courteous job seeker makes a good impression (Copyright © istock.com).

Absenteeism and lack of punctuality are two major complaints of employers who accept students as interns.

Most people are strongly influenced by visual impressions. Health care professionals, including interns, should follow the following dress and grooming guidelines:

1. Conservative—out of consideration for patients
2. Clean—for the safety and consideration of others
3. Safe—for the benefit of self and others
4. Healthy—to provide a good example of wellness

Some facilities are more formal than others, and what is appropriate in one may be unacceptable in another. Follow the directions you receive during your orientation. As a student intern, it is better to be more rather than less conservative, even if the employees seem to be casual about their appearance.

Courtesy is another factor in making a good first impression. Much more than simply using good manners, courtesy refers to being considerate and helpful. It means respecting the feelings of others and showing appreciation for the help you receive.

Introduce yourself to anyone you don't know, and be courteous to everyone at your site, whether you work with them or not.

⊖ JOURNALING 2-11

Describe a time when someone made a negative impression on you when you first met. Did your impression change after you got to know the person? Why and how? Did it take a long time to change?

Learn All You Can

Your classroom experience has provided you with occupational knowledge and skills. But there will be a lot more to learn when you start your externship because each facility has its own policies, rules, and procedures. Add to this the need to know the proper operation of equipment, location of supplies, and correct way to fill out forms.

Start by learning about the job. Ideally, your supervisor should introduce you to the facility and the employees with whom you'll be working. Your on-site orientation should include the following:

* Tour of the facility
* Location of supplies, files, anything you will need
* Safety rules
* How to use equipment
* Job description or list of your duties

If you approach your externship with a "can-do" attitude and apply the same skills that helped you succeed in school, you can learn and master your job systematically and effectively.

Use Your Note-Taking Skills

Your supervisor and co-workers will be important sources of useful information. Just as you took notes in class, you can profit from taking notes on your externship. Some note-taking situations will be formal, such as structured orientation sessions and employee training programs. Informal situations include receiving explanations and demonstrations from your supervisor and other staff. Taking good notes will prevent you from asking the same questions over and over, something that others will find annoying. Other benefits of taking notes at your externship site are listed in Box 2-13.

Recall that a key factor in effective note-taking is careful listening: clear your mind of distracting

BOX 2-13

Benefits of Taking Notes in the Workplace

- It helps you to concentrate on what you are hearing.
- It reinforces what you hear, through the act of writing it down.
- It creates a record of information you can study later.
- It enables you to put together a personal reference guide.
- It demonstrates to your employer and co-workers that you care about your work and want to learn.

BOX 2-14

Unsure? Ask for Guidance About:

- Direct patient care in which the physical safety of both you and the patient is at risk
- Use of equipment, chemicals, and other materials that can be hazardous if handled incorrectly
- Administrative responsibilities in which errors can jeopardize the facility's standing with a regulatory agency
- Coding and billing tasks in which errors can cause rejection of payment by insurance companies, Medicare, and other agencies

thoughts, focus on what the speaker is saying, and ask questions to clarify anything you don't understand.

Keep a Journal

Consider keeping a journal in which you record your thoughts, experiences, and feelings. (Caution: Do not record any patient names in your journal.) Describe significant situations and what you can learn from them. For example, describe incidents in which you are either involved or that you simply observe that cause you to think or feel strongly. Write about your reactions, how you believe the situation was handled, and how you handled—or would have handled—the situation. Your journal is also a good place to write out your externship goals and record your progress. Finally, you can include a task log in your journal in which you record the new skills you are acquiring.

Ask Questions

The potentially negative consequences of workplace errors make the ability to ask appropriate questions an essential professional skill. Whenever possible, use resources, observe, and think through situations to find the answer for yourself. If you cannot find the answer, there isn't time to do research, or if the situation is urgent, don't hesitate to ask an appropriate person for help. See Box 2-14 for situations in which asking for guidance can be critical.

Knowing *when* to ask questions is important. In situations that are not urgent, choose a convenient time for the other person. It is also important not to

ask questions about patients in the presence of anyone else, including other patients. Remember that the patient's right to privacy is protected by law.

⭐ EXPERIENTIAL EXERCISES

Start preparing a list of questions or information you think you will need as you begin your externship. Take the list with you during your first few days to note the answers you receive by being told, observing, or asking.

Create a Workplace Reference Guide

Your reference guide can be paper or digital. The important thing is to include information that will help you succeed on your externship. The following are items you might find useful:

* The name and telephone number of the person to contact if you must be absent or late
* Materials given to you during orientation or training sessions
* Notes taken during training sessions
* Schedules: holidays, vacation, meetings, and weekly schedules if they vary
* Facility staff directories and important phone numbers
* Maps and floor plans if you work in a large facility
* Notes from meetings attended
* Printed instructions and other how-to information
* Instructions about what to do in case of an emergency
* Procedures to follow during inclement weather

Use Your Reading Skills

Printed materials are the source of important job-related information. The following examples highlight a few of the most common ones:

* **Employee manuals.** These contain policies and rules regarding employee conduct, holidays and vacations, and other topics related to the employer-employee relationship. As an intern, some policies may not apply to you, but you should ask your supervisor if you can review the manual.
* **Policy and procedure handbooks.** Facilities create manuals to provide standard instructions for routinely performed tasks. Although it may not be necessary for you to read the entire manual, you should study the sections that apply to your duties. Pay special attention to procedures to follow in emergency situations.
* **Regulatory and approval agency standards.** Health care facilities are regulated by a variety of government and private agencies. Following the standards and rules set by these agencies is critical in determining the success—even the survival—of a facility. See Box 2-15 for a list of important regulatory agencies.
* **Instructions and technical manuals.** Being able to read and follow instructions (often called *documentation*, especially when applied to computer software) is an important job skill. Misusing equipment or performing a procedure incorrectly can result in serious consequences, including injury to the intern and/or patient.
* **Professional publications.** These include general health care newsletters and journals and those that apply to your specialty. They help you keep up-to-date in your field, which is essential in health care.
* **Library.** Many large facilities, such as hospitals, have libraries with resources you may find of interest.

Do note that you should *not* read patient charts, unless given permission or direction as part of your duties. They contain protected confidential information.

Use Your Observation Skills

There may be important things you need to know about your externship site that no one will think to tell you. They are not written down anywhere and may not even be discussed. Everyone simply takes them for granted. Here are some examples of customs and expectations:

* **Level of formality:** Does Dr. Patricia Abrams want the staff to call her "Dr. Abrams" or "Dr. Pat"?
* **Amount of at-work socializing among employees:** Does everyone go out to lunch to celebrate birthdays and holidays, or do individuals who have become friends at work plan these events on their own time?
* **Organizational values:** What are the most valued employee/intern characteristics?
* **Management styles:** Are student interns closely supervised or given lots of freedom?
* **Methods of communication:** Does your supervisor prefer all requests in writing?
* **Daily customs:** Who goes to lunch first?

You can learn the organizational culture and discover how to fit in as an intern by observing carefully and asking questions. At the same time, it is advised that student interns maintain some professional distance and avoid getting involved in office politics or employee cliques. It is also best to avoid developing close friendships or dating employees until your externship has ended.

Observe in order to learn from the staff. Note how they perform their work. Pay special attention to employees who seem especially competent and effective in their work.

You may notice that some of the procedures and methods used at your externship site are different from those you learned in school. Often a certain procedure can be performed in a variety of different, but correct, ways. Some experienced professionals develop preferences or acceptable (in terms of safety and effectiveness) shortcuts. Your facility may have

---

BOX 2-15

Important Regulatory Agencies

* Occupational Safety and Health Administration (OSHA): Oversees worker safety
* Clinical Laboratory Improvement Amendments (CLIA): Regulates laboratory testing on humans
* The Joint Commission: Evaluates the quality and safety of care for more than 15,000 health care organizations

specific reasons for using a different method. If you observe an employee using a method with which you are unfamiliar, increase your learning by asking the person to explain why it was done that way. Then use the method that is most comfortable for you *and* meets facility requirements. Never suggest that an employee is wrong because he or she is not doing something the way you learned it in school. The only exception is if you believe a law or safety measure is being violated. Under these circumstances, it is usually best to speak first with the employee. Then, if necessary, speak with your supervisor. And never feel pressured just because you are an intern to perform a task in a way you know to be unsafe.

Dealing with Criticism

Always keep in mind that the main purpose of your externship is for you to *learn*. You have just completed your classroom training, and no one expects you to perform perfectly at all times. You may make mistakes or not handle situations ideally. In these cases, you may receive criticism from your supervisor or the staff members, or even a patient. Consider this criticism as an opportunity to learn.

No one likes to be criticized, and it is natural to react emotionally. Dismissing the criticism as unfounded, becoming angry, or taking the criticism to heart and feeling worthless are common reactions. These reactions are natural but not very helpful. A more constructive response is to pay attention to the message, examine the criticism, and consider it carefully. Then decide, honestly, if any or all of it applies to you. If it does, you can choose to benefit from it and work on self-improvement. If it does not, consider talking over your feelings with the person who gave the criticism to see where the misunderstanding lies.

Becoming a Competent Intern

LEARNING OBJECTIVE 15: BECOMING A COMPETENT INTERN

- Explain why believing in your self-worth is important.
- Give examples of integrity in the workplace.
- Explain the importance of being responsible on your externship.

- Discuss ways of getting along with others in the workplace, including your supervisor.
- List the six steps that are useful for solving problems.
- List ways the student intern can contribute to cost control at the externship site.
- Explain how personal management habits influence your externship experience.

Employers have contributed to surveys about the competencies they value in their employees. As an intern, you can work on developing these competencies. Doing so will help you best contribute to the success of your externship, as well as prepare you for a future job.

Believe in Your Self-Worth

Positive feelings about oneself are essential to enhancing the life force in self and others.
—Mattie Collins

Believing in your self-worth means that you value yourself and your actions. You consider both to be important and deserving of respect. You understand that you and your work truly make a difference. These beliefs provide the foundation for all other career competencies, because they generate the self-confidence necessary to ask questions, learn new skills, and build positive relationships with others.

⭐ EXPERIENTIAL EXERCISES

1. List five things you like about yourself.
2. List five accomplishments that give you pride.
3. List five things you believe will make you a good intern.

Demonstrate Integrity

Integrity means being guided by sound moral principles, such as sincerity and honesty. Let's look at some examples of workplace behavior that demonstrate integrity.

* Admit when you make a mistake. Covering up errors in the health care environment can have serious consequences.
* Conduct yourself ethically. This means conforming to established standards for moral and correct behavior. In addition to ethical

BOX 2-16

BOX 2-16

Demonstrate Loyalty to Your Externship Site

- Dedicate your time on the job exclusively to work. Personal tasks and telephone calls should be limited to the lunch hour or break time.
- Do not use the site's computer to send personal emails or to surf the Internet at any time. Remember, anything that occurs online can be traced back to you.
- Never take anything that belongs to the employer. Don't contribute to the rising cost of health care by increasing the site's expenses.
- Do not speak badly or complain about your supervisor or the facility. If you have problems, seek solutions by discussing legitimate concerns directly with your supervisor.

BOX 2-17

Avoid Unintentional Breaches of Confidentiality

- Never discuss patient issues with anyone other than health care professionals who are directly involved in the care of the patient, and confine discussion to matters pertaining to this care.
- Limit allowable discussion to locations where you won't be overheard.
- When speaking with patients about personal matters, do so in a voice that only they can hear.
- Take care when speaking to and about patients on the telephone not to be overheard by others in the area.
- Leave patient-related matters at the externship site. Although it is natural to want to share your work with family and friends, any reference to patients and "interesting cases" is illegal.
- Clear computer screens containing patient records when you leave the computer.
- Don't leave paperwork or files containing patient information on reception counters and other areas where they can be viewed by unauthorized individuals.
- Do not discuss a patient's health information with anyone, even a patient's spouse or relative, without the written permission of the patient.

standards that apply to society as a whole, each health care profession has a code of ethics that serves as a guide for proper conduct. You should become familiar with the code for your profession.

* Develop a strong work ethic. This means taking a positive approach to your duties and giving each task your best effort. As an intern, you have responsibilities just as the paid employees do.
* Be loyal to your employer. You may not be paid as an intern, but the employer has agreed to take the time to help you continue your training. See Box 2-16 for examples of ways to demonstrate loyalty.

⭐ EXPERIENTIAL EXERCISES

1. Obtain a copy of the code of ethics for your profession.
2. Read the code and describe if and how it addresses human dignity, loyalty, honesty and sincerity, and responsibility to patients.

Respect Confidentiality

You have an ethical and legal responsibility to respect patient confidentiality, including both oral and written communications. You must be willing to monitor your work habits and conversation to make sure this important patient right is constantly guarded. Serious or habitual disregard of this principle can be a cause for dismissal from your externship site, as well as fines and disciplinary action against the facility.

All health care facilities have developed policies and procedures to ensure that medical privacy is maintained. It is essential that you learn and strictly follow these policies to prevent problems for yourself and for your externship site. See Box 2-17 for suggestions to help you avoid unintentional "leaks" of private information.

In addition to patient confidentiality, you have an obligation to protect the privacy of the facility where you are doing your externship. You also need to respect your own privacy. This means that personal problems don't belong at work and should not be discussed there, not with staff members and *never* with patients.

Be Responsible

As an intern you will be performing tasks that contribute to the workplace, and the employer will be depending on you. Acting responsibly means that your actions include the following:

* Be on time. If you haven't already visited the site, make a trial run before the first day of your externship so you'll know what time to leave home to arrive on time. Then be sure to arrive at the site on time every day, return promptly from lunch and breaks, and get to meetings on time. Absences should occur only for real emergencies. Have backup plans for child care, transportation, and anything else that could interfere with your attendance. *If you are going to be absent, call your supervisor as much in advance as possible.*
* Complete all tasks. This includes returning equipment and supplies to their proper places for the next person who needs them.
* Strive for accuracy. Examples of the many health care tasks in which accuracy is critical include patient charting, medical coding and billing, filling out compliance reports and lab reports, preparing sterile fields, and providing patient education.
* Help out when needed, even when it's not your job. The unexpected must be anticipated in health care. Co-workers are sometimes absent, emergencies occur, and situations can quickly change from routine to urgent.
* Follow through with everything you are directed or have offered to do. If you cannot perform a task or need assistance, let your supervisor know so the task can be reassigned or help recruited.

 WHAT IF?

What if the medical assistant who works in a busy pediatric office fails to autoclave the instruments as directed? As a result, the physician cannot perform minor elective surgery scheduled for a young patient. What would be the impact on the patient, parents, physician, and medical assistant?

Work Effectively with Others

Failure to work well with others is a major cause of employee dismissal because it reduces the health care facility's capability to provide high-quality

FIGURE 2-10 Workers collaborate and discuss creative solutions (Copyright © istock.com).

service. Your externship will provide you with the opportunity to practice good interpersonal and teamwork skills (Figure 2-10).

Providing good health care requires the cooperation of many specialized individuals. In addition, new types of professionals, in response to medical advances and increasingly complex delivery systems, continue to join the team. Whatever your occupational field, you will be working with a variety of people who will bring different personalities, work styles, personal goals, and skill levels to the job. Your challenge will be to work in harmony with them all because each one is important to successful care delivery.

Working with Your Supervisor

How well you get along with your supervisor can make the difference between looking forward to each day and benefiting from your externship or dreading the thought of showing up. Take the time and effort to get to know this important person.

Just as instructors have their own teaching and classroom management styles, supervisors also are characterized by a variety of management styles. These are shaped by the supervisor's personality, beliefs about management, personal experiences, and the organizational culture in which they work. Table 2-4 contains examples of different management styles.

Your work style may not match the management style of your supervisor. This is not uncommon. Consider these differences as challenges rather than obstacles. A number of constructive ways to work effectively with your supervisor in spite of differences include the following:

1. Keep communication open. One of the worst things you can do is avoid someone with whom

TABLE 2-4
Common Management Styles

Management Style	Examples of Supervisor's Actions
Micromanages	Closely monitors your work. Frequently checks on you and wants regular progress reports.
Believes interns and employees work best on their own	Doesn't appear to pay much attention to your work unless something goes wrong.
Likes a friendly work environment	Conversation is warm and friendly. Interested in your family and other aspects of your personal life. Birthdays and holidays are celebrated in the workplace.
Maintains a businesslike environment	Keeps most conversation work-related. Co-workers who become friends engage in social activities outside the workplace.
Disorganized or too busy to keep order	Loses reports you've turned in. Forgets scheduled meetings. Doesn't give you promised follow-up in a timely way. (Caution: Don't assume that because your supervisor is disorganized, he or she will tolerate *your* disorganization and accept actions such as completing assignments late.)
Values and practices order	Rarely misses deadlines and expects you to meet them too, correctly and efficiently. Keeps lists, calendars, and orderly files.
Communicates directly	Lets you know how you are doing. Offers suggestions and criticism as needed. You know where you stand.
Communicates indirectly (or not at all)	Doesn't want to hurt your feelings. Avoids confrontations. May not tell you if you are doing something incorrectly or not to his or her liking. (Caution: May complain about you behind your back, thus depriving you of the opportunity to learn and resolve the problem.)

you disagree or have difficulty. Cutting off contact is likely to increase distance and decrease understanding.

2. Don't complain to the employees at your externship site. This does not resolve problems and can actually create new problems: lowered morale among those who hear your complaints, lost work time, decrease in the quality of service to patients, and worsened relationships with the supervisor who hears about the grumbling through the grapevine.

3. Be empathetic. Your supervisor may have pressures and problems that explain his or her actions.

4. Ask questions to learn your supervisor's priorities and find out what is most important. Box 2-18 contains examples of questions to ask your supervisor.

5. Ask for clarification if you are unclear about your duties or exactly what is expected of you.

6. Realize the bottom line is this: you must work with your supervisor, and this means adapting to his or her style. Do your best to make the situation positive. Focus on learning as much as possible from both the supervisor and the situation.

BOX 2-18

Questions to Ask Your Supervisor

- What are your expectations of me?
- What do you most value in an intern?
- How can I best contribute to the success of the organization and/or facility?
- How often would you like me to report to you?
- What is the best time to report to you, ask questions, and receive progress reports about my work?

Think about What You Are Doing

Health care interns, as well as employees, must keep their minds in gear, continually observing and thinking as they perform their duties. You cannot perform daily work automatically in a "robot mode." You must ask yourself questions, think about the meaning of what you see, and use this information to determine the most appropriate action to take. Your externship work will be important, and the potential consequences of failing to be alert and thinking can be serious.

 WHAT IF?

Mr. Cardenas, who doesn't understand English well, is scheduled for a lab test that requires him to follow certain directions the day before the test. The medical assistant gives him a written instruction sheet in English.

Solve Problems Effectively

A problem well stated is a problem half solved.
—Charles F. Kettering

Every day we are confronted with situations that require us to solve problems and make decisions. You should expect to practice these actions during your externship, both at home and in the workplace. Having an organized way to approach problems makes it easier to find effective solutions. One commonly used method consists of six steps:

1. Define the problem.
2. Gather information.
3. Brainstorm alternative solutions.
4. Consider possible results and consequences.
5. Choose a solution and act on it.
6. Evaluate the results and revise as needed.

Good problem-solving skills involve both reasoning and creativity. Start by examining what you believe to be the problem. Try to see it from different angles. Mentally walk around the problem, looking at it from all sides.

Try using brainstorming to come up with possible solutions. This means thinking of as many ideas as possible, from the sensible to the crazy. Think creatively. Original methods often provide the solutions to problems.

While creativity generates ideas, reasoning helps you to put the ideas together in ways that work. It also helps you to test potential outcomes mentally. Use it to check "What would happen if ..." scenarios for the possibilities you have brainstormed.

Before you approach your supervisor with a problem, think it through. Do your best to come up with solutions to suggest. This demonstrates your initiative and willingness to take an active part in solving workplace problems.

EXPERIENTIAL EXERCISES

1. Choose a real problem you would like to solve and go through the six-step process.
2. Describe and evaluate your results.

Practice Cost Control

Cost control is a major concern in health care today. The United States spends more of its total income on health care than any other nation. How can you help control these costs during your externship—and later as an employee? There are a number of ways. They may seem insignificant, but if practiced by everyone, they help make a difference.

* Work carefully and thoughtfully so tasks don't have to be repeated by you or anyone else.
* Don't waste supplies. Use what is needed and no more.
* Learn how to use supplies correctly. For example, follow the instructions when using lab test kits.
* Take care of equipment. Follow directions, use it carefully, and report any problems promptly.
* Never take supplies or use services for your personal use.
* Use work time for work.

Manage Yourself

Managing your personal habits effectively will help you succeed on your externship. The major components of self-management include:

* Attitude
* Personal organization
* Time management
* Stress reduction techniques

Failure to maintain control in these areas can negatively affect your work in a number of ways, as shown in the following examples:

* Arriving late can disrupt the schedules of patients and co-workers.
* Running out of energy before the workday is over can delay the completion of important tasks.
* Repeatedly calling in sick because of stress-related illnesses may force others to fill in for you, disrupts schedules, and/or leaves tasks undone.
* Failure to prioritize tasks can result in missing deadlines.
* Feeling tired can reduce your ability to concentrate and complete work assignments accurately.

This does not mean, however, that your life should be entirely devoted to work. In fact, just the opposite is true. You need to take time out to attend to your own needs. The key is to achieve a balance between your needs and those of others in your life: supervisor, co-workers, patients, family members, and friends. If you continually ignore your own needs, you can deplete your physical, mental, and emotional resources. The result will be that you have nothing left to give others.

At your externship site, self-management means the ability to work without constant supervision. Working without being reminded and told what to do will help you achieve a reputation as an excellent intern. If you are unclear about what you are supposed to be doing, ask your supervisor. Never simply sit around, spend lots of time visiting with others, or engage in personal matters such as emailing friends or talking on your phone.

⭐ EXPERIENTIAL EXERCISES

1. Start now to prepare backup plans for your life during your externship. Consider transportation, child care, and/or any personal responsibilities that could interfere with your attendance.
2. Start now to develop organizational strategies that will help you balance your professional and personal lives.
3. Consider which of your self-management skills need improvement, and develop a plan to improve them.

Focus on the Goal

LEARNING OBJECTIVE 16: FOCUS ON THE GOAL

■ Describe ways to handle difficult situations that students may encounter on their externship.

In spite of your best efforts to learn and benefit from your externship, difficulties may arise. These can range from the annoying to the intolerable. Some problems can be handled with your own resources. Others require the assistance of others to resolve. In either case, approach problems with the intention of finding solutions. Choose actions that are appropriate for the situation and that will build your professional reputation.

Some situations must simply be tolerated. For example, simple patience may be required when working with people who have annoying habits. Actions such as refusing to work with them and/or complaining to others behind their backs may hurt you professionally and ruin your chances for a good recommendation from your supervisor. On the other hand, if you note serious situations, such as unsafe or illegal actions, taking place—and not being corrected—you will want to report this to your school and request a different externship site.

The following are examples of problems that students may encounter on their externship:

1. *You are asked to perform duties that fall outside your scope of practice, tasks for which you were not trained, or tasks that are illegal.*

   Fortunately, this problem is rare. Unfortunately, when it does happen, it places the student in a difficult situation. The best advice in these cases is "don't." Even if you are pressured by your supervisor or are assured that it is okay and "everyone does it," this is too big a risk to take. Report this situation to your school.

2. *You find it difficult to get along with your supervisor.*

   Begin by taking an honest look at your own behavior to see whether there is something you are doing—or not doing—to contribute to the problem. Speak privately and frankly with your supervisor about how important your externship success is to you. Tell him or her that you want to have a good working relationship. Ask if there is anything you need to do to improve your performance.

   When trying to communicate with your supervisor, keep in mind that your purpose is to promote mutual understanding and get the information needed to perform your duties effectively. It is not to prove you are right or to tell your supervisor off—actions that will most likely make the situation worse. Look for ways to relieve your stress without venting your frustration at your supervisor.

3. *You observe low employee morale. The employees at your externship site are unhappy and complain a lot. You'd like to get along with everyone and fit in, but the conversation and atmosphere are getting you down.*

   This can be a tough situation because you are there only temporarily, and it is unwise to become involved in negative conversation and office politics. Do your best to avoid participating in complaint sessions.

4. *There's too much to do and you can't finish all your work.*

Start by reviewing your work habits. Are you taking too much time to complete each task? Are there some tasks that you are still learning? Are you practicing good time management skills? You may be able to draw on the experience of your supervisor and/or the employees to help you increase your efficiency. Talk with your supervisor about prioritizing your work. If you can't complete everything, which tasks are the most critical? What help is available?

5. *Patients do not want to be attended to by a student intern.*

Some patients will insist on being seen by someone they know: the physician, a long-time medical assistant, and so on. Don't take this personally. Patients may be in pain, upset, or experiencing difficult medical conditions.

After Your Externship

LEARNING OBJECTIVE 17: AFTER YOUR EXTERNSHIP

- Describe ways to show your appreciation to the externship supervisor.
- Explain how to evaluate your externship experience.
- Explain how you can document your externship experience in your resume.

Showing Your Appreciation

In addition to verbally thanking your supervisor and everyone else who helped you, write a thank you letter to your supervisor after completing your externship. Include a statement about what

you learned and how he or she helped you to achieve your goals.

Be sure to ask your supervisor if he or she would write you a letter of recommendation. This is important, especially if this is your only experience in the health care field. Keep this in mind as you do your externship: the skills and professionalism you exhibit here can influence your future employment prospects.

Some students are hired at their externship sites, although students should not expect to be offered a job—nor should they ask for one. Some sites prefer to continue offering opportunities to students from local schools and therefore cannot hire every good student who works with them.

Evaluating and Documenting Your Experience

Use your journal and task log to write a summary of what you learned. Marianne Ehrlich Green, author of *Internship Success*, suggests that students consider the following questions:

1. Did you meet your learning objectives [goals]? Explain how.
2. What was your most important contribution?
3. What new skills did you develop?
4. What were the highlights of your externship?

When asking yourself these questions, consider areas that need improvement and how you plan to improve them.

Include your externship experience in your resume in the Education section. You can write a brief description of what you learned, the skills you practiced, or anything else that supports your job objective. Make copies of your letter of recommendation to include with your resume or to put in your professional portfolio.

CASE STUDY **2-4**
Advice from a Professional

Students in the medical assisting class at Goodhealth College are attending their first externship workshop conducted by Ms. Gutierrez, the school's externship coordinator. To help the students prepare for their first days at their externship sites, Ms. Gutierrez has invited Betty Stanford, a nurse with 42 years of experience, for a question-and-answer session.

Q What advice would you give students who are starting their externship?

A The basics are still very important for success. Things like professional appearance. In the last 10 years or so, trends like tattoos have become a problem because some older patients find them objectionable. They don't understand they are just a fashion statement and no longer have the negative connotations they had years ago. Another style that's a problem is low-cut blouses and tops on female employees. These are seen just about everyplace these days, but they just aren't appropriate on the job in health care.

Q Along with appearance, what other recommendations would you offer?

A It's important to show an interest in your duties. Students should want to learn, and they can do this by asking questions—and then following up. By this I mean writing the information down and making an effort to learn and remember it. We had a student recently who would ask questions and then fail to pay attention. She ended up doing the work her way, which unfortunately wasn't always correct.

Q There are instances in which students with recent training believe their current education actually makes them more qualified than experienced health care workers. Have you run into this problem?

A Yes. This know-it-all attitude can be a problem with students. What they don't realize is that much of their learning will be based on years of experience on the job. They need to do their best to perform efficiently and correctly, while also being willing to learn.

Q What other advice do you consider essential for success in a health care externship?

A In a few words: be prepared to meet the needs of others. And I don't just mean your patients. I used to work in the ER. When there was a seriously injured accident victim, for example, I was not only helping the patient, but I was also dealing with family members and friends and working with other hospital personnel. There were lots of things to consider, and they all dealt with people. Regardless of the situation, good social skills are really a must.

QUESTIONS FOR THOUGHT AND REFLECTION

1. Why do some people find tattoos objectionable?
2. What message might be communicated by female students who wear revealing, low-cut tops when working at their externship site?
3. How do you plan to learn from the experience of others when doing your externship?
4. If you think you know how to perform a procedure in a better way than what you see employees doing at your site, what should you do?
5. What are possible consequences if students neglect people skills and focus only on their practical skills while on their externship?

Down a Dark Road

Paul worked in construction for many years before deciding it was time to hang up the hammer. The climbing, bending, and reaching were starting to get to him, and he wanted to be able to enjoy his later years without the injuries he witnessed in older workers.

Paul wasn't ready—or financially able—to retire, so he spent some time thinking about what he wanted to do next. As a teen, he had considered the medical field, but his family didn't have money for college, so he had followed his hobby of building things and went into construction with his Uncle Frank. Now in his fifties, Paul thought it might be interesting to check out a health-related career. He ended up enrolling in a medical assisting course and discovered that he really enjoyed the technical aspects of the program.

Being the oldest student in his class bothered him a bit. His study skills were pretty rusty, and concentrating on reading took some effort. But he made it through his program and was happy to be assigned to a large orthopedic clinic near his home for his externship.

As the only clinic in the area specializing in orthopedics, the clinic was a busy one. Paul's supervisor, Ms. Adams, only had time to greet him and give him a very brief description of his duties. Paul spent the first couple of days trying to orient himself. As in school, it seemed like everyone was younger than he was. This made him self-conscious and hesitant to ask questions about his duties and how he was to perform them. He believed that at his age, he should be able to figure things out for himself. He tried observing the employees and thinking about what he had learned in school. The confusing thing was that much of what went on at the clinic was either unfamiliar to him or done in ways he had not been taught. Still too embarrassed to ask for help, he did what he believed were his assigned tasks as best he could, keeping to himself much of the time.

Paul believed that his work had been satisfactory, but a couple of weeks into his externship his supervisor called him into her office and informed him that some of his work was unsatisfactory—that he was not following the protocols of the clinic. At this point, Paul became upset, raising his voice and telling Ms. Adams, "I can't believe you're telling me this! I've tried hard to figure out what I'm supposed to do here—and how. I really believe I've done my best."

Ms. Adams replied, "That may be—that you've tried. But if you were having trouble, why didn't you ask for help? You never said anything, so we just assumed you were doing okay. Unfortunately, that's not the case."

QUESTIONS FOR THOUGHT AND REFLECTION

1. Whose responsibility was it to explain Paul's duties when he started his externship?
2. Whose responsibility was it after the first week?
3. What could Paul have done to make his experience at the clinic more positive?
4. What do you think he should do now?

Bibliography

1. Bonewit-West K, Hunt S, Applegate E. (2009). *Today's Medical Assistant: Clinical and Administrative Procedures.* St. Louis, MO: Elsevier.

2. Berkeley UC. *Teaching Library Internet Workshops.* Retrieved July 28, 2015, from http://www.lib.berkeley.edu/TeachingLib/Guides/Internet/SearchEngines.html.

CHAPTER 3

Finding Your First Job

- Understand how the skills needed to succeed in school are related to the skills needed to succeed on the job.

- List three actions you can take to get the most out of your health care training.

- Describe what employers and patients expect from health care professionals.

- Identify the skills and attitudes you need to develop more fully.

- Know what skills you have to offer an employer.

- Use a variety of resources effectively to locate health care job leads.

- Create a product—your professional self—that you can offer with confidence to prospective employers.

- Develop a professional appearance that is appropriate for the health care field.

- Begin professional networking activities.

- Write an effective resume and appropriate cover letters.

- Fill out employment applications correctly and accurately.

- Secure good references who will support your job search efforts.

- Create a professional portfolio that supports your qualifications.

- Identify the needs of potential employers.

- Prepare to answer interview questions in ways that demonstrate what you can offer an employer.

- Demonstrate appearance and behavior that create a positive first impression.

- Communicate courteously and effectively.

- Use your portfolio to support your qualifications.
- Deal appropriately with difficult situations, including illegal questions.
- Write appropriate thank-you letters to interviewers.
- Develop appropriate criteria for determining whether to accept a job offer.
- Calculate the total value of a compensation package.
- Accept or turn down job offers properly.
- Describe how to deal with and learn from the experience if you are not selected for a job.

Your Career in the Health Professions

Your First Step on the Road to Success

Today is the first day of the rest of your life.

Congratulations! By choosing to study for a career in health care, you have taken the first step toward achieving a productive and satisfying future. You have made a significant commitment to yourself and your community.

By enrolling in an educational program, you have demonstrated your ability to set your sights on the future, make important decisions, and follow through with action. You have proven that you have the strong personal foundation on which you can build the skills and habits needed to ensure your success in school and in your career.

JOURNALING 3-1

List the reasons you enrolled in a health care program. What positive characteristics do these reasons show about you?

Connecting School and Career

LEARNING OBJECTIVE 1: CONNECTING SCHOOL AND CAREER

- List ways that study skills, such as note-taking, writing, and taking tests, are useful in life and on the job.

- Describe the work habits you want to develop while you are in school.
- Explain how good time management can help you succeed in life and in a health care career.

The process of becoming a health care professional began the day you started classes. In addition to providing you with opportunities to learn important technical skills, your education will help you acquire the attitudes, personal characteristics, and habits of a successful professional. This is because what you think and do while in school will determine the quality of the professional you will become. Students who practice good work habits in school generally carry those same habits into the workplace (Figure 3-1).

You can apply the organizational, personal, and study skills discussed in future chapters to achieve success in school, during the job search, and on the job. Let's look at four examples:

1. **Time Management**

   For busy people, time is one of their most precious possessions. Your success in school depends heavily on how well you organize your time. Effective use of time is also an important health care job skill. Many health care professionals are responsible not only for their own time, but also for planning other people's time. Administrative medical assistants, for example, may be in charge of the physician's daily appointment scheduling. Insurance coders and billers must submit claims on time to avoid rejections and financial losses. Nurses who care for patients must plan to complete their tasks during their shifts.

2. **Communication**

   Expressing yourself clearly and listening attentively are important for speaking in class and asking and answering questions as well as for

FIGURE 3-1 Appropriately dressed and attentive veterinary technician students take notes during a demonstration. Dressing professionally, arriving to class on time, and completing homework accurately are a few ways to develop good work habits (Copyright © istock.com).

establishing and maintaining relationships with your instructors and classmates.

A critical part of the job search is the interview in which you combine your ability to think and use verbal skills effectively. Good communication skills are necessary in health care because most positions involve interaction with others, including patients, co-workers, supervisors, and the general public.

Physical and occupational therapy assistants are examples of the many health professionals who provide patient education. The effectiveness of their explanations of exercises and self-care techniques influences their patients' rehabilitation progress.

3. Taking Notes

You may think of note-taking as being limited to use in lectures, but this skill is used extensively outside the classroom. During the job search, it will be important to record information about job openings, interview appointment dates, and times and directions to facilities accurately. After interviews, you may want to make notes about the job requirements, additional information you need to send to the prospective employer, and other important facts.

Note-taking is also an important health care job skill. Many professionals are responsible for interviewing patients and taking patient histories. Another specialized form of note-taking is called charting, or making notes on medical records in either written or electronic form. The notes include information about symptoms, treatments, and medications prescribed. These medical records not only affect patient care, but they also are legal documents. They must be clear, accurate, and complete.

4. Taking Tests

You may think you have escaped taking tests once you leave school, but testing is not limited to the classroom. The truth is that life is full of tests. Job interviews are a form of testing designed to assess your ability to present yourself and your qualifications. To legally work in many health care occupations, such as licensed practical nurse, radiologic technologist, and physical therapist, you must pass a professional exam. Other occupations, such as medical assistant, have voluntary tests to obtain certifications that improve your chances of getting a job. In fact, many employers only hire certified medical assistants.

Once on the job you are, in a sense, being tested every day. Although you may not think of your regular tasks as tests, they are applications of what you have learned, and your ability to perform them correctly will be noted by your patients, co-workers, and supervisor. The annual employee performance evaluation is a type of test in which your supervisor writes a report about your work and then meets with you to discuss it. Learning to perform "when it counts" is a valuable skill and represents the ultimate ability to take and successfully pass a test. The mother of an infant wants to know that the health care professional giving the injection has "passed the test" and is qualified to safely perform the procedure.

CASE STUDY 3-1
Control of Time, Control of Life

Sam was late again. He had overslept and couldn't find his car keys. On top of everything else, he discovered that he didn't have clean clothes ready for the day. He dreaded the look—and possible lecture—he would get from his boss, physical therapist Angie Johnson.

The tough part was that Sam loved his job as a physical therapist assistant and didn't want to lose it. He had worked hard, actually struggled at times, to complete his program at Wellness College, and he didn't want to lose everything now because he of his tardiness.

Feeling stressed as he drove to work, he went over in his mind how hard it seemed for him to stay on top of things in his life. He noticed that many of his friends and classmates seemed to have things under control, and he wondered why everything seemed so hard for him.

Today felt like the last straw. He was tired of being rushed and worried and decided to see if Angie had any advice. After all, she was well aware of his problem. Maybe if he talked with her, she would realize that he was serious about improving.

There were already patients waiting in the office when he arrived, so he knew Angie would already be annoyed with his tardiness. Everyone got to work, however, and by lunch time the office was on schedule. Sam asked Angie if they could talk in her office. "Sure," she answered. "In fact, we have to talk about your work habits."

Once in her office, Angie told Sam that, in spite of being good with patients, it didn't help her when he wasn't there on time to begin the day with the early appointments. "Sam," she said, looking directly at him, "you've got to get yourself organized or you're not going to make it in this office—or in this field, for that matter."

Sam looked down at his hands and said in a soft voice, "I know, Angie, and that's what I wanted to talk to you about. I love this job and I want to be good at it, but I just can't seem to get my act together. I thought maybe you'd have some suggestions."

"Well," she said, "you seem to have a lot of trouble with time management. Tell me, do you write lists and prioritize your tasks so that you get the most important things done first?"

"No," said Sam. "I just keep stuff in my head and do what seems right at the time."

Angie asked Sam how he was able to finish his homework and the studying needed to pass his exams at school.

Sam laughed. "I pulled at lot of late nights—even some all-nighters. There always seemed to be other stuff to get done, so a lot of times I didn't sit down to study till maybe 10 or so at night."

Angie thought for a few moments and said, "We may have identified part of the problem, and it has to do with prioritizing. When you say you had "other stuff to get done," I want you to think about it—was it more important than studying? Keep in mind that you had a big investment in school and that you did want to work in physical therapy. Do you like your job here?"

Sam sat up in his chair. "Absolutely. I really like working here."

"I thought so," said Angie, "and you are good at it. But you've got to get in control of your time, arrive at work promptly, and"—she smiled—"make time to do your laundry. We'll start by talking about prioritizing. I'm also going to recommend a couple of books on time management that I think will help you."

Sam was so appreciative that he had found someone to help him—his boss, no less. He promised himself that he would do his best to learn about and practice time management and personal organization. He had so much to gain.

QUESTIONS FOR THOUGHT AND REFLECTION

1. What made Sam finally seek help for his tardiness and disorganization?
2. Why do you think Angie was willing to help him?
3. How would learning to prioritize improve Sam's life?
4. Do you think Sam will be successful with time management? Why or why not?

Down a Dark Road

Until today, Christie had been pleased with herself and her life. Just six months ago she completed her nurses training and passed the state licensing exam. Now, at age 22, she is a registered nurse and has a job at a nursing home.

While in school, she studied hard and took pride in the grades she received in most of her courses. She especially enjoyed anatomy and physiology and classes on nursing procedures. But as she told her friend, Nadine, one day on the phone, "I just don't understand why all the emphasis on communication skills. It seems like the instructors are always going on about it. Good grief, I'm great at communicating."

"That's true," said Nadine. "You always have something interesting to say—the latest news and gossip."

"Right! In fact, I've got something good to tell you about right now. Remember Gerry, the girl I told you about in class—I thought she was carrying on with Jim? Well, I heard she's pregnant."

"Get out!" exclaimed Nadine.

"No kidding! But listen, I've got to go. My next class starts in 15 minutes."

Once on the job at the nursing home, Christie applied what she believed to be her "good communication skills" by befriending other staff members, chatting with the patients, and sharing juicy stories to keep everyone entertained. She noticed that not everyone seemed interested in spending much time visiting with her, but she figured these people were simply too busy working or not the friendly type.

Christie thought things were going just fine until today when Sarah Caldwell, the nursing director, called Christie into her office. "Christie," she said. "I've got to talk with you about how you are communicating with the other staff and patients."

"You must be kidding," exclaimed Christie. "I'm one of the best communicators around here. Some staff don't even talk—"

"Christie!" interrupted Sarah. "I'd like to know how you are defining 'communicate' because what I'm hearing about you certainly does not fit my definition, especially for a professional."

"I like people. I like to talk. I like to share the news," Christie explained.

"Well, the 'news', as you call it, that you are sharing often involves personal information about patients—as well as about staff members. Patient confidentiality is critical in health care. It is required both legally and morally. You simply cannot share information with anyone who is not on the patient's care team. And even then, it must be discussed in private, out of the hearing of others."

For once, Christie didn't know what to say. She wasn't sure she agreed with Sarah. After all, what kind of an impersonal place would this be if people couldn't share what they knew? She told Sarah she would think about what she had said.

"I certainly hope so," said Sarah. "In other ways, you are a good nurse, but if this doesn't stop, it is grounds for dismissal. I won't have a choice."

Christie didn't say anything, but a thought did pass through her mind: maybe her instructors were right when they encouraged her to work on her communication skills.

QUESTIONS FOR THOUGHT AND REFLECTION

1. What is wrong with Christie's definition of "good communication"?
2. What could be the consequences for the nursing home if Christie continues to share confidential information about others, especially the patients?
3. Other than confidentiality, what other essential part of good communication does Christie seem to be missing?
4. What do you think Sarah Caldwell's definition of communication might be?
5. How does Christie's situation demonstrate how "soft skills" such as communication can be as important as technical skills?

Maximizing Your Education

- Develop a positive attitude about learning and using your school experiences to practice what you will need to succeed on the job.
- Practice asking questions that help you better understand your subjects.
- Investigate the resources your school has to offer and use the ones that can help you.
- Carry out your responsibilities as a student.
- Dedicate yourself to learning as much as you can from your school experiences.

You are making a significant investment of time, effort, and money in your education. A worthy professional goal is to do everything possible to become the best health care professional possible. Both you and your school have responsibilities to ensure that this happens.

Your Rights as a Student

Making mistakes is inevitable. Not learning from them is inexcusable.

1. Make Mistakes

You may think this sounds a little strange. After all, aren't you supposed to do the best you can, earning the highest grades possible? Yes, but many students see grades as ends in themselves, rather than as signs of having mastered the skills they will need in the future. Good grades do not always guarantee mastery, nor do you receive grades for all the skills that will determine your future success.

Many students want to know "what's on the test" so they can focus their efforts on learning only what they will be tested on. But think about it—can you possibly be tested on everything you will need to know and do to perform your job? If you were, all class time would have to be devoted to testing, leaving little or no time for learning! Studying only what you need to pass tests and earn grades may make you a "good student," but a good student is not necessarily a good health care professional.

Compare your educational experience with learning to ride a bike. First, you use training

FIGURE 3-2 The time to learn—and even make a few mistakes—is while you are in school. You want to be competent on the job when you work with patients like this woman, who depends on your knowledge (Copyright © istock.com).

wheels, go slowly, and tip over once in a while. Eventually you become a proficient cyclist, ready for the big race. School offers you a rehearsal for professional life, providing you with opportunities to learn from mistakes that would be unacceptable if you were to make them on the job. A health care professional may have made mistakes when she practiced working with a classmate in lab, but she learned from them and is now able to use correct techniques to help her patients (Figure 3-2).

2. Ask Questions

You are attending school to benefit from the knowledge and experience of your instructors. So take advantage of this opportunity by being an active participant in your classes. Don't be an invisible student. If there is something you don't understand, ask questions. There would be no need for you to attend school if you already knew the information presented in your program.

Never be afraid of "looking stupid" and hesitating to admit you don't understand or are confused. Failure to ask questions not only decreases the chances of maximizing your education, it prevents you from learning a critical health care skill—how to ask good questions. Consider, for example, the serious consequences for a medical assistant who is not sure of drug dosages or the steps in a procedure but is afraid to ask the supervisor for

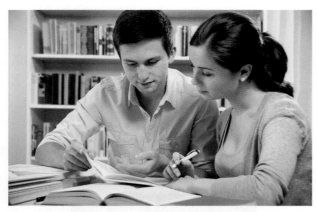

FIGURE 3-3 Being a student in the health care field is not easy. If you find yourself falling behind in class, it is important to seek assistance from counselors and tutors (Copyright © istock.com).

direction. In these situations, risking the well-being of patients is indeed stupid, whereas asking questions demonstrates intelligence.

Of course, you should not use questions to substitute for reading your textbook or studying the assigned material before each class meeting. This results in the misuse of class time and is unfair to students who are prepared. A related on-the-job example is employees who arrive late and unprepared for meetings, thus wasting their co-workers' time. Develop habits now that show consideration for others.

3. Take Advantage of School Resources

Every school wants every student who enrolls to graduate, and considerable resources are spent on services to support this effort. Find out now what services are available to you, the hours they can be accessed, and whether appointments are necessary. Two of the most important services that all students should become familiar with are the library (or resource center) and career services.

If you are having personal problems or academic difficulties, ask whether your school provides counseling and/or tutoring (Figure 3-3). Some schools refer their students to outside agencies that offer assistance for problems such as dealing with domestic abuse and finding reliable child care.

The school catalog is an often overlooked source of information that can help you succeed in school. Spend a few minutes becoming informed by reading the catalog and other printed information produced by your school. On the job, you will likely be expected to read organizational handbooks and procedure manuals. Getting in the habit of reading informational literature is a good job skill.

? WHAT IF?

What if a classmate with whom you are becoming friends confided in you that her husband was abusing her physically? How would you advise her?

★ EXPERIENTIAL EXERCISES

1. Take a tour of your school and list the resources available for students.
2. Read a copy of your school catalog and highlight important policies that apply to you.

Your Responsibilities as a Student

1. Attend All Scheduled Learning Activities

Health care educational programs feature a variety of learning opportunities including lectures, lab sessions, guest speakers, field trips, and hands-on experiences in health care facilities. These activities are designed to help you understand and master all the knowledge and skills necessary for your future work.

Learning to perform essential tasks, such as giving injections, requires you to spend time and put forth effort under the guidance of your instructors. Now is the time for learning, not when you are faced with your first patients.

Employers routinely request information about a student's attendance record. Good attendance is considered a valuable job skill because health care services are driven by time requirements. The success of a clinic or hospital and the well-being of patients depend on treatments, procedures, and surgeries completed in a timely way.

2. Apply Your Best Efforts to Learning

As a student, it is your responsibility to complete all reading, writing, and lab assignments and to participate actively in class. To be successful in your future work, you must now focus on your studies, work hard, and be persistent. Your willingness to do the "shoulds" when you would rather be doing the "wants" will be a major determinant of how well you do in school. Being a college student is not always easy. Keeping your long-term career goals in mind will help you find the self-discipline to stick with it.

3. Ask for Help When You Need It

Take responsibility for requesting assistance. Ignoring problems will not solve them; they often only get worse. Don't wait until you are hopelessly lost in a class and cannot possibly be ready for the upcoming final exam before asking for help. Remember that asking for help when you need it is a sign of strength, not weakness, and it is one of the actions that distinguishes a graduate from a dropout.

The flip side of asking for help is being willing to give it. Offer your assistance to others in the school community. Volunteer to hand out papers for the instructor. Give a student who lives in your area a ride to school. Tutor a classmate who is struggling with a subject you find easy.

You have chosen a profession that is based on giving service, and this is a habit you can start practicing now in all areas of your life.

← JOURNALING 3-2

List any obstacles that might interfere with your school attendance (e.g., problems with child care). What can you do now to overcome these obstacles?

? WHAT IF?

You find yourself struggling in one of your classes. You attend class and do the homework as best you can, but you just don't understand the material. Who would you turn to for help?

CASE STUDY 3-2
Fed Up

Karolyn has just about had it. She is tired of her friend and classmate, Julie, asking for help. It started with their anatomy homework. At first, Karolyn didn't mind. She enjoyed learning about the body and was doing well in the class. She liked Julie and wanted to help her succeed.

After finishing their anatomy class, with Julie just scraping by, the request came for help with medical terminology, and it was for more than just tutoring this time.

"Karolyn," Julie begged, "if you could just let me see your homework. Jimmy was sick last night, and I just didn't have a chance to do the assignment."

Karolyn felt sorry for Julie. She was a single mom and there always seemed to be problems with her kids: the babysitter didn't show up; someone was sick; they bothered her when she was trying to study. So the first few times, she gave her a copy of the medical terminology homework. After all, the purpose was just to memorize a list of terms. What harm could it do if Julie learned them in a way other than doing the fill-in exercises that comprise most of the homework?

It was when they got to the hands-on courses that Karolyn started to wonder if she was doing Julie any favors. Or doing *anyone* any favors? If Julie didn't master the material and understand exactly why and how they were doing certain procedures, would she be safe in the workplace? Would Karolyn want to be in the hands of a medical assistant who gives an injection without knowing something

about the underlying muscles? Or why this drug is being given?

These questions bothered Karolyn, and she decided to discuss the situation with her friend, Stephanie, a nurse at St. Francis.

"I see what you mean, Karolyn," said Stephanie. "And frankly, you are right. Someone who performs patient procedures, especially invasive ones like injections, and doesn't really understand what they're doing could be dangerous. I really wouldn't want someone like that on my team."

"I know," said Karolyn, "this is really a tough one. Julie seems to want this so much, but she just isn't doing the work."

"It's hard when it's a friend, I know," said Stephanie. "But you've got to take a broader view. What does it mean to the community if our health care professionals just get by in school without really knowing what they are doing? It could be dangerous."

Karolyn sighed. "You're right. I'm just going to have to do the right thing."

The next day, Karolyn told Julie she could no longer share her homework assignments and "help" her with tests. Julie was upset and accused Karolyn of not being her friend. Karolyn tried to explain why she decided that Julie must study and do her own work, but Julie was not interested in hearing what Karolyn had to say. They both completed their medical assisting program, but they are no longer friends.

1. Did Stephanie give Karolyn good advice?
2. Do you think Karolyn was right in refusing to continue helping Julie?
3. Was it worth losing Julie's friendship for Karolyn to be honest with her?
4. What kind of medical assistant do you think Julie will be?

Down a Dark Road

Julie, who we met in the previous case study, does not give up. She finds another student to befriend and starts in with her requests for "help" with class, "help" with the homework, and "help" with the tests. She ends up finishing her program after just barely passing her finals, and she does okay on her externship by being friendly with the supervisor.

She is able to find a job at a local clinic and things go well for the first few days; however, Julie realizes that there is much she doesn't know. In school, she depended on others rather than figuring out how to learn for herself. She tries this same strategy at work, frequently interrupting her co-workers with questions about how to do this or that; where to find information she needs; how to determine proper drug dosages; and on and on.

It is the drug dosage requests that draw her physician-employer's attention. He is concerned that she doesn't seem to have mastered this important skill. In fact, it was Karolyn back in school who did the computations that got Julie through that portion of the class. Dr. Kent calls Julie into his office.

"Julie, I've been told that you seem to always be unsure of the drug dosages you are to administer to patients. Tell me about this."

Julie responds, "Well, Dr. Kent, I'm only a recent graduate and I really need more time to master all the details of this job."

Dr. Kent says, "Julie, this knowledge is part of the medical assisting program at your college. This is something you should have learned about in school and practiced on your externship. When I hired you, I knew you were just starting out, but I expected you to have mastered certain skills, and this was one of them."

"Well," says Julie, "I think your expectations may have been a bit unreasonable."

"I will say that drug dosages can be confusing, and I understand that you might be nervous about making mistakes with pharmaceuticals. But this isn't the only thing. I've received a lot of complaints from my staff about your constant questions when they are working. It seems to have gotten out of control and is affecting some of their work."

"You know what, Dr. Kent?" Julie says. "If this is the kind of unfriendly atmosphere you've got in this office, I don't think it's a place I want to work." And she stomped out the door. Dr. Kent sighed and called in his office manager. "Louise," he said, "I think we're going to need to look for another medical assistant."

QUESTIONS FOR THOUGHT AND REFLECTION

1. How did the "favors" from Karolyn and others contribute to Julie's failure on the job?
2. Was Dr. Kent right in being concerned about Julie's lack of knowledge? Why or why not?
3. Was Julie's response to Dr. Kent appropriate?
4. What must Julie do if she wants to have a career in health care?

Planning for Your Future

LEARNING OBJECTIVE 3: PLANNING FOR YOUR FUTURE

- Start researching your occupational field and jobs for which you might qualify.
- Explore the needs of potential employers.
- Consider the needs of patients and how you might fulfill these needs.
- Make a list of what you are looking for in your first job and in your career.
- List the advantages for you of a career in health care.

Your future job search can be compared to marketing, a multi-step process that begins with an idea for a product and ends with the sale of that product. When you apply for a job, you are presenting yourself as a product: the combination of your skills, characteristics, and talents.

You can start developing your own personal marketing plan now as you begin you health care studies. The first step is market research, studying the needs of customers. *Your* customers will include your future employers and patients. Now is the time to find out about their needs. You are investing time, effort, and money in the development of yourself as a product just as a business would, so it makes sense to make sure you are creating a product that is both wanted and needed.

What Do Employers Want?

In recent years, employers in all industries have expressed concerns that entry-level workers are not adequately prepared for the modern workplace. Employers are looking for job candidates who not only are qualified technically, but who also bring essential supporting skills such as the ability to communicate effectively, work cooperatively with others, accept responsibility, and solve problems (Figure 3-4). These "soft skills" are especially critical in the health care industry because it is service-based and depends heavily on the quality of its personnel.

National Health Care Standards

A project of special interest to future health care professionals is the National Health Care Skill Standards, a list of entry-level worker competencies.

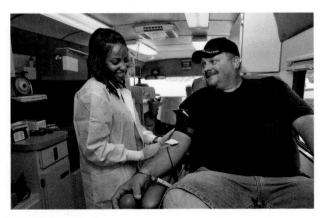

FIGURE 3-4 A phlebotomist communicates with a donor while collecting blood (Copyright © istock.com).

BOX 3-1

Examples of the National Healthcare Foundation Standards and Accountability Criteria

Health care workers will:
- Apply speaking and active listening skills
- Summarize basic professional standards of health care workers as they apply to hygiene, dress, language, confidentiality, and behavior
- Exemplify professional characteristics
- Employ safe work practices and follow health and safety policies and procedures
- Apply ethical standards in health care
- Demonstrate respectful and empathetic interactions with diverse age, cultural, economic, ethnic, and religious groups
- Recognize methods for building positive team relationships
- Apply behaviors that promote health and wellness
- Utilize and understand information technology applications in health care

Box 3-1 contains examples that apply to all health care occupations. You can see that they are not limited to technical skills, such as taking blood pressure, but include the ability to communicate and work on teams. Some employers report that these types of skills are as important as technical skills in the provision of good health care.

 EXPERIENTIAL EXERCISES

1. The next time you visit your own doctor, dentist, or other health care provider, ask what he/she believes is necessary to succeed in health care work.
2. If this person is also an employer, ask about what characteristics he/she looks for when hiring.

WHAT IF?

What if you don't know much about the employers in your area and what they are looking for when they hire? How could you find out more about them?

Professional Organizations

Many of the professional organizations that represent specific health care occupations have statements outlining the characteristics needed to work successfully in their fields.

 EXPERIENTIAL EXERCISES

Find the website of the professional organization for your chosen occupation. What personal characteristics are needed to succeed? What qualities do you think you need to work on to be successful in this occupation?

What Do Patients Want?

Patients do not care how much you know until they know how much you care.

Patients want to receive competent care delivered with consideration and respect. When seeking health care, people are often at their most vulnerable. They fear what might be discovered during a diagnostic test or that they will experience pain during a necessary treatment. The self-esteem of patients can be threatened by a feeling of powerlessness that often accompanies illness and injury.

Many patients want to participate in making decisions about their care. They have the right, both ethically and legally, to be fully informed about their condition, treatment options, and possible outcomes. Health care professionals must give clear explanations in everyday language and offer patients the opportunity to ask questions. At the same time, patients want and have the legal right to confidentiality.

Over the years, the U.S. health care system has undergone changes that have brought special challenges for both patients and health care professionals. In the past, many people had the same doctor throughout their lives. They belonged to the same community, and a sense of trust developed over the years.

Patients today may see a different physician each time they visit their health care facility. They may face a serious illness or life-threatening condition in the care of a stranger, adding to the stress of an already difficult situation. As a health care professional, you can demonstrate a caring attitude that helps create a bond of trust with patients by being attentive, listening carefully, and practicing empathy. Studies have found that even if a health professional excels in one area, poor

---

BOX 3-2

Examples from The Patient Care Partnership of the American Hospital Association

Patients have the right to:
- Be treated with compassion and respect
- Receive information about the benefits and risks of treatments
- Have their privacy protected
- Participate in making decisions regarding their care, including the right to refuse treatment
- Have their health goals and values taken into account as much as possible

---

communication skills or the appearance of not caring can cause patients to view that person negatively National Consortium for Health Science and Technology Education, (www.healthscienceconsortium.org).

Many of today's patients are from different ethnic backgrounds, some of whom have beliefs about health care practices that differ from traditional Western medicine. Patients also come from various economic and social groups. They may have lifestyles or personal beliefs with which you disagree, but they all want and deserve your best efforts.

See Box 3-2 for a formal list of patient rights.

? WHAT IF?

What if you just arrived at an urgent care facility with a suspected broken arm? You were out for a fun day biking with friends when you hit a hole in the pavement and fell. Your arm is very painful, and you are worried about whether you can work if you end up in a cast. Describe how you feel and how you would want to be treated by the health care professionals.

EXPERIENTIAL EXERCISES

1. Make a list of your personal qualities that you believe will help you succeed in your health care career.
2. Now make a list of attitudes and habits you would like to change to increase your chance of success.
3. Take some time to observe people you believe are successful in their careers. Do they have qualities in common?

What Do You Want?

If you don't know where you're going, chances are you'll end up somewhere else.

In addition to exploring the needs of your "customers"—your future employers and patients—an important part of planning is to identify what *you* want. You must consider you own needs and desires as you create your professional self. The clearer you are about your career goals and expectations, the greater the chance you have of achieving them.

Beginning now to think about your goals and priorities will also keep you alert to employment possibilities. Observe, ask questions, and read about your occupational area. Many fields in health care today have newly created positions and expanded responsibilities for traditional jobs. A wide variety of choices may be available for new graduates.

> **JOURNALING 3-3**
>
> Why did you choose a career in health care? What do you hope to accomplish? What do you hope to contribute?

CASE STUDY 3-3
Planning Ahead

Rosa Gonzalez is the first child in her family to go to college. Her parents have worked hard to support their family and encouraged their children to take advantage of all educational opportunities. However, money is scarce and Rosa has a part-time job to help pay for school expenses. It is not easy working and going to school, but she believes that it is through a good education she will be able get ahead in life. She wants to not only train for a career in health care but also to serve as an example for her younger brothers and sisters.

Rosa is studying medical assisting. She wants to do well so her parents will be proud of her. Her career goal is to work as a back-office assistant with a plastic surgeon, helping the physician with outpatient procedures. Her interest in plastic surgery began when she saw the miraculous work performed on a young cousin who was disfigured after being burned in a fire.

Early in her program Rosa did some research and found that there were only a few plastic surgeons in her town and they all preferred to hire assistants with previous work experience. Rosa decides not to let this information discourage her and creates a plan of short- and long-term goals to help her achieve her career dream.

While in school, Rosa asks her instructor to recommend books and articles about plastic surgery and allow her to spend extra practice time in the lab so she can reach a high level of competence with sterile technique, surgical instruments, wound care, and related skills. At the same time, Rosa works hard in her classes, asking for help when necessary and completing all homework assignments.

Upon graduating, Rosa decides to look for a job with a general practitioner or pediatrician who does minor surgery in the office. Her entry-level job goals are to gain experience with sterile technique, standard precautions, surgical assisting, and patient care. She knows that this experience will help her reach her goal of someday working with a plastic surgeon.

QUESTIONS FOR THOUGHT AND REFLECTION

1. Why do you think Rosa wants to serve as an example for her siblings?
2. What would have happened if Rosa had not researched her career goal before she completed her medical assisting program?
3. How do Rosa's short-term goals serve as stepping stones for reaching her long-term goal?
4. Do you think Rosa will achieve her goal of working with a plastic surgeon? Why or why not?

Down a Dark Road

Greg worked in roofing and construction from the time he graduated from high school. He got a job with a company owned by a buddy's father and worked his way up from doing cleanup to full-time work as a roofer. He liked the physical nature of the work, being outside most of the day, and having a beer with his fellow workers at the end of the day.

One fall day as his work team was trying to finish a job before the rainy weather worsened, Greg slipped from a steep incline and fell onto a cement patio. He broke his leg and fractured two vertebrae in his back. He recovered the use of his legs although he was in pain a good deal of the time. His roofing and construction days were over.

Being unable to work posed a huge problem for Greg. He and his wife, Kathy, had two children to support, and Kathy's job was only part-time and did not provide any benefits. On the advice of a friend who worked at a local clinic, Greg looked into a career in health care. Although the idea of working inside all day wasn't appealing to him, it seemed as though there were many job openings in health care and the work was steady.

He and Kathy talked it over, and she encouraged him. "You know," she said, "my friend Louise has been working for Dr. Lewis for years as a medical assistant and really likes the work." Greg had some doubts. "Don't you think there might be lifting and helping patients? My back might not take that kind of work."

"Well," said Kathy, "I did talk with Louise about that and she said that there are *administrative* medical assistants. There are also people in the office who do billing and other kinds of paperwork."

"Gosh," said Greg. "I've never done that kind of work. I don't know if I'd be any good at it."

Kathy reassured him. "Honey, I know you can do whatever you set your mind to."

Greg had his doubts, but he enrolled in a medical office administration program at the local college. Kathy's friend Louise gave him some help with his studies, and he managed to complete the program with passing grades. The family's finances were approaching the point of desperation, and he knew he was obligated to finish his program and look for employment.

Greg worked hard at finding a job. He pursued every lead and presented himself well at interviews. It wasn't surprising, then, that he had a job just a few weeks after graduation greeting patients and doing front-office work for a local doctor. His outgoing personality made him popular with patients, but he found the appointment scheduling, data entry on the computer, and other paperwork tedious and not to his liking. Sitting all day in a small area made him feel closed in and uncomfortable. He stayed with the job and did his best because he didn't want to let his family down, but he was never happy with his work and knew inwardly that someday he would have to find something else.

QUESTIONS FOR THOUGHT AND REFLECTION

1. What do you think of Greg's reasons for studying medical assisting?
2. What effect did Kathy and Louise have on Greg's decision?
3. What could he have done to learn more about the job?
4. Do you think he should have explored other career options?
5. Is there anything Greg can do now to improve his situation?

The Nature of Work in Health Care

People are generally happiest and most productive when their work provides them with more than material rewards. Health care is a complex, ever-changing field that offers both opportunities and challenges. Here are some of the major sources of satisfaction you can expect.

1. Meaningful Work

Good health is a basic need for both human survival and happiness. Working to promote health gives you the chance to make meaningful contributions to the well-being of others. Whether you provide direct patient care or perform supporting activities, your work directly affects patients, and the quality of your work can truly make a difference in their lives.

2. Opportunity to Serve

People seek the services of health care professionals when they need help. They come with the hope that you can assist them in solving their problems, and they entrust themselves in your care.

3. Career Stability

The need for health care will always exist, even if job titles change over time. The reorganization taking place in today's health care delivery system is causing continual shifts in the need for specific occupational positions. A decrease in the number of jobs for one position is often balanced by an increase in another. If you are willing to be flexible, you can add the experience and/or training to qualify for new positions.

4. Interesting Work Environment

Health care is changing rapidly, both scientifically and organizationally. Advances in our understanding of how the body works, along with discoveries about the causes and treatments of disease, are reported almost daily. Computers and technology have increased our ability to collect and organize information as well as diagnose and treat disease. Your work will provide a steady stream of new information to learn and apply.

5. Opportunities for Advancement

You are likely to have opportunities for advancement if you are willing to continue learning and add to your skills. Many jobs offer on-the-job training, and many occupational specialties, such as nursing, have career ladders. These are a hierarchy of jobs that require different levels of knowledge and skills. The higher-level positions almost always require further education and additional certifications or licenses.

Looking Ahead to Your First Job

While it is important to try to meet your personal needs when seeking employment, you must also have realistic expectations. You will need to compare your work preferences with the needs of employers to see how well they match.

Students sometimes have unrealistic goals for the positions they hope to fill immediately after graduation. Recent graduates are qualified for entry-level positions. You can avoid frustration and disappointment if you understand the workplace and adjust your expectations. Box 3-3 contains a list of what you should look for in your first job.

BOX 3-3

Expectations for Your First Health Care Job

- Apply what you learned in school
- Gain self-confidence
- Work with a variety of people
- Acquire additional knowledge
- Increase your skill base
- Explore specialties within your field of interest
- Network with other professionals
- Demonstrate your abilities

Setting Career Goals

Entry-level jobs, performed well, can be the first step leading to positions that meet all your hopes for a fulfilling career. Adjusting your short-term expectations doesn't mean giving up your long-term goals. In fact, purposeful planning now can help you arrive where you want to be in the future. Find out now what skills are needed to achieve your future goals and look for opportunities to learn as many of them as possible during your studies, externship, and first job.

For new health care professionals who are well-prepared and who contribute enthusiastically to the success of their employers, entry-level jobs can serve as launch pads for career success. Serving the needs of others can provide you with opportunities to meet your own needs.

CROSS CURRENTS WITH OTHER SOFT SKILLS

ADOPTING A POSITIVE ATTITUDE: A good attitude will go a long way toward your school success (pp. 2-11)

SETTING GOALS AND PLANNING ACTION: Goals help you achieve academic and career success (pp. 286-291)

INTERACTING SUCCESSFULLY: Good communication skills will help you work better with your instructors and classmates (Chapter 9)

MANAGING YOUR TIME AND ORGANIZING YOUR LIFE: Balancing school, work, and other life responsibilities are essential skills for students (pp. 11-18)

Beginning the Job Search

The Search Is On

Employment is nature's physician and is essential to human happiness.

—Galen

Congratulations! All the studying, assignments, labs, and clinical experience are about to pay off. You are now ready to focus on the job search and reaching your goal of working in the health care field. Completing your education and graduating represent important personal achievements. Your attitude played a large part in your success. In the same way, attitude will play an important role in helping you get the right job.

The Big A: Attitude

Remember that your own resolution to succeed is more important than any one thing.

—Abraham Lincoln

Attitude is the single most important factor in determining whether a student finds a job. Keep in mind that you have control over your attitude. You can approach any situation either positively or negatively. Some people are nervous and fearful about looking for a job. They worry about lacking the qualifications needed by employers and see each interview as a chance to be rejected. A more positive approach is to look at the process from the employers' point of view. Think about it: health care facilities cannot function without good employees. Employers must fill positions with well-trained individuals who can help them serve their patients. *You* are a recently trained person ready to fill one of these positions.

In this chapter, we compared starting a new career with marketing a new product. You are now ready to begin marketing yourself to prospective employers. Knowing what skills and competencies you have is the first step in presenting yourself successfully as the person who fits an employer's needs. Students sometimes don't realize just how much they have learned and underestimate their abilities. Being aware of your accomplishments will build your self-confidence and help you present yourself positively at interviews.

 JOURNALING 3-4

What do you hope to learn and gain from your first job?

 EXPERIENTIAL EXERCISE

Write a description of yourself in which you explain what you have to offer prospective employers. Include your skills and personal characteristics that will make you a valued employee.

Focus Your Search

To find out what one is fitted to do, and to secure an opportunity to do, is the key to happiness.

—John Dewey

Knowing *where* to market yourself is the next step in carrying out a successful job search. This means identifying the type of job and facility in which you'd like to work. Keep in mind that it is sometimes necessary to set short-term goals to achieve long-term career success. When seeking an entry-level position, you'll do better if you are open to a variety of possibilities. School career services personnel report seeing students lose good opportunities by setting limits that are too restrictive. For example, some students don't want to have long commutes. But passing up a good position at an excellent facility by refusing to consider jobs just outside your immediate area may not be a good career move. Driving an extra 10 minutes may, in the long run, be worth the extra investment.

 EXPERIENTIAL EXERCISE

Create a list of your work preferences that includes the following: type of facility and population served, specialty, work schedule, type of supervision, work pace, amount of interaction with others, range of duties.

 WHAT IF?

You need to start looking for a job, but you've never worked in health care and don't know what to look for in an employer.

Making a Commitment to the Job Search

You can't try to do things; you simply must do them.

—Ray Bradbury

> **LEARNING OBJECTIVE 4: MAKING A COMMITMENT TO THE JOB SEARCH**

- State how much time graduates should plan to spend on their job search.
- List the activities involved in a successful job search.
- Describe job search time management techniques.

Obtaining a job has been compared to actually working at a job. It can take a lot of time and effort. You'll be most successful if you dedicate a portion of each day to your search and be on call to follow up quickly on leads. Employment professionals recommend that job seekers spend between 20 and 40 hours a week on job search efforts. See Box 3-4 for a list of activities related to your job search. Failure to spend enough time on these activities is one of the major reasons why people fail to get hired.

> **JOURNALING 3-5**
>
> How strong is my commitment to finding a job? How much time and effort am I willing to spend?

BOX 3-4

Job Search Activities

- Preparing skills inventories and examples
- Networking
- Putting together a support team
- Finding leads
- Conducting searches on the Internet
- Writing and revising your resume
- Assembling your portfolio
- Writing letters
- Contacting references
- Creating a reference sheet
- Preparing for and attending interviews
- Writing thank-you notes

Time Management Tips for Your Job Search

Prioritize. The job search should be your main focus, apart from your family. Looking for a job *is* your job. Determine which job search activities are most productive and spend the majority of your time on them.

Keep a Calendar. Missing—or even being late for—an interview is a sure way to lose a job even before you are hired. Take care to note all appointments and follow-up activities accurately and to check your calendar daily.

Plan a Weekly Schedule. Decide what needs to be done each week and create a to-do list to serve as a guide to keep you on track.

Plan Ahead and Be Prepared. Suppose that one morning you are notified that a hospital where you want to work is scheduling interviews for later the same day. You don't want to miss out because you haven't completed your resume or don't have a clean shirt to wear. Make sure your car is in good running order or that you have other reliable transportation.

Plan for the Unplanned. The unexpected tends to strike at the worst possible moment. Keep an extra printer cartridge on hand. Have extra copies of your resume printed. Leave early for interviews in case you get lost. Better yet, take a dry run a day or two in advance to learn the route. Check out alternate routes in case of traffic.

> **? WHAT IF?**
>
> *Your school has called to say they have scheduled an interview for you tomorrow. However, you have been busy with family responsibilities and don't feel ready. What should you do?*

Setting Up Job Search Central

> **LEARNING OBJECTIVE 5: SETTING UP JOB SEARCH CENTRAL**

- List the supplies you may need for your job search.
- Explain what job search records should contain.
- Describe the purpose and contents of a job lead log.

Job Central Checklist

- Telephone
- Telephone directories, including Yellow Pages
- Computer, printer, and supplies
- Dictionary
- Good-quality paper for resume and cover letters
- Matching envelopes
- Extra copies of resume
- Note paper or thank-you cards
- Calendar, planner, or electronic planner
- Job search notebook

■ Explain how the telephone, fax machine, and computer can be used as job search tools.

Set up a space for your job search activities. Gather up your resources and supplies in one location. Check the list in Box 3-5 to see if you have what you need.

Your Job Search Records

Keep records of copies of applications you have submitted, list of professional contacts, employee contact information, names of the facilities and individuals where you interviewed, etc. Use a three-ring binder to give you the flexibility to add pages and keep everything organized or create computerized folders and files.

Job Lead Log

A job lead log consists of pages, either paper or computerized, on which you record all job leads and contacts. See Box 3-6 for suggested information to include.

If you have more than one version of your resume (for example, different objectives to match specific jobs), indicate on your lead log which version you sent, or you can place a copy of the resume on the next page in your binder or refer to the computer file name. This way, you'll know how to respond if you get a call for an interview. It will also ensure that you take the correct resume to the interview. (More information about interviews and what to take with you appears later in this chapter.)

Students who prefer to use a computer for tracking can set up an Excel spreadsheet or other form, such as a table in Word, to record their job search activities.

Job Lead Log

- Source of the lead (school, personal contact, Internet, etc.)
- Facility name
- Contact person
- Address
- Phone number
- Fax number
- Email address
- Website

Regardless of the method you choose, design something that is easy for you to use and be sure to keep it up-to-date.

Dialing for Jobs

The telephone can be one of the job seeker's best friends. It can also be a barrier if not used properly. Employers form an impression of you based on your telephone manners, so be sure they hear you at your best. The following suggestions for making calls will apply to your telephone habits on the job as well as during the search to get a job:

1. Be prepared with pen and paper for taking notes.
2. Prepare what you plan to say ahead of time and be as brief as possible without rushing and speaking too quickly.
3. Be courteous, never pushy. If the receptionist cannot connect you to the person you wish to speak with, leave a clear message and ask for a good time to call back.
4. Speak clearly and distinctly. Don't mumble or use slang or nonstandard speech that the listener may not understand.
5. When making appointments or gathering important information, listen carefully and repeat to make sure that you have the correct date and time, address, suite or office number, and so on.
6. Always thank the other party and end the call graciously.

It is important that your school, potential employers, and other contacts be able to reach you in a timely way. Be sure the telephone number you distribute is accurate and includes your area code. If you have an answering machine, call your number to make sure it is working properly. The outgoing message should be simple and professional. Avoid the use of music, jokes, and clever remarks. This also applies to your email address. If it's too cute or strange, it may send the wrong message to any potential employer who sees it. Instruct everyone who might answer the telephone about proper telephone manners and how to write down a message. Every contact represents you, and employers don't have time to deal with rude adults or untrained children.

Online Communication

Many employers advertise job openings online. They also request, or even require, that applications and resumes be submitted electronically. If you don't have a computer or Internet capability, ask your school if these are available to students.

Communicating by Fax

Although fax machines are becoming less common, some employers may ask you to fax your resume. If you don't own a fax machine or a computer that has fax capability, find a print, postal, or business supply store that provides this service. Some schools will fax student resumes to potential employers. When sending documents by fax, the print on the original should be clear and dark for maximum quality transmission. Be sure there is at least a 1-inch margin on all sides so nothing gets cut off.

When faxed resumes are requested, it is best to follow the employer's instructions. Mailed resumes may arrive too late to be considered. Demonstrate that you are resourceful and can follow instructions. If you don't hear from the employer in a couple of days, call to make sure your resume was received.

Setting Up a Support System

■ List the tasks that members of your support system can do.

■ Describe proper etiquette when working with your support system.

Your job search will be easier and more pleasant if you have people available who care about your success and are willing to help you. They can provide technical support or offer friendly encouragement. Could you use some help with any of the following tasks?

* Proofreading your resume and other written materials
* Role playing with you to practice interviewing
* Discussing postinterview evaluations
* Helping you to keep things in perspective and not get discouraged

You may want to work with just one other person who is qualified to help you in many areas, or you might enlist the help of several "specialists." Be sure the people you choose are qualified to spot spelling and grammatical errors and are comfortable giving you constructive feedback. They should know when you need a push and when you need a hug. Consider drawing from friends, family members, classmates, school personnel, and health care professionals. If you have a mentor, this person might be an excellent choice. Be considerate of everyone's time, be prepared when you have meetings with them, and show appreciation for their help.

The career services department at your school provides specific help and support to students as they conduct their job search. Find out what services are provided. In addition, some schools and communities have job clubs or support groups for people seeking employment. Consider using these resources to supplement your support system. They can offer additional viewpoints, encouragement, and helpful suggestions.

Understanding the Job Market

- List the conditions that affect job markets.
- Describe the factors that influence health care jobs.
- Explain where you can find job market information.
- Explain why contacting employers directly can be a good strategy.

Employment conditions vary from one geographic location to the next, and economic conditions change over time. Consider the following factors when planning your job search strategies:

* Local employment customs
* Current economic conditions
* Current employment rate
* Trends in health care delivery
* Medical advances
* Changing government regulations

Local and employer customs vary in what is considered acceptable dress for the workplace. In some places, health care providers dress casually, with males sporting long hair and even wearing an earring. In other areas, anyone who showed up for work looking like this would be sent home to change.

Local and national economic conditions affect the job seeker. When the economy is strong and unemployment is low, job seekers have the advantage. When the economy slows down, competition heats up and it becomes more difficult to find a position.

Health care occupations are also affected by state and federal laws. The demand for certain occupations is influenced by the reimbursement (payment for services) policies of both government and private insurance carriers. Know what's happening in your area as well as national trends. Ask your career services department at school for information. Look in the business section of your local newspaper for articles about the economy and local employment trends. Health care trends and major facilities are often featured. Reading articles about major health care employers enables you to present yourself at interviews as a candidate who has taken the time to learn about the employer.

Many newspapers publish weekly or monthly sections dedicated to employment. They contain articles about resume writing, lists of local agencies that assist job seekers, and announcements of job fairs. News magazines such as Newsweek, Time, US News and World Report, and BusinessWeek contain many articles about health care topics, and the Internet provides access to a wide variety of topics from literally millions of sources. For example, the Bureau of Labor Statistics maintains a website with reports on employment trends and the national labor market.

★ EXPERIENTIAL EXERCISE

Use your research skills to write a report that includes the following:
1. Unemployment rate in your area
2. Major health care employers
3. Current hiring trends in health care
4. Current conditions that affect your occupation
5. Influence of all this information on your job search strategies

Locating Job Leads

- Explain how your job search time should be allocated.
- How do economic conditions affect the job search.
- List and describe the sources of job leads.
- Explain how to best use career services at your school.
- Explain who to include in your network.
- Describe how to best take advantage of career fairs.
- Explain how professional organizations can help with the job search.

Increase your chances of finding the job you really want by using a variety of lead sources. Don't limit yourself to the one or two methods you find easiest or most comfortable to use. Employment experts recommend that no more than 25% of your time be spent on any one job search method (Figure 3-5).

When the economy is slow and there are few job openings, networking and developing personal contacts can be the most effective methods for finding a job. It's possible you won't find the "perfect job" under these economic conditions. Looking for an opportunity to gain experience may be the best strategy. When the economy is booming or there is a

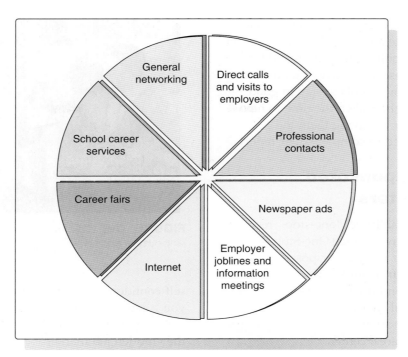

FIGURE 3-5 Use a variety of job lead sources to increase your chances of finding the right job for you.

shortage of qualified workers in your field, you are likely to have a larger selection of opportunities. Under these conditions, you may find that responding to job postings and directly contacting potential employers are effective methods. It is a sure thing that you will experience all types of job markets during your career. The economy and employment levels run in cycles, and you must be prepared to deal with changing conditions.

 WHAT IF?

You live in a small town where there are few medical facilities. How can you increase your chances of finding a job?

Career Services at Your School

The staff at your school wants you to succeed. The goal of health care educators is to train future workers, and a sign of *their* professional success is when a graduate becomes satisfactorily employed. Schools have special personnel who are trained to help students find jobs. These people work to develop relationships with local employers. Employers may contact your school about job openings before they are advertised. How can you be among the graduates who are recommended by your school?

* Get to know the career services staff. Introduce yourself early in your program. Don't wait until you are beginning the job search. Seek their advice about how you can best prepare ahead for successful employment.
* Treat school staff with the same courtesy and respect you would an employer. They cannot risk the school's reputation with employers by recommending students who are rude or uncooperative.
* Maintain an excellent attendance record. Schools report that this is the question asked by nearly every employer about students.
* Participate in career development classes or workshops. Attend every session and complete all assignments. Conduct yourself in practice interviews as if they were the real thing.
* Follow up on all leads you are given, even if you don't think the job is for you. Attend all interviews scheduled for you. Failure to show up embarrasses your school and may result in the employer refusing to consider candidates from your school in the future. And even if the job isn't the one for you, the employer may know about one that is.
* Keep your school informed about how to contact you.

* Let the school know when you are hired. Many agencies that regulate and accredit schools require annual reports to monitor graduation and job placement rates. These act as school report cards and are important for schools to stay in good standing. If the staff has taken the time to help you, return the favor by giving them the information they need to complete their reports.

Government-Sponsored Resource Centers

Governments have established "one-stop" resources for job-seekers. They may be called One-Stop Resource Centers, County Career Centers, or possibly another name in your area. Staff members are well-informed about employment conditions, as well as specific employers, in their local areas. Ask your school about these resources or go to www.careeronestop.org for the location of your nearest center.

Networking

Many people learn about job openings and become employed through personal and professional contacts. Don't be shy about asking for their advice about where you might apply or about the job search in general. People who are successful in their careers are generally happy to help newcomers. Do show consideration for their time and send a thank-you note when they put forth effort on your behalf. It is critical that you follow up on any leads given to you by professional contacts. Failure to do so is not only rude, it also may result in the withdrawal of their support.

In addition to professional contacts, general networking can be an effective way to get the word out about your search efforts (Figure 3-6). Let the people in your life know you are seeking employment. By telling 10 people who each know 10 other people, you create a network of 110 people who know you are looking for a job. Of these 110, it is likely that a few work in health care. When speaking with others about your career goals, present yourself positively and express enthusiasm about your field. People want to feel confident about passing your name along.

Direct Employer Contacts

Calling, visiting, or writing to specific employers to inquire about job openings can be successful strategies. These actions demonstrate motivation and

FIGURE 3-6 Informal networking can lead to potential employment contacts (Copyright © istock.com).

self-confidence, the very qualities that can help win you a job. They are also a way to discover the estimated four fifths of jobs that are never advertised—the "hidden job market."

If you are sending a cover letter and resume, find the name of the person who makes the hiring decisions for his or her department. If you are calling a small medical office, this may simply mean getting the name—with correct spelling!—of the physician. In the case of a large facility, you may have to do more inquiring by phone to find the right person.

Craft a letter that briefly explains why you would be a good employee for this particular employer. The letter should communicate enthusiasm, interest, and a desire to help the employer. Of course, this means that you know something about the employer: specialty or services offered, typical patients, etc. Include your resume with the letter. Follow up in a few days with a phone call.

Calling employers by phone to inquire about job openings can be especially helpful if you are relocating. Explain that you will be moving and are unfamiliar with the area. If the facility contacted has no openings, ask whether they can refer you to anyone else in the area.

Personally visiting facilities that have jobs for which you might be qualified can be a productive. It gives you a chance to introduce yourself to at least one staff member and personally distribute your resume. Ask who does the hiring, leave your resume, and express your appreciation. While you should be dressed as if you were attending an interview, *do not ask* for one at this time if you don't have an appointment.

Large medical facilities, such as hospitals, often coordinate hiring through their human resource office.

All resumes and applications must be submitted to this office. It can be worthwhile to also contact or visit the department where you wish to work. Ask for the supervisor and, if available, let him or her know that you have applied for work through human resources and are very interested in working in that department. Explain why you want to work there and ask that your application be given consideration. If the supervisor is not available, ask to make an appointment. Don't be discouraged, however, if you are unable to make direct contact. Health care professionals today are extremely busy and may not have the time. If they don't, send a letter or email that expresses your interest.

> ### JOURNALING 3-7
>
> 1. Do I conduct myself professionally at all times, including in the classroom?
> 2. Will people who know me feel confident recommending me for jobs?
> 3. Are there habits or behaviors I need to improve so people will recommend me?

Your Externship Site

Students who perform well during their externship are sometimes offered jobs at the site. Some employers even create new positions for graduates who impress them with their attitude and skills. Although it is *not* appropriate to ask your clinical site for employment before completing your training there, you should work as if this were your goal. Even if the site is unable to offer you a position, your supervisor can serve as a valuable reference and may recommend you to another employer.

Career and Job Fairs

Some schools, community agencies, and large health care facilities organize activities to connect job recruiters and job seekers. In a single day, you can meet dozens of potential employers. You can gather information, ask questions, and submit your resume. Check your local newspaper for events in your area. Call large health care organizations in your area or check their websites about career fairs or open houses. You can also find upcoming career fairs across the nation on websites such as nationalcareerfair.com.

Here are suggestions for taking full advantage of job fairs:

* Dress as you would for an interview.
* Prepare a list of questions, such as the following, in advance:
  1. What types of jobs does your facility offer?
  2. How can I get more information?
  3. What are the most important qualifications you look for when hiring employees?
  4. Can you give me a written job description?
  5. What is the application procedure?
  6. Who do I contact to set up an interview?
* Take copies of your resume.
* Smile, make eye contact, and introduce yourself to recruiters. Thank them for any information they give you. Leave graciously by telling them it was nice meeting them.
* Take something in which you can collect brochures, job announcements, and business cards. A small notebook is helpful for taking notes.
* As soon as possible after the fair, organize what you collected and use your job lead log pages to record the people you met and what you learned.
* Prepare a list of follow-up activities, such as people to call and resumes to send.

Professional Organizations

Some professional organizations include job search tips and job postings on their websites. These organizations are also a good place to network. See Box 3-7 for examples of professional organizations.

BOX 3-7

Allied Health Professional Organizations

* American Dental Assistants Association
  www.adaausa.org
* American Massage Therapy Association
  www.amtamassage.org
* American Association of Medical Assistants
  www.aama-ntl.org
* Medical Association of Billers
  www.physicianswebsites.com
* American Academy of Procedural Coders
  www.aapc.com
* American Health Information Management Association
  www.ahima.org
* National Pharmacy Technician Association
  www.pharmacytechnician.org

Employment Ads

Newspaper classified ads are much less used than in the past, they are still included in today's newspapers. You can see what types of jobs are available in your area. Writing a cover letter and mailing or faxing a resume may be worth the time and expense it takes. Every action you take increases your chance of finding the right job.

In addition to the newspaper, many professional journals contain employment ads targeted to their members.

JOURNALING 3-8

Am I taking advantage of all sources of job leads? Are there any I need to explore further?

Using the Internet

LEARNING OBJECTIVE 9: USING THE INTERNET

- Describe the ways you can use the Internet in your job search.
- Explain the purpose of The Riley Guide.
- List examples of employment websites.
- Explain how the Internet provides networking opportunities.
- List ways to best use the Internet.
- Create and use and Internet tracking form.

The Internet greatly expands your job search possibilities by being available worldwide 24 hours a day. It offers a wide range of how-to information, facts about specific occupations and employers, and job postings. So much information is available, in fact, that it's easy to get lost in cyberspace.

Getting Started

An excellent place to start learning about using the Internet for the job search is The Riley Guide. Available both in print and online, it has provided free, updated career and employment information since 1994. (www.rileyguide.com) Developed by a librarian, the website serves as a gateway to hundreds of other websites on all phases of the job search. Other good sources that have been in business for some time are Quintessential Careers (www.quintcareers.com) and Career Builder (http://careerbuilder.com).

General Research

Studies have shown that only a small percentage of applicants are actually hired as the result of posting a resume on one of the large employment websites as there is simply too much competition. The Internet, however, can be a valuable job search tool. You can read about health care trends, the general economy, and advances in medicine. You can scan job postings to see what characteristics employers mention most, get information about major facilities, and see samples of good resumes.

To access general information, enter key phrases such as "health care trends," "future of health care," "health care providers," and "health care employment" into a search engine. Government agencies such as the Department of Labor (www.dol.gov) and the Bureau of Labor Statistics (www.bls.gov) have information about the national job market, laws that affect employees, and resources for job-seekers.

Health Care Facility Websites

Many large health care facilities have websites that include photos, maps, information about the services they offer patients, and statements of their goals and overall mission. If you don't know the address, use a search engine and enter the name of the company or facility. Many organizations now list their current job openings along with online applications. In fact, some facilities accept *only* electronic applications.

Employment Websites

Job openings are listed on hundreds of websites. Although some are easier to use than others, most sites organize jobs by occupational fields, such as health care, and geographic location. Box 3-8 lists both general and health care specific employment websites.

You can view the job listings on these sites without registering. If you wish to post your resume, however, you must register by supplying information such as your name, address, and telephone number. You then select a username and password to access your account each time you visit the website.

In addition to these general health care sites, there are many specialty websites that feature jobs in one career area, such as dental assisting. Links to these websites are available at www.quintcareers.com/healthcare_jobs.html.

Keep in mind that new websites are continually being developed and old ones are merging, being deleted, or being moved to a different "address." Some of the addresses given in this book and in others may have changed by the time you try them, and it is certain that new websites will have been created.

 EXPERIENTIAL EXERCISE

Using websites that list job openings, find and list 10 jobs for which you might be qualified.

Networking

The Internet provides opportunities for sharing information and ideas with others through mailing lists and newsgroups. Mailing lists (also known as Listservs and email discussion groups) operate through email. Each list is devoted to a specific topic: occupations, hobbies, health conditions, and so on. Once you have subscribed, you receive email messages to which you can respond. Your email is then sent to all other subscribers. Mailing lists offer a way to learn what other job seekers are doing and what's happening in your field around the country. Comprehensive directories of the thousands of mailing lists are available from CataList (www.lsoft.com/lists/listref.html). Another source of mailing list groups is available from Yahoo! at http://groups.yahoo.com.

Newsgroups offer another way to network online. A newsgroup is basically an online discussion group for a specific topic. Anyone can join and participate by reading and posting messages. Messages that address the same topic are called a "thread" and each time a different topic is introduced, a new thread is started. See "groups.google.com" for a list of groups.

If you decide to use either mailing lists or newsgroups, it is important to learn the proper "netiquette" for participating. Experts suggest that you read a group's messages for at least 2 weeks before submitting anything so that you'll know the type and quality of material that is expected. It is also recommended that you check the "Frequently Asked Questions" or FAQs section, if available, to avoid asking something that has already been covered. When you do send messages, keep them short and to the point.

Web forums are another form of online discussion group offered through a variety of websites. You only need an email address and web browser to participate. You can ask questions, such as, "How's the job climate in San Antonio?" and someone from that area may answer. Lists of discussion groups are available on the Internet. Using a browser, enter the keyword "forum" and a topic of interest to get a list of ongoing forums.

One important rule is to never send advertising or use these groups to ask for a job. You may, however, find someone in the group who you can contact personally via email for possible assistance, just as you would other professional contacts.

See Box 3-9 for Internet success tips.

 EXPERIENTIAL EXERCISES

1. Read the article "How to Use the Internet in Your Job Search" at http://rileyguide.com/jobsrch.html.
2. Write a list of the information or suggestions you found most useful.

Internet Tracking Form

If you use the Internet to find information, post your resume, participate in groups, and record your activities.

 EXPERIENTIAL EXERCISES

Create an Internet tracking form that includes the following: name and address of the website, your username and password, the date you posted a comment or your resume, and a section for additional information and comments.

Job Titles

Regardless of the source—Internet, professional journal, or newspaper—look under every category that might contain jobs for which you are prepared. For example, graduates of health information programs may be qualified for the following positions:

coding specialist, health information technician, medical records coordinator or supervisor, and patient records technician. New job titles are constantly being created to describe the many activities performed in the modern health care facility.

CASE STUDY 3-4

Melva Duran, the director of career services at a large career college, answers students' questions at a workshop she is presenting for soon-to-be graduates.

Student: With so many job-seekers out there, how can graduates increase their chances of being noticed by employers?

Mrs. Duran: I think many graduates make the mistake of simply submitting a resume or application. When using the Internet, they may believe that once they've pushed the send button, it is up to the employer. But I have found that this just isn't enough. Graduates need to follow up. Unless requested otherwise in the job posting, this might be a phone call. It can be brief—something like, "I noticed your job posting on the Internet and I've sent an application online. I wanted to let you know I'm very interested in the job and am wondering when you'll be making a hiring decision."

I even had a major health care employer tell me that after he receives resumes, he waits a day or two to see if he receives any follow-up. Then he only reviews the resumes of applicants who have followed up!

Student: You mention the Internet. Are you finding that many graduates are getting jobs by posting their resumes?

Mrs. Duran: Actually, the large job sites often attract too many resumes—there is just so much competition. So I recommend to students that they browse the job postings to identify where the jobs are and find potential employers. Then they should go in person with their resumes.

Student: So you believe applicants should go personally to places of employment?

Mrs. Duran: Oh, yes, I think that's even better than a phone call—and certainly better than simply sending a resume electronically. They should do both—send a resume and then follow up. If they notice a large, local employer that seems to have jobs available, they should go to the facility. When talking to a contact person, they should state their interest in employment, ask about current hiring and future jobs that might be available, and ask if there is anything else they should do to apply for jobs.

Student: How about cold calling—do you recommend it?

Mrs. Duran: Absolutely! In fact, I've had good success with this method when graduates have trouble getting hired. I advise them to dress professionally and go to buildings that have potential employers. This is a better and faster approach than calling on the phone. Employers may be looking to hire and this saves them time and money spent on posting the job. Even if they don't have an opening, they often take the resume and call later.

This should be a soft sell—that is, don't be pushy and don't ask for an interview on the spot. On the other hand, do be prepared for an interview because that can happen!

Student: Are you suggesting that job-seekers should not make telephone calls to seek openings?

Mrs. Duran: No, not at all. With the telephone, you can obviously contact more potential employers.

Student: What is the best way to conduct a phone search?

Mrs. Duran: It's critical when calling to conduct yourself professionally. Second, it's important to speak with someone who has hiring authority. In a physician's office, this is not likely to be the receptionist in a doctor's office, so you need to ask for the office manager.

Student: Many of us are nervous when making these calls. What is the best way to go about it—what should graduates say?

Mrs. Duran: First state your name and say that you are a graduate of the _____ program at _____ school. Then say something like, "I would like to get my resume to you for any jobs you might have now or in the future."

If they are willing to receive your resume, it is best if you drop it off in person. This gives you a chance to see the facility, even if briefly and only the front office, and it gives someone there the chance to see you. So be sure to dress professionally! Before hanging up, ask for the address and any special directions.

QUESTIONS FOR THOUGHT AND REFLECTION

1. Which advice from Mrs. Duran do you find most helpful?
2. What is her advice about using the Internet?
3. Why does she recommend making direct contact with employers?
4. How can you best prepare to make a good impression on the phone? In person?
5. What does she mean by a "soft sell"?

Down a Dark Road

Jacob was frustrated and angry when he entered the office of Mr. Gonzalez, director of career services at Health Career College. Jacob graduated two months before he stopped by to see Mr. Gonzalez and still hadn't received a job offer. In fact, he hadn't even had an interview.

"Hi, Jacob," Mr. Gonzalez greeted him. "I haven't seen you in awhile. What's going on?"

"Not much, to be honest," Jacob told him. "I'm not happy. I finished my externship two months ago, and you guys haven't found me a job yet."

Mr. Gonzalez looked at Jacob for a moment and then said, "Well, I think there's been a misunderstanding. Our job is to *help* our students in their job search. We don't *get* them jobs."

"Look," says Jacob, "When I enrolled at this school I was told that the majority of students who graduated from my program get placed. I paid a lot of money to go here, and the least you can do is find me a job."

"Let me ask you, Jacob, did you attend any of my job search workshops?" "Honestly, by the time I graduated, I'd had enough of school," Jason said. "I really didn't feel like coming back for more classes."

"I'm sorry you feel that way," responded Mr. Gonzalez. "The workshops are designed to help students carry out an effective job search. Let me ask you a few questions."

"Here we go," grumbled Jacob, as he flopped down into a chair.

"What have you done so far to look for a job?" Mr. Gonzalez asked.

"A lot! I went to those online job sites and looked for jobs for pharmacy techs," said Jacob. "But most of them were too far away, or didn't look very interesting, or didn't pay enough. I can't take just anything, you know. I've got student loans to pay."

"How about networking? Or visiting pharmacies where you might like to work?" asked Mr. Gonzalez.

"I thought I *was* networking by being a student here," explained Jacob. "My instructors know me; you know me. I didn't have time while I was a student to go out and meet a bunch of people. I thought that was *your* job. Go meet employers and find us jobs."

"Jacob, I'm afraid that you're going to have to take more responsibility for conducting your own job search," said Mr. Gonzalez. "We can give you leads and connect you to employers who are interested in our graduates. But you haven't been in touch with us at all—not to attend the workshops or ask for help. That's our job, but you have to be willing to do your part."

"Well, I needed time to relax and just hang out after I graduated. And I can see it wouldn't have done any good anyway if *you're* not going to get me placed in a job I like—and that pays well."

QUESTIONS FOR THOUGHT AND REFLECTION

1. What mistakes is Jacob making in his job search?
2. What part do you think his attitude is playing in his failure to find a job?
3. What do you think about how Mr. Gonzalez handled being confronted by Jacob?
4. Do you think Jacob will have a successful career as a pharmacy technician? Why or why not?

Writing Your Resume

Production: The Second "P" of Marketing

You have to take life as it happens, but you should try to make it happen the way you want to take it.
—Old German Saying

LEARNING OBJECTIVE 10: PRODUCTION: THE SECOND "P" OF MARKETING

- List the five P's of marketing.
- Explain how finding a job is like marketing a product.
- Describe how visualization and affirmations can help you succeed.

You read about the first step in the marketing process: planning. There are actually five steps in an effective marketing plan, listed in Box 3-10, and we will start this chapter with the second P: production. In

BOX 3-10

The Five P's of Marketing

1. Planning	4. Presentation
2. Production	5. Promotion
3. Packaging	

production, you use the information gathered from market research to design and put together a product that meets the needs of the customer. Recall that your market research was finding about what patients and employers want and need from health care professionals.

Your goal is to become competent and professional. You must master the skills needed for your future occupation, along with practicing the attitudes and behaviors that will make you a valuable member of the health care team.

Henry Ford is quoted as saying, "Whether you think that you can, or you can't, you are right." The tendency for people to get what they expect is known as the self-fulfilling prophecy. Our beliefs about

Concept   Action   Reality

Create an image   Act on image   Become the image

Imagine yourself on the job. Picture how you look and what you are doing.

Do what it takes to achieve your goal—study, develop good work habits, complete your clinical experience.

You are a successful health care professional.

FIGURE 3-7 Become what you visualize. (From Haroun L, *Career Development for Health Professionals: Success in School and On the Job*, ed 4, St. Louis, 2016, Saunders.)

ourselves—what we can achieve—are more important than any other factor. You can apply the principle of expecting success as you begin your career journey. All achievements begin as ideas, and what you picture mentally can become your reality. Positive images of you succeeding in school and on the job are powerful motivators (Figure 3-7 and Box 3-11).

In addition to visual suggestions, your self-talk influences your success—or lack of it. We are continually holding conversations with ourselves that either give us encouragement ("I know I can pass this test.") or put ourselves down ("I'll never be able to get this report finished."). By taking control of the pictures and words in your mind, you can apply their power to help you create the life you want.

A powerful concept you can apply to your life is to act as if you already are what you hope to become. Practice behaviors now that you know will be expected on the job. For example, because accuracy and efficiency are important characteristics for the health care professional, complete all class assignments as if the well-being of others depended on their accuracy. Working effectively with others as part of a team will

be required in your work, so start using every opportunity to develop your teamwork skills. Cooperate with your classmates and instructors.

JOURNALING 3-9

Describe yourself as a health care professional. What do you offer the employer? How do you add value to the health care team?

EXPERIENTIAL EXERCISE

Try using the following affirmations to increase your confidence:
- I have many qualities of value for my future employers.
- I have a plan for preparing to become a successful health care professional.
- I am on my way to a great future.

BOX 3-11

Using Visualization

1. Find a quiet, private place where you won't be disturbed.
2. Close your eyes.
3. Imagine yourself as a (occupation of your choice).
   A. Create the details. Attempt to make the image as real as possible.
      I. What are you wearing?
      II. Who are your co-workers?
      III. What is the setting? A hospital? A physician's office? A business office?
      IV. What are you doing? Interacting with a patient? Performing a procedure? Working on a computer?
   B. Create positive thoughts and feelings for yourself in the scene: You are competent. You work well with patients and co-workers. You like what you are doing.
4. Try to keep your scene going for a few minutes. Make it as specific as possible and keep filling in the details. The idea is to have a clear, firm image of yourself successfully carrying out the duties of your chosen profession.

Packaging: The Third "P" of Marketing

LEARNING OBJECTIVE 11: PACKAGING: THE THIRD "P" OF MARKETING

- Explain why appearance is important for the health care professional.
- List the characteristics of appropriate appearance for the health care professional.
- Explain why a healthy appearance and good hygiene are important for the health care professional.
- Explain how safety factors affect the dress and grooming of the health care professional.

Even an excellent product may not sell if it is poorly packaged. Companies know this and invest a lot of time and money to make their products visually appealing to customers. Most of us package ourselves to impress others or to fit into a specific social group. Americans spend billions of dollars annually on clothing, cosmetics, accessories, and hair care in an effort to create what we believe to be a pleasing appearance.

Appearance is especially important in the health care field because many patients form their opinions about the competence of health care professionals based on their appearance. Your effectiveness in meeting patient needs can be influenced by your appearance because patient satisfaction increases when health care professionals "look like they know what they are doing."

Appropriate Dress

What is expected of health care professionals? They should be fairly conservative in dress and grooming. It is best to avoid fashion trends such as brightly colored hair, tattoos, and body piercing. At the same time, some employers are more accepting of these trends. The problem is that for some patients, they may be interpreted as signs of rebellion, immaturity, and lack of common sense. Others are offended or even frightened.

Even clothing that is not extreme may be inappropriate for work. Dressing for work is different than dressing casually for recreation or for social functions. What is perfect for a party may be totally out of place for a job interview or for the job itself.

? WHAT IF?

You have tattoos that cannot be covered by clothing. Do you think this will be a problem with employers?

Healthy Appearance

Strive for an appearance that radiates good health. An important responsibility of the health care professional is to promote good health and this is partly achieved by example. If you smoke or are overweight, putting you at risk for serious health problems, this would be a good time to adopt new healthy living habits. Other conditions, such as teeth that need dental work, badly bitten fingernails, and dandruff indicate a lack of self-care, and this is inappropriate in a profession that encourages the practice of good personal health habits (Figure 3-8). The way you present yourself reflects your approach to life and your opinion of

FIGURE 3-8 As a health professional, it is important to maintain good dental hygiene (Copyright © istock.com).

yourself. Failure to care for yourself can project a lack of self-confidence and undermine patient faith in your effectiveness.

Good Hygiene

Issues of cleanliness and hygiene are important for professionals whose work requires them to touch others. Patients must feel assured that they will benefit from, and not be harmed by, any procedures performed. It is natural to want the professional to look clean and neat and be free of unpleasant odors. For example, while the hands of the dental assistant may be clean and gloved, a dirty uniform or shoes (or even shoe strings!) give an unfavorable impression to the patient who may wonder whether proper attention was given to sterilizing the equipment and cleaning the work area.

 WHAT IF?

A friend and fellow graduate has been looking for a job but has received no offers. You think it might be his hygiene habits: body odor and bad breath. How might you help him?

Safety

Health care professionals must consider the safety and comfort of both patients and themselves.

Perfumes and scented personal products cannot be tolerated by many patients. Long fingernails, flowing hair, and large dangling earrings may be attractive and appropriate for a social event, but in a health care setting they can scratch patients, contaminate samples, get caught in equipment, or be grabbed by a young patient. Safety on the job cannot be compromised to accommodate fashion trends. Some clothing customs are determined by one's culture, such as head coverings and flowing skirts. These customs may also have to be modified to ensure the safety of both you and the patient.

JOURNALING 3-10

Is there anything about my appearance I want to improve in preparation for work in health care? Examples: fashion trends, health habits, cleanliness and hygiene, safety issues. What can I do to create a professional image?

(**Note:** If you are not sure about any aspects of your appearance or grooming, speak privately with your instructor or someone else you trust.)

Presentation: The Fourth "P" of Marketing

LEARNING OBJECTIVE 12: PRESENTATION: THE FOURTH "P" OF MARKETING

- Define the purpose of the professional resume.
- List the benefits of planning your resume while you are in school.
- List the ten resume building blocks.
- Describe the contents of each of the building blocks.
- Plan and prepare your professional resume.

Your resume, a written outline of your qualifications for work, is an important tool for presenting yourself and what you have to offer to prospective employers. The main purpose of a resume is to convince an employer to give you an interview. The focus of the rest of this chapter is on learning about the content of the resume and how you can use it as a guideline to create your professional self. Starting to plan your resume now will help you:

1. Recognize what you already have to offer an employer.
2. Build self-confidence.
3. Motivate yourself to learn both the technical and nontechnical skills that contribute to employment success.
4. Identify anything you might want to improve about yourself.
5. Know ahead of time what kinds of experiences will enhance your employability.
6. Get a head start gathering information and collecting examples to demonstrate your value and skills.

Your Resume as a Guide to Success

Begin with the end in mind.

—Stephen Covey

Thinking about your resume before the end of your educational program turns your resume into a checklist of "To Dos" for creating a product—your professional self—that you'll be able to offer with confidence to prospective customers: health care employers. The various components of a resume, listed in Box 3-12, are explained in this chapter, along with suggestions on how to make them work for you while you are still in school.

Building Block #1: Career Objective

The career objective is a brief description, often only one sentence long, of the position or job title you are seeking. You may also include a brief statement of what you can offer the employer:

BOX 3-12

Resume Building Blocks

1. Career Objective
2. Education
3. Professional Skills and Knowledge
4. Work History
5. Licenses and Certifications
6. Honors and Awards
7. Special Skills
8. Volunteer Activities
9. Professional and Civic Organizations
10. Languages Spoken

* Obtain a position as an administrative and clinical medical assistant where I can contribute by applying up-to-date skills
* Occupational therapy assistant in a pediatric facility

It is wise to have reasonable expectations for your first employment positions. Set positive long-term goals but be realistic when starting out. Your first job is your chance to work with real people who have real problems. The wider the range of jobs you are willing to accept when first entering the field, the better your chances of obtaining employment.

As you go through your training, learn as much as possible about the various jobs for which you might qualify. You may be unaware of jobs that closely match your interests. It is not uncommon to rewrite objectives more than once before beginning the actual job search.

 WHAT IF?

You enjoy your classes but are having a hard time being specific about the kind of job or facility you want. Where could you get more information to help you decide?

⭐ **EXPERIENTIAL EXERCISE**

Write at least two sentences that describe your objective for your first job in health care.

Building Block #2: Education

The education section contains a list of all your education and training, with emphasis on health care training.

Start your list with the school you attended most recently. Include grade point average and class standing (not all schools rank their students by grades) if they are above average. Do your best academically so you can present a strong education section. Here is an example of the health care portion entry:

Mental Health Technician Certificate, 2010
Wellness College, Salem, OR
* Graduated with Top Honors
* Grade point average 3.7 on a 4.0 scale
* Received Perfect Attendance Award
* Completed CPR training
* Organized musical program presented by students at Christmas to local extended-care residents

Workshops completed 2011-2012
Sunnyville Psychiatric Institute, Salem, OR
* Review of Research on Depression (25 hours)
* Suicide Prevention Measures (20 hours)
* Managing Assaultive Patients (25 hours)

 EXPERIENTIAL EXERCISE

List the schools you have attended, starting with the most recent. Include name of program(s) completed; degree(s), diploma(s), and/certificate(s) earned; grade point, if above average; awards and honors; additional training; special projects.

Building Block #3: Professional Skills and Knowledge

Professional skills and knowledge refer to the skills and knowledge that contribute to successful job performance.

The way you organize this section depends on your educational program and the number and variety of skills acquired. You can list them individually if there are not too many (such as "Take vital signs") or as clusters of related skills (such as "Perform clinical duties").

Listing individual skills or clusters of skills is a good idea if your previous work experience is limited and you want to emphasize the recent acquisition of health care skills as your primary qualification. It is also helpful if you have trained for one of the newer positions in health care that is not familiar to all employers. For example, "Patient Care Technician" is a relatively new multi-skilled worker who can be employed in a variety of health care settings.

Even if you decide not to include a skills list on your resume (it is optional), maintaining a list for yourself will remind you of what you know and have to offer an employer. Employers report that many recent graduates don't realize how much they know and therefore fail to sell themselves at job interviews.

Find out if your school provides lists of program and course objectives and/or the competencies you will master. Some instructors give their students check lists to monitor the completion of assignments and demonstration of competencies. Other sources of information include handouts from your instructor, such as syllabi and course outlines; the objectives listed in your textbooks; and lab skill sheets. You will

BOX 3-13

Examples of Professional Skills and Knowledge

- Set up dental trays for common procedures
- Accurately complete medical insurance claim forms
- Create presentations using PowerPoint
- Teach a patient to use different ambulatory devices

BOX 3-14

Examples of Transferable Skills

- Work well with people from a variety of backgrounds
- Provide good customer service
- Resolve customer complaints satisfactorily
- Perform accurate word processing
- Demonstrate empathy
- Apply ethical standards
- Apply active listening skills

be amazed by how much you are learning! See Box 3-13 for examples of skills.

 EXPERIENTIAL EXERCISE

Create an inventory of the skills you are learning in your program. Update the inventory as you complete your classes.

Building Block #4: Work History

The work history is list of your previous jobs, including the name and location of the employer, your job title and duties, and the dates of employment.

You can benefit from this section of your resume even if you have no previous experience in health care. There are three ways to do this. The first is to review the duties and responsibilities you had in each of your past jobs. Which ones can be applied to health care work? Skills that are common to many jobs are called transferable skills. See Box 3-14 for examples of transferable skills.

Identifying transferable skills is especially important when you are entering a new field in which you have little or no experience. There is a type of resume that emphasizes skills and abilities rather than specific job titles held. It is called a "functional resume," and the format is described later in this chapter. Start compiling a list of your own transferable skills.

The second way to maximize the value of the Work History section of your resume is to state what you achieved in each job. In a phrase or two, describe how you contributed to the success of your employer. When possible, state these achievements in measurable terms. If you can't express them with numbers, use active verbs that tell what you did. Here are some examples:

* Increased sales by 20%
* Designed a more efficient way to track supplies
* Worked on a committee to write an effective employee procedure manual that is still in use
* Trained five employees to use office equipment correctly

A third way to add value to this section is to include your externship experience. Although you must clearly indicate that this was a part of your training and not paid employment, it still serves as evidence of your ability to apply what you learned in school to practical situations. For many new graduates, this is their only real-world experience in health care; however, some students fail to realize the impact their performance can have on their career. Remember that clinical supervisors represent future employers. (In some cases, they *are* future employers because some students are hired by their externship sites.) Their opinion of you can help successfully launch your self-marketing efforts or cause them to fizzle, so commit to doing your best during your clinical experience.

(**Note:** Do *not* be concerned if your work experience is limited or you can't think of any achievements.) You may have finished high school recently or perhaps you spent several years working as a homemaker. Employers understand that everyone starts with a first job and you are receiving training to qualify you for work, and homemakers, as well as mothers and others who care for family members, gain experiences that are valuable to employers (Figure 3-9). Examples include caring for others, time management, and handling family finances.

WHAT IF?

The jobs you've held were all entry-level. You can't think of any real achievements in any of them.

FIGURE 3-9 Working in food service requires organization, time management and people skills, all of which are desirable skills that employers seek in new health care workers. Think about the skills you developed in previous job roles and how they transfer to the health profession (Copyright © istock.com).

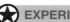

EXPERIENTIAL EXERCISE

List the jobs you've had in the past. Include the name and location of the employer; dates of employment; and your job title, duties, and achievements.

Building Block #5: Licenses and Certifications

Some professions require you to be licensed or have specific types of approval before you are allowed to work. Nursing is one example. Others include physical and occupational therapy and dental hygiene. Some professions have voluntary certifications and registrations, such as those earned by medical assistants. The kind of approvals needed vary by state and profession. Most licenses and certifications require certain types of training and/or passing a standardized exam. It is important that you clearly understand any professional requirements necessary or highly recommended for your profession.

Learn about the requirements for the occupation you have chosen. Ask your instructors about review classes, books, and computerized material. Check with your professional organization. Become familiar with the topics on the exams and plan your studies accordingly. Knowing the format of the questions (multiple-choice, true-false, etc.) is also helpful.

1. Describe the licensing and certification requirements for your occupation, including those that are voluntary.
2. What type of test(s) must you take?
3. What study and review materials are available?

BOX 3-15

Examples of Awards and Honors

- Parent Volunteer of the Year for James Madison Middle School (2010)
- Recognition for successful senior center fundraiser
- Perfect Attendance Award, Wellness College, 2013

Building Block #6: Honors and Awards

The section on honors and awards is optional. Your school may offer recognition for student achievements and special contributions. Community and professional organizations to which you belong may also give awards. Acknowledgments received for volunteer work can also be included in this section. See Box 3-15 for examples.

Investigate what you might be eligible for and use these rewards as incentives for excellent performance. Keep in mind, however, that although awards are nice to report, they are not essential for getting a good job.

 EXPERIENTIAL EXERCISE

Investigate and list awards for which you might qualify or have already earned.

Building Block #7: Special Skills

Special skills are those that don't fit into other sections but do add to your value as a prospective employee. Examples include proficiency in desktop publishing and the ability to use American Sign Language (Figure 3-10).

Research the needs of employers in your geographic area. Do you already have special skills that meet these needs? Would it increase your chances for employment if you acquired skills outside the scope of your program—for example, to become more proficient on the computer? If (and only if!) time permits,

FIGURE 3-10 Many skills, such as sign language, enhance the value of the health care professional. What skills do you already have that you can use in your future work? (Copyright © istock.com).

you might decide to attend workshops in addition to your regular program courses, do extra reading, or take a course on the Internet.

 EXPERIENTIAL EXERCISE

Record special skills you have that might be applicable to a job in health care.

Building Block #8: Volunteer Activities

Include volunteer activities on your resume if they relate to your targeted occupation or demonstrate desired qualities such as being responsible and having concern for others. If you are already involved in volunteer activities, think about what you are learning or practicing that can help you on the job. If you aren't, consider becoming involved if you have a sincere interest and adequate time. Adult students face many responsibilities outside of class, and the additional activities mentioned in this chapter should be taken as suggestions, not must-dos. Mastering program content should be your first priority.

 EXPERIENTIAL EXERCISE

List any volunteer activities you might use on your resume.

Building Block #9: Professional and Civic Organizations

Professional organizations provide excellent opportunities to network, learn more about your field, and practice leadership skills. Participation in civic organizations, groups that work for the good of the community, promotes personal growth and demonstrates your willingness to help others. Consider joining and participating actively in a professional or civic organization while you are in school. See if your school or community has a local chapter.

 EXPERIENTIAL EXERCISE

List professional and civic organizations you might include on your resume. Include offices held, committees served on, etc.

Building Block #10: Languages Spoken

In our multicultural society, the ability to communicate in a language other than English is commonly included on the resume. Find out whether many patients speak a language other than English in the area where you plan to work. Consider acquiring at least some conversational ability or a few phrases to use to reassure patients. Patients benefit greatly, during the stress of illness or injury, when health care professionals know at least a few phrases of their native language. Also consider learning about the customs, especially the ones related to health practices, of ethnic groups in your community.

 EXPERIENTIAL EXERCISE

List languages you speak other than English, including your ability level in speaking, reading, and writing.

 JOURNALING 3-11

As I put together my resume content, do I feel more confident about what I have to offer an employer?

Portfolios

LEARNING OBJECTIVE 13: PORTFOLIOS

- Define professional portfolio.
- List the items that might be included in a portfolio.
- Describe how a portfolio should be organized and put together.

Although resumes are the principal method for job seekers to present their qualifications to potential employers, portfolios can be used to supplement the resume. A portfolio is an organized collection of items that document your capabilities and qualifications for work.

Start planning your portfolio while you are taking classes. As you complete each course, save assignments that might be suitable for your portfolio. Select those that demonstrate your abilities. Store them in a folder or large envelope so they stay in good condition.

In addition to written assignments, there are nontraditional ways to showcase your abilities. The items you collect need not be limited to evidence of your technical skills. For example, it is appropriate to include documentation of other activities, such as organizing an event for charity. No standard list of items to put in your portfolio exists although your school may have prepared a list for students. In any case only accurate and neat work should be included. The following are examples of portfolio contents:

1. Assignments
   * Accurately filled out insurance form
   * Accounting forms
   * Perfectly typed/word processed letter
   * Lab reports
   * Sample medical history form filled out
   * Charting entries
   * Research report
2. Certificates of Completion or Achievement
   * Verification of having completed courses, seminars, and workshops
   * Proof of skill mastery, such as CPR, first aid, or the Burdick electrocardiographic (EKG) procedure, or documentation of the number of successful performances of an important procedure, such as venipunctures, injections, and x-rays
   * Documentation of speed, such as for word processing or data entry
   * Recognition of special achievements, such as honor or merit roll or perfect attendance
3. Grade Records or Transcripts
   * Consider including these if your grades are above average. If they started out as average or even below-average and then improved as you advanced through your program, you might use them to demonstrate your persistence and progress.

4. Employer Review or Evaluation
   * You can include these from your previous employment if they demonstrate attitudes or skills applicable to work in health care. A positive review from your clinical supervisor can be very valuable because it is recent and relates directly to health care.
5. Recognition of Contributions
   * Thank-you letters
   * Verification of participation in activities such as walk-a-thons to raise money for worthy causes
6. Attendance Record
   * Excellent addition if you have very good attendance
7. Honors and Awards
8. Licenses or Certifications (copies)
9. Photographs
   * Use these to document activities in which you had a major role, such as organizing a fund-raising activity or planning and coordinating a school picnic.
10. Letters of Recommendation

⭐ **EXPERIENTIAL EXERCISE**

Use the key words "professional portfolio" to locate information on the Internet about preparing a professional portfolio. Write a summary of your findings.

Promotion: The Fifth "P" of Marketing

LEARNING OBJECTIVE 14: PROMOTION: THE FIFTH "P" OF MARKETING

- List various ways to network professonally.
- Explain the purpose of professional references.
- Give example of appropriate professional references.
- Explain how a job interview is an opportunity to promote yourself.

Think about how companies use promotional campaigns to give new products maximum exposure. They advertise—sometimes endlessly, it seems!—on television, in magazines and newspapers, and on the Internet to spread the word to as many consumers as possible about how the product will fulfill their needs. You will conduct a similar campaign as you conduct your job search. As with your resume and portfolio, you can begin to prepare now. Networking, references, and the job interview are the three main ways to promote yourself during the job search.

Networking

Networking is meeting and establishing relationships with people who work in health care. It is an effective way to learn more about your chosen career. At the same time it gets the word out about you and your employment goals. Examples of networking opportunities include professional meetings, career fairs, class field trips to health care facilities, and guest speakers who come to your school.

There are many ways to begin networking: at a professional meeting, introduce yourself to other members; after hearing a guest speaker in class, ask questions; at a career fair, ask a local employer for advice about what to emphasize in your studies. Be sure to follow-up with a phone call or thank-you note to anyone who sends you information or makes a special effort to help you.

Another benefit of networking is building your self-confidence as you introduce yourself to people. You can improve your speaking ability and increase your ability to express yourself effectively. These are valuable skills you will use when attending job interviews. Start to create a web of connections to help you develop professionally and assist you in your future job search and career.

← **JOURNALING 3-12**

What opportunities do you have now for professional networking?

⭐ **EXPERIENTIAL EXERCISES**

1. Use the search term "career networking" to find websites with information about this important job search tool.
2. Write a short report listing five reasons to use networking. Include the names and addresses of the sites where you find the information.

References

References are people who will confirm your qualifications, skills, abilities, and personal qualities. They endorse you as a product. Professional references are not the same as personal or character references. To be effective, professional references must be credible (believable) and have personal knowledge of your value to a prospective employer. Your best references have knowledge of both you and the health care field. Examples include your instructors, externship supervisors, and other professionals who know the quality of your work. Previous supervisors, even in jobs outside of health care, also make good references.

→ JOURNALING 3-13

Are you the kind of person a reference would feel comfortable recommending for a job? What can you do to increase your chances of finding good references?

★ EXPERIENTIAL EXERCISE

1. Make a list of potential professional references.
2. Contact each person on your list and ask if he/she is willing to serve as a reference.

Job Interview

Job interviews provide the best opportunities to promote yourself to prospective employers. Interviewers often ask for examples of how you solved a problem or handled a given situation. Start thinking about how you would answer these questions and begin to collect examples from your work as a student, such as from your externship experience, that will demonstrate your capabilities. Start preparing for your future interviews as opportunities to shine, at ease and confident that you are presenting yourself positively like the applicant in Figure 3-11.

FIGURE 3-11 How is the job candidate demonstrating self-confidence as she meets the employer? What can you start doing now to ensure you attend future job interviews with confidence (Copyright © istock.com)?

CASE STUDY 3-5

Emily worked for many years in sales, spending most of it in the clothing departments of retail stores. She always enjoyed the work, especially working with customers and helping them select something they would enjoy wearing.

A few years ago, Emily was in a car accident and injured her back. She recovered from major injuries, and her employer, Sharpe's Department Store, was eager to have her back. However, when Emily returned to work, she found standing all day too difficult. She stayed on the job for a month, but the steady pain interfered with her ability to do her job well. By the time she returned home each day, she was too worn out to do anything but sit in front of the television.

Reluctantly, Emily gave her notice to Sharpe's and, after taking a couple of weeks off to rest, started investigating a

career change. "I really want—in fact I need—to work," she told her friend Jennie. "I can't just sit home all day."

Jennie was Emily's best friend. She worked for a health insurance company. "Why don't you look into some kind of office work?" she suggested. "I'm at a desk most of the day," she explained. "You could get up and stretch your back once in a while, but you wouldn't have to stand all day like you did at Sharpe's."

"Well, I never thought I'd want to sit all day," Jennie responded. "But life threw me a curve ball here—I guess I'm going to have to think about some changes."

After exploring career options, Jennie enrolled in the medical administrative assistant program at BeWell College last month. The program appealed to her because it sounded like she wouldn't just sit at a desk all day, but could look for a front office job where she would have contact with patients. Working with people was one of the things she had enjoyed most while working in sales.

After a slow start at BeWell—she had to work on improving her study skills—she did well in her classes, completing them last month. She began her externship at St. Francis Family Clinic two weeks ago, and she's started thinking about looking for a job.

"I'm pretty nervous about it," she told Jennie as the two enjoyed a visit over coffee. "I haven't had to look for a job in years! And I hear a lot of it is done online these days. Remember when we typed up a little resume and just took it by whoever was hiring?" she said.

"Yeah, our age is showing now, isn't it?" laughed Jennie.

"You know, the other day I happened to meet Mr. Bard, the director of Human Resources at St. Francis. He stopped by the table where I was having lunch with my supervisor, Olivia. She introduced us," Emily said.

"Emily, I know what a people person you are. I bet I know where you're going with this!" said Jennie.

"Yep—I'll see if I can get an appointment with him. He seemed like a nice guy. Maybe he'll have some good advice for a rusty old job seeker like me," she laughed."

Mr. Bard agreed to meet with Emily. He liked her go-to spirit and confidence in asking for his advice. They met one afternoon in his office.

Emily: "How much of the application process at this clinic is done electronically?"

Mr. Bard: "Actually, we accept only electronic applications. We also prefer that resumes be submitted electronically, either typed into the electronic application or sent as an attachment. There are a couple of reasons for this. One is that people who work here must have computer skills so the application process requires that they demonstrate these skills. The second reason is so we can maintain an electronic database of applicants. If someone submits an application and resume today, we may not have a job that matches his or her skills. But an opening may come in a month. We can electronically review the resumes that we've scanned into our database and quickly identify potential candidates."

Emily: "Does this mean that applicants shouldn't bother to prepare printed resumes?"

Mr. Bard: "Not at all. They should still have them. In fact, they should always bring extra copies to an interview in case they're needed."

Emily: "Do you recommend any particular type of resume?"

Mr. Bard: "No, the standard resumes—chronological and functional—are still acceptable. One thing a resume should demonstrate is the applicant's computer skills. Its appearance is important, too—proper alignment, consistent fonts, that kind of thing. Resumes should also show that candidates have thought about where they want to go in their careers."

Emily: "How do applicants access an application for this clinic?"

Mr. Bard: "They can go to our website. We list all current job openings on the site along with our general application. For applicants who don't have computers, we have one they can use in the human resources office."

Emily: "Mr. Bard, I have to get back to work, but I'm so appreciative of the time you spent answering my questions. If it's okay with you, I'd like to share what you told me with my classmates at BeWell. Those of us on externship have a workshop next week at the school."

Mr. Bard: "That would be fine. Please do share anything you think is worthwhile."

QUESTIONS FOR THOUGHT AND CONSIDERATION

1. What do you think of Emily's idea to "interview" Mr. Bard?
2. What did you learn from his answers?
3. Why are employers asking for electronic versions of applications and resumes?
4. Do you think Emily will succeed in her job search? Why or why not?

Down a Dark Road

Laura had decided before she even entered high school that she wanted to live "the good life" when she grew up. For her, this life would include living or traveling in Europe, driving a sports car, and having nice clothes. She was raised in an upper-middle-class neighborhood by loving parents, and her chances of receiving a quality education and the ability to earn a good living seemed possible.

Unfortunately, Laura had a personal trait that caused many problems: she couldn't be told anything. She had a natural talent in music, but she insisted to her piano teacher that it was a waste of time to learn to read music. She could just listen and repeat what she heard. Many of the subjects she was required to take in high school were, in her opinion, a waste of time. As she told her friend Nicole, "I just can't see spending my time learning stuff I'll never use."

Unfortunately, she used this tone with her teachers and as a result, was forced to transfer to three different high schools before she finally graduated. It had been a struggle, but she did earn a diploma.

Not knowing what she wanted to do to attain "the good life" she still had in mind, Laura spent her first year out of high school cashiering in a fast food restaurant and stocking shelves in an electronics store.

As summer came to an end, her mother advised her, "Laura, you really need to starting thinking about your future."

"Mom, please. I don't know what I want to do. And if you don't mind, I really don't want to think about it right now. It's just too stressful," Laura said.

"Well," her mom told her. "One of these days you'll have to start taking care of yourself, so I suggest you put some thought into it."

The next day, Laura complained to her friend Nicole. "I don't see what the rush is about my future. Why is my mom getting all excited about it?"

Nicole said, "I guess I'm lucky. I've known for a long time that I wanted to be a nurse, and I like the classes I'm taking, even though some of them are a little challenging. Anatomy, for example. But it's stuff I need to know."

"Yeah, you're lucky that way—knowing what you want to do. I just know I want to make good money—and not have to work too hard," explained Laura. "And I want to travel. The other day I was reading about cruise ships. I wonder what kind of job I could get on a ship?"

"I guess you could be like a waitress or something," said Nicole.

"That doesn't sound very appealing," said Laura. "Working in the burger place is bad enough."

"Hey, I just thought of something," said Nicole. "Last week I was talking to a girl in the massage therapy program at school. She said something about jobs on cruise ships. It seems that massages are a service they offer the passengers."

"Hmmm ... that's something I hadn't thought of," said Laura.

Laura spent a little time thinking about what Nicole said and decided to look into the massage therapy program at the school Nicole attended. The program wasn't terribly long and Laura liked the idea of not spending too much time in school. Her mother had doubts about Laura's dreams of "money and travel working on a cruise ship" but was glad that Laura had at least come up with a plan for her future.

The required classes for massage therapy surprised Laura. She thought it would be mostly hands-on and not require much reading or written tests. The worst part was being told what to do by her instructors. The dress code really annoyed her. Laura, who is slender with long blonde hair, liked the look of rather tight, revealing clothing and 4-inch heels. She had been warned that this attire was not appropriate for a job in health care, especially in massage therapy, and therefore was not appropriate for school. Laura believed the dress code is "stupid" and "unfair" and continued to dress as she wishes. She really didn't believe that halter tops and low slung pants were a big deal. What's the problem with short shorts if you have good legs?

QUESTIONS FOR THOUGHT AND CONSIDERATION

1. What is your opinion of Laura's reasons for wanting a career as a massage therapist?
2. Why is dressing appropriately and professionally especially important for massage therapists?
3. What would you suggest Laura do about her attitude toward learning and education?
4. Do you think the school will allow Laura to continue her massage therapy education? Why or why not?

Pulling It All Together

LEARNING OBJECTIVE 15: PULLING IT ALL TOGETHER

- Explain why it is best to create your own resume.
- List the advantages of using word processing software to prepare your resume.
- List the ten steps for assembling your resume.

- Describe the three types of resumes.
- Explain who would best benefit from each type of resume.
- Understand the importance of perfect grammar and spelling in the resume.

You are now ready to gather the information in your Resume Building Blocks to construct a finished product. The steps described in this section will help you create a document that best highlights your qualifications.

There is no one best way to write a resume. Everyone has different talents and experiences. Even students who complete the same program at the same time come from a variety of backgrounds that can be presented in different ways. For example, a young person who graduated from high school shortly before beginning a dental assisting program will more likely benefit from emphasizing different experiences than a classmate who worked in sales for 20 years before entering the same program.

There are also local customs and employer preferences regarding resumes. Seek the advice of your instructors, school career service personnel, and professional contacts. They keep in touch with employers and can offer sound advice.

You may be tempted to use a standard resume format. Filling in the blanks on a "one-type-fits-all" resume may seem to be a fast and easy way to complete this task; however, the time spent customizing your resume can pay off in several ways. For example, you will:

1. Better recognize and review your own qualifications
2. Respond to employers' specific needs
3. Be prepared to support your claims with examples
4. Demonstrate your organizational skills
5. Show your initiative and creativity

(**Note**: Your school may require or recommend that you use a format it has developed.)

The best way to put together a resume is with word processing software because you can:

* Try different layouts and formats
* Change and reorganize content quickly and easily
* Check for (most) spelling errors
* Change your objective or skill clusters to address specific employer needs
* Use special features such as bolding and different letter sizes and styles
* Send your resume as part of an email and/or post it on the Internet

 WHAT IF?

You want to put together a good resume, but you aren't very skilled with word processing software.

10 Steps for Assembling Your Resume

■ List the 10 steps for assembling your resume.
■ Choose the building blocks for your resume.
■ Decide on the best order for the building blocks.
■ Understand the purpose of the personal statement.
■ Determine the best layout for your resume.

Following a step-by-step process will help you assemble a resume to fit your needs. Box 3-16 summarizes the steps that are explained in the following sections.

Step One: Prepare the Heading

It is not necessary to write the word "Resume." Instead, clearly label the top of the page with your name, address, telephone number(s), and email address. Center your name on the page. Placing it on the far left side makes it more difficult for the employer to find if it is placed in a stack of other resumes or in a file. Capitalizing, bolding, and/or using a slightly larger font (letter) size than the rest of the document helps it to stand out. Be *sure* that all numbers are correct.

BOX 3-16

10-Step Checklist for Assembling Your Resume

1. Prepare the heading
2. Add the objective
3. Select the best type of resume for you
4. Decide if you want to include a Summary of Qualifications section
5. Choose which Resume Building Blocks to include
6. Plan the order of your Building Blocks
7. Decide whether you want to add a personal statement
8. But leave out personal information
9. Plan the layout
10. Create an attractive and professional-looking document

JAIME RAMIREZ
3650 Loma Alta Lane
San Diego, CA 92137
(619)123-4567
jrnurse@aol.com

The following format is an option if your resume is long and you are trying to save space:

JAIME RAMIREZ
3650 Loma Alta Lane San Diego, CA 92137
(619)123-4567 jrnurse@aol.com

Step Two: Add the Objective

The objective, from Resume Building Block #1, should be near the beginning of the resume so prospective employers can quickly see whether there is a potential match between your goals and their needs. This part of the resume may change slightly if you are trying to match your objective with the stated needs of each employer. Your objective will not change if you have specific requirements you are not willing to change, if you have written a very general objective that meets a number of job targets, or if your objective simply states a job title such as "surgical technologist."

Consider writing a targeted objective when applying for a specific job. This type of objective mirrors the employer's language and draws attention to how you fit that particular job. The following example shows how to write a targeted objective:

Job Post: "X-ray tech with strong patient relations skills for orthopedic practice. Great opportunity to join an established team environment."

Key Words in the Post: X-ray tech, patient relations skills, orthopedic, team

Targeted Objective: Position as an X-ray tech in an orthopedic office where I can apply my excellent human relations skills working with patients and fellow workers.

Step Three: Select the Best Type of Resume for You

The three basic types are chronological, functional, and combination. They provide different ways to present your work history and professional qualifications. Your particular background determines which type you should choose.

Chronological Resume

The chronological resume emphasizes work history. It shows the progression of jobs you have held and how you have gained increasing knowledge and experi-

ence and/or responsibility that applies to the job you want now. This type of resume is recommended if you have:

* Held previous jobs in health care
* Had jobs in other areas in which you had increases in responsibility or a strong record of achievements
* Acquired many skills that apply to health care (transferable skills)

In the chronological resume, each of your past jobs is listed, followed by the duties performed and your achievements. The Work History section is well-developed and likely to be longer than most other parts of your resume.

Functional Resume

The functional resume emphasizes skills and traits that relate to the targeted job but which weren't necessarily acquired through health care employment. They can be pulled from both work and personal experiences. For example, if you cared for a sick relative for an extended period of time or perhaps were a child care provider, this is an experience you might include. Once you have identified and listed qualifications that fit your target jobs, organize them into three or four clusters with descriptive headings. Figure 3-12 shows three clusters developed by a graduate who wants to find a job in health information technology. She has drawn from her experiences as a parent, active member of her community, and bookkeeper.

Functional resumes are recommended if you:
* Are entering the job market for the first time
* Have held jobs unrelated to health care
* Have personal experiences you can apply to health care work

The Work History section of a functional resume consists of a simple list of job titles with each employer's name, city and state, and your dates of employment. A functional resume may take more time to develop than a chronological one, but the extra effort can pay off because it allows you to highlight the qualifications that are your strongest bid for employment.

Combination Resume

The combination resume, as its name implies, uses features of both chronological and functional resumes. The details of the job(s) held in or closely related to health care are listed, along with clusters of qualifications or a list of supporting skills. This resume is appropriate if you:

COMPUTER SKILLS

- Created electronic spreadsheet to track fund raising for Lewison Elementary School PTA

- Taught self to effectively use leading brand software programs in the following areas: word processing, database, spreadsheets, and accounting

- Set up and managed electronic accounting system for family construction business

- Teach computer classes at Girl Scout summer day camp

ORGANIZATIONAL SKILLS

- Created system to monitor all church collections and fund-raising projects

- Initiated and developed computer career awareness program for Girl Scouts

- Secretary for college HIT student organization

- Completed HIT associate degree program with record of perfect attendance while working part-time and managing family life

CLERICAL/ADMINISTRATIVE SKILLS

- 7 years bookkeeping experience

- Keyboarding speed of 78 wpm

- Excellent written communication

WORK HISTORY

Bookkeeper 2008-Present
Buildwell Construction Company, Yuma, AZ

Bookkeeper 2003-2008
Perfect-Fit Cabinetry, Yuma, AZ

Secretary 1999-2003
Caldwell Insurance Company, Yuma, AZ

FIGURE 3-12 Work History section of a functional resume for a recent graduate seeking a health information technology (HIT) position. The graduate does not have experience in this field, so she has clustered other skills that support work in HIT, such as bookkeeping and tracking details.

* Have held jobs in health care, and
* Have related qualifications you gained through other, non-health care jobs and experiences, or
* Have held a number of jobs in health care for which you performed the same or very similar duties.

Let's look at how a recent occupational therapy assistant graduate who worked for 2 years as a nursing assistant and for 3 years as a preschool aide creates a combination resume. She decides to:

* Include a list of the duties she performed in the nursing assistant job

* Create clusters to highlight her teaching and interpersonal skills, both important in occupational therapy
* List skills from her teaching and other experiences under each cluster heading

Figure 3-13 illustrates how she organized her material to best show her qualifications.

Choosing the Best Resume for You

Review your skills and experiences and use the guidelines in this section to choose the best type of resume

NURSING ASSISTANT   2005-2010
GoodCare Nursing Home, Denver, CO

- Encourage patients to achieve their maximum level of wellness, activity, and independence

- Demonstrate interest in the lives and well-being of patients

- Assist patients with prescribed exercises

- Organize and participate in activities with patients

- Help patients carry out basic hygiene and dressing

TEACHING SKILLS

- Teach swim classes to all ages at YMCA

- Conduct CPR instruction for the American Heart Association

- Organize holiday programs and outings for nursing home residents (volunteer)

- Planned and supervised craft and play activities for preschool children

- Tutored ESL students at Salud College while in OTA program

INTERPERSONAL SKILLS

- Provided daily care for parent with Alzheimer's disease for 18 months

- Answered telephone, directed calls, and took messages for busy sporting goods manufacturer

- Received Connor Memorial Award for graduating class for making positive contributions and assisting classmates at Salud College

WORK HISTORY   **Preschool Aide** 2002-2005
Bright Light Preschool, Denver, CO

                       Swim Instructor 2002-Present
YMCA, Denver, CO

                       Receptionist 1999-2002
Sportrite Manufacturing Co., Denver, CO

FIGURE 3-13 Work History section of a combination resume for a recent graduate seeking an occupational therapy assistant position. She details the one health care-related job she has held while organizing other skills that support the new career into clusters.

for you. If you decide to use a chronological presentation, copy what you prepared for your Work History in Building Block #3.

If a functional resume would serve you better, use the following guidelines to create the clusters:

1. Consider the current needs of employers. Check your local help-wanted ads and job announcements, the National Healthcare Foundation Standards, and information from your professional organization.

2. Identify the skills and traits that will contribute to success in your occupation.

3. Review your work history, externship experience, personal experiences, volunteer activities, and participation in professional organizations.

4. Create three or four headings for clusters that support your job target and give you an opportunity to list your most significant qualifications. The following list contains examples of appropriate clusters for health care occupations:

* Communication Skills
* Organizational Skills
* Teamwork Skills
* Interpersonal Relations
* Computer Skills
* Clerical Skills

5. List specific skills under each heading.

Step Four: Summary of Qualifications

Decide whether to include a Summary of Qualifications Section. This is an optional section. Here you can list skills that support you as a job applicant but which don't fit well in other sections. Placed near the beginning of your resume, it highlights how you will benefit the employer and encourage the reader to look over the rest of your resume. In other words, it can serve as an appealing introduction to you and your resume.

You may have decided to use a chronological resume but have additional experiences that don't belong in the Work History section. Perhaps you are using a functional resume but have single experiences worth mentioning that don't fit any of the headings. Here are some examples:

* Excellent time-management skills
* Ability to work calmly under pressure
* Proven problem-solving ability
* Cost consciousness
* Enthusiastic team player
* Work well without supervision
* Enjoy learning new skills

A qualifications section can also serve as a summary of highlights to draw attention to your most significant features. Such a summary might look like this:
Eight years' experience working in health care.
Up-to-date administrative and clinical medical
    assisting skills.
Current CPR certification.
Fluent in spoken Spanish.
Ability to communicate with patients of all ages.

(**Note:** If you have created clusters and are using them in a functional or combination resume, you may not want a Qualifications section. The important thing is not to repeat information in your resume.)

Step Five: Choose Which Resume Building Blocks to Use

Your resume should be comprehensive, but you don't want to repeat information. For example, if you are using a functional format and have listed a special skill in one of your clusters, don't list it again under another heading. Group as much as fits well into each Resume Building Block instead of having many headings with just one item listed. Think about which items fit together. The following are the most appropriate to combine:

1. Licenses and certifications can be placed in their own section, in the Education section, or listed as a Professional Qualification.

2. Honors and awards earned in school can be listed under Education. If you have a variety of awards, it might be better to highlight them by listing them in their own section.

3. Memberships can go under Education if they are related to school groups or your health care professional organization. If you have been active in the organizations and want to state what you've done or are involved in several organizations, they might better go in their own section.

4. Externship experience can be listed under either Education or Work History. Wherever you place it, include some information about the duties you performed. For career changers and recent graduates, this may be a significant part of your work history. Be sure to indicate clearly that the work was unpaid and part of an educational program.

5. Languages you speak other than English can be listed under Qualifications, Special Skills, or Languages Spoken.

Deciding which headings to use and where to place content depends on the amount of content, how directly it relates to the kind of job you want, and your own organizational preferences. Suppose you speak two languages other than English. If they are spoken by many people in your geographic area, they are likely to be valuable job qualifications and might be listed in a Summary of Qualifications. If they are not commonly spoken in your area, they might best be listed under Languages—skills you want to show but that may not be directly related to the job.

Step Six: Plan the Order of Your Building Blocks

Place the sections that contain your strongest qualifications first. For example, if you are changing careers and recent education is your primary qualification, place this section before Work History.

Step Seven: Decide If You Want to Add a Personal Statement

In their book on career planning, Dave Ellis and coauthors suggest adding a positive personal statement at the bottom of your resume (Ellis, 1997). This is an opportunity to make a final impression and add an original touch. It is a way to say "Here is something personal and interesting about me that might help you, the employer." If you decide to write a personal statement, be sure it is a sincere reflection of you and not just something that sounds good. And be sure it relates to your job target. Here are some examples:

"I enjoy being a part of a team where I can make a positive contribution by using my ability to remain calm and work efficiently under stressful conditions."

"I get great satisfaction working with people from a variety of backgrounds who need assistance in resolving their health care problems."

If you decide to include a personal statement, review your reasons for choosing a career in health care along with what you believe are your best potential contributions to prospective employers. It's a good idea to have someone such as your instructor review your statement.

Step Eight: Leave Out Personal Information

Don't include personal information such as your age, marital status, number of children, and health status and *never* include false statements about your education or experience. If these are discovered later, they can be grounds for dismissal from your job.

Although it is important to have a Reference Sheet (list of references with their contact information) available for potential employers who request it, it is not necessary to write a statement such as "References Available Upon Request."

Step Nine: Plan the Layout

Each section of your resume, except the heading at the top and personal statement (optional) at the end, should be labeled: Objective, Education, Work History, and so on. Headings can be flush (aligned) with the left margin, with the content set to the right:

OBJECTIVE XXXXXXXXXXXXXXXXXXXX
      XXXXXXXXXXXXXXXXXX
EDUCATION XXXXXXXXXXXXXXXXXXXXXX
      XXXXXXXXXXXXXXXXXX

Alternatively, you can center your headings and list the information beneath and flush left:

OBJECTIVE
XXXXXXXXXXXXXXXXXXXXXXXXX
XXXXXXXXXXXXXXXXXXXXXXXXXXXXX
EDUCATION
XXXXXXXXXXXXXXXXXXX
XXXXXXXXXXXXXXXXXXXXXXX
XXXXXXXXXXXXXXX

The design should be based primarily on whether you need to use or save space on the page. However you choose to lay out your resume, strive for a balanced, attractive look. See Box 3-17 for examples of various ways to use capitalization and boldface.

Step Ten: Create an Attractive and Professional-Looking Document

Selecting and organizing content can take time and effort so don't waste your efforts by failing to attend to the details of appearance. A poor appearance can land a resume in the wastebasket without even a review. The following tips will help you achieve a professional look:

Leave enough white space so the page doesn't look crowded. Double-space between the sections.

Limit your resume to one page, unless you have more information than will fit. Write "More" or "Continued" at the bottom of the first page and your name and contact information and "Page 2" at the top of the second.

BOX 3-17

Using Special Elements

WORK HISTORY	Medical Transcriptionist 2001-Present Hopeful Medical Center Better Health, NJ
OR	MEDICAL TRANSCRIPTIONIST 2001-Present Hopeful Medical Center Better Health, NJ
OR	**Medical Transcriptionist** 2001-Present Hopeful Medical Center Better Health, NJ

BOX 3-18

Resume Checklist

_____ Dates and numbers are complete and accurate

_____ Your phone number(s) and email address are included

_____ The objective is clear

_____ Content supports the objective

_____ Content is organized in order of importance

_____ All important qualifications are included

_____ Information is not repeated

_____ Spelling is perfect

_____ Grammar is correct

_____ Layout is consistent

_____ The page is attractively laid out

Capitalize headings.

Use bullets to set off listed items.

Try using boldface for emphasis.

Make sure your spelling and grammar are perfect.

Leave at least a 1-inch margin on all sides.

Use good quality paper in white, ivory, or very light tan or gray.

Make sure the print is dark and clear.

See Box 3-18 for a resume checklist to ensure you have a comprehensive and quality resume that represents you well.

See Figures 3-14, 3-15, and 3-16 for examples of completed resumes.

Distributing Your Resume

LEARNING OBJECTIVE 17: DISTRIBUTING YOUR RESUME

■ List the people and places where you might distribute your resume.

Make the best use of your printed resume by distributing it to people who have or may have job openings—employers—and people who might know about jobs. Here are some suggestions to get you started:

* Employers who place "Help Wanted" ads or post job openings on the Internet or elsewhere

* Employers who have unadvertised openings you have heard about from other sources

* Your networking contacts

* Friends and relatives

* Anyone who indicates that he or she knows someone who might be hiring

* Your school's career services department

Keep enough copies of your resume on hand to respond to unexpected opportunities. Take copies to interviews (even if you have sent a copy in advance), career fairs, and the Human Resources departments of health care facilities. Have plenty on hand if you decide to drop in on employers.

It is usually not recommended, however, that you send resumes to dozens of employers in the hope of locating one that has a job opening. One exception is when there are more job openings than applicants. When there is a shortage of applicants, you are more likely to receive responses. A second exception is when you are moving to a new area. Sending a large number of resumes, along with a cover letter explaining that you are relocating, may be more economical and productive than calling many potential employers.

❓ WHAT IF?

You feel shy about handing out your resume. You don't want to "bother" people with it.

New Developments in Resumes

LEARNING OBJECTIVE 18: NEW DEVELOPMENTS IN RESUMES

■ Explain how to reformat your resume to send or post it online.

■ List cautions and suggestions to follow when posting your resume online.

The capacities of the computer to sort and organize data, along with the speed and convenience of the Internet, have resulted in new forms of resumes and ways for job searchers and employers to connect.

RUDY MARQUEZ
1909 Franklin Blvd.
Philadelphia, PA 19105
(610) 765-4321   MAmarquez@aol.com

OBJECTIVE	Position as a clinical medical assistant in an urgent care setting

QUALIFICATIONS

- 13 years experience as a certified medical assistant
- Current certifications in CPR and Basic Life Support
- Proven ability to communicate with patients and staff
- Proactive employee who anticipates office and physicians' needs
- Fluent in Spanish and Italian

WORK HISTORY

Medical Assistant   2005-present
Founders Medical Clinic   Philadelphia, PA
- Perform clinical and laboratory duties
- Assist physicians with exams, procedures, and surgeries
- Reorganized patient education program, including selection of updated brochures, videos
- Provide patient education and present healthy living workshops
- Train and supervise new medical assistants

Medical Assistant   1999-2005
North Side Clinic   Pittsburgh, PA
- Performed clinical and laboratory duties
- Developed system for monitoring and ordering clinic supplies that resulted in annual savings of over $25,000
- Received commendation for providing outstanding patient service

Medical Assistant   1997-1999
Dr. Alan Fleming   Erie, PA
- Assisted Dr. Fleming with procedures and minor office surgeries
- Prepared treatment and examining rooms
- Took vital signs and administered injections
- Performed routine laboratory tests
- Handled computerized recordkeeping tasks
- Assisted in researching and purchasing new office computer system

EDUCATION

Associate of Science in Medical Assisting   1997
Emerson College of Health Careers, Erie, PA

Recently Completed Workshops and Continuing Education Courses
- Health Care Beliefs of Minority Populations
- Medical Spanish
- New Requirements for Maintaining Patient Confidentiality

ORGANIZATIONS

American Association of Medical Assistants (AAMA)
Pennsylvania Association of Medical Assistants
Philadelphia Lions Club

FIGURE 3-14 Example of a Chronological Resume. This type of resume, which lists a detailed work history, is recommended for applicants who already have experience working in health care.

HEATHER DIETZ
10532 Cactus Road
Yuma, AZ 85360
(520) 321-7654   thedietz@linkup.com

OBJECTIVE	Entry-level position in health information management in which I can apply up-to-date knowledge and skills. I especially enjoy applying my organizational skills and working on challenging tasks that must be complete and accurate.
EDUCATION	Associate of Science in Health Information Technology 2009 Desert Medical College Yuma, AZ

COMPUTER SKILLS
- Created electronic spreadsheet to track fund raising for Sage Elementary School PTA
- Taught self to efficiently use leading brand software programs in the following areas: word processing, database, spreadsheets, and accounting
- Set up and managed electronic accounting system for family-owned construction business
- Teach computer classes at Girl Scout summer day camp

ORGANIZATIONAL SKILLS
- Created system to monitor all church collections and fund-raising projects
- Initiated and developed computer career awareness program for Girl Scouts
- Secretary for college HIT student organization
- Completed HIT associate degree program with perfect class attendance while working part-time and managing family life

CLERICAL/ADMINISTRATIVE SKILLS
- 7 years bookkeeping experience
- Keyboarding speed of 78 wpm
- Excellent written communication skills

WORK HISTORY

Unpaid Internship at St. John's Medical Center, Yuma, AZ   2009
Medical Records Department

Bookkeeper   2003-2007
Buildwell Construction Company, Yuma, AZ

Bookkeeper   1998-2003
Perfect-Fit Cabinetry, Yuma, AZ

Secretary   1995-1998
Caldwell Insurance Company, Yuma, AZ

ORGANIZATIONS

Desert Medical College Health Information Technology Student Organization, Secretary
Sage Elementary School PTA, Treasurer
Faith Community Church, Member of Social Service Committee

FIGURE 3-15 Example of a Functional Resume. This type of resume, which lists skills that support a health care job, is recommended for applicants who have not worked in health care.

1234 Graduate Lane
Collegeville, CA 90123
June 6, 2010

Samantha Ernest, Office Manager
Good Health Clinic
922 Wellness Avenue
Cassidy, CA 91222

Dear Ms. Ernest:

I was excited to see your ad in the Cassidy Times on June 5 for a medical assistant. As a recent graduate of Medical Career College, I believe I can make a positive contribution to your health care team. In addition to submitting my resume for your review, I would like to point out how I believe I meet your needs for this position.

Your requirements:	How I Meet Them:
75% clerical duties	I enjoy and am proficient in front office duties. I received top grades in all my administrative classes. I understand the importance of efficiency, accuracy, and confidentiality when performing clerical functions in the medical office. I have very good written and oral communication skills.
25% clinical duties	I have up-to-date skills in all medical assisting back-office procedures.
Computer literate	I have basic computer literacy skills, can work in a Windows environment, and am proficient in Medical Manager, Word, and Excel.

I am an energetic, detail-oriented person with good interpersonal skills. I understand the need to maintain high-quality patient relations in today's health care environment and know I am capable of providing efficient, caring service.

Good Health Clinic has an excellent reputation in Cassidy and it would be a privilege to have the opportunity to discuss my qualifications with you in person. I will call next week to schedule an appointment or you can contact me at (760)123-4567. Thank you for your time and consideration.

Respectfully,

Gwen Graduate

Gwen Graduate

FIGURE 3-16 Example of a Combination Resume. This type of resume is recommended for applicants who have some experience working in health care but who also want to highlight other skills that support their target job.

E-Resumes

You will need to modify your resume if you are sending it to an employer electronically, if it will be scanned, or if you are posting it on an Internet site. This is to ensure that it transmits and scans properly. You will note that some changes require you to do exactly the opposite of the directions given in the previous sections to create an attractive printed resume! You will simply have an additional version.

For a resume to copy and paste into online forms or to post in online resume databases, start by converting your resume to what is called "plain text." If you created your resume using MS Word (on either a PC or a Mac), use the "Save As" command and choose the plain text format (the ending will be .txt). This format strips your document of all special formatting—things like bullets, bolding, and italics. The instructions embedded to create these "special effects" do not translate well electronically, and your resume can become scrambled or interspersed with odd-looking characters.

Once you have created a plain-text version, do the following (Susanireland.com):

1. Proof it for oddly wrapped lines, scrunched up words, and similar problems that can happen when text is converted.
2. Delete "continued" or "page 2" if these exist.
3. Use caps to emphasize words that otherwise would have been bolded or italicized—your name, for example.
4. Replace bullets with standard keyboard symbols such as * + − ~ (These may have converted to little boxes or other odd characters.)
5. If you need to add spaces, use the space bar, not the Tab key.
6. If you use quotation marks anywhere, these only convert if they are straight, not curly (also called smart). Check your word processing program to see how to do this.

Just as with the original version of your resume, it is critical that this version be free from errors. Once sent or posted online, it is there for potentially millions of people to view.

Posting Your Resume on the Internet

There are many types of websites on which you can post your resume. Some are general employment sites, such as www.monster.com. Others are specific to health care, and still others are employer websites that allow—or even require—you to apply electronically for specific job openings. Deciding whether to place your resume on the Internet and which type of website to choose depends on your job target and the kind of employer you are seeking. While many websites allow job searchers to post their resumes for free, they charge employers to place "Help Wanted" ads online and to view the resumes in their databases. Therefore, larger organizations are the ones most likely to pay for this service. A physician's office or small clinic may not be able to justify the expense for its relatively small number of hires. Organizations with many employees, such as Kaiser Permanente or even a single hospital, may have their own websites and online application capabilities.

Spend some time considering whether to post your resume on the Internet. Although posting on a large website makes your resume available to millions of viewers, you are also competing with millions of other job seekers. Experts suggest that posting your resume on a few carefully chosen sites is worth some of your time but is not as likely to help you find a job as methods such as networking and applying to specific employers.

In general, experts recommend that you should not pay to have your resume distributed. Many of these "services" simply send out mass emails containing the resumes of everyone who pays them. The resumes may or may not match the jobs posted (if indeed, the targeted employers even have job openings) and it is reported that resumes are often sent without contact information, such as your name and telephone numbers, so employers cannot reach you even if they are interested in learning more about you.

The following suggestions can help you choose an appropriate website (Dickel, 2004):

* Do not use websites that won't allow you to review at least a sample of their job lists before you provide personal information or your resume.
* Read the privacy policy! Some websites sell or give your information to other businesses. NEVER put your social security number on your resume.
* Check the wording. Do the lists provided include real jobs or are they examples of what the website claims to be trying to fill?
* Check for currency. Are there dates on the jobs listed? Are they recent?
* Look for information about who sponsors the site. Do they have credentials and/or experience in the job search industry?
* If you do not get any responses to your resume within 45 days, remove it.

As a courtesy to those who are looking for applicants, remove your posted resume once you become employed. Also, your new employer may see your resume online and wonder if you are still looking for a better deal.

Introducing Your Resume: Cover Letters

Always send a cover letter with your resume, whether it goes by conventional mail or electronically. The purpose of a cover letter is to provide a brief personal introduction. It should be short, informative, persuasive, and polite. The fact that you write a letter can be persuasive in itself. It shows that you took the time and made the effort to consider why and how you meet this particular employer's qualifications.

Cover letters can be customized for different circumstances. Before discussing the different types, let's look at a few how-tos common to all cover letters:

1. Use a proper business letter format.
2. Be sure your spelling and grammar are error-free.
3. Direct your letter to a specific person whenever possible. Look for a name in the employment ad, ask your contact for the name of the appropriate person, or call the facility and ask. If you are writing in response to an unadvertised position, having a name on your correspondence is especially important. Letters without names can get misdirected or discarded. Busy facilities don't have time to determine to whom to direct your inquiry.
4. Write an introduction. State who you are, why you are writing, who referred you or what ad you are responding to, and what position you are applying for. Employers may have more than one position open so don't assume they will know which job you are applying for.
5. Develop the body of the letter. Explain why the employer should interview you; that is, what you have to offer and how you can help him or her.

Summarize your qualifications for the job. Do your best to match them with what you believe the employer is seeking. At the same time, don't simply repeat the same information that is on your resume.
6. Include a closing paragraph. Ask the employer to call you for an interview or state that you will call for an appointment.
7. If you are sending your cover letter electronically (in the body of an email, for example), keep the format simple: don't use bolding, bullets, or other special features and avoid using tabs to indent text.

Letter for an Advertised Position

When you respond to employment ads, show how you meet the employer's needs. Use language in your letter that mirrors the words used in the ad or job announcement (Figures 3-17 and 3-18).

⭐ EXPERIENTIAL EXERCISES

1. Locate a posting for a job of interest.
2. Write a cover letter that responds to the stated requirements and preferences of the employer.

Letter for an Unadvertised Opening

You may learn about unadvertised job openings through your school or from your networking contacts. Before writing the letter, learn as much as possible about the job. Sources of information include the person who told you about it, the employer's website, or an inquiry call to the facility. Mention your source of information in the introduction of your cover letter. (Be sure to obtain permission from the contact person before using his or her name!)

Letter of Inquiry

There may be a facility where you would like to work, but you don't know if it has any job openings. Perhaps you have a friend who is happily employed there and has recommended it as a great place to work. Or it may have a reputation for excellent working conditions and educational and promotional opportunities. When you are not responding to a specific job opening, state your general qualifications that meet the current needs in health care. Explain why you are interested in working at the facility. Learn as much as possible about the facility so you can be specific about why you

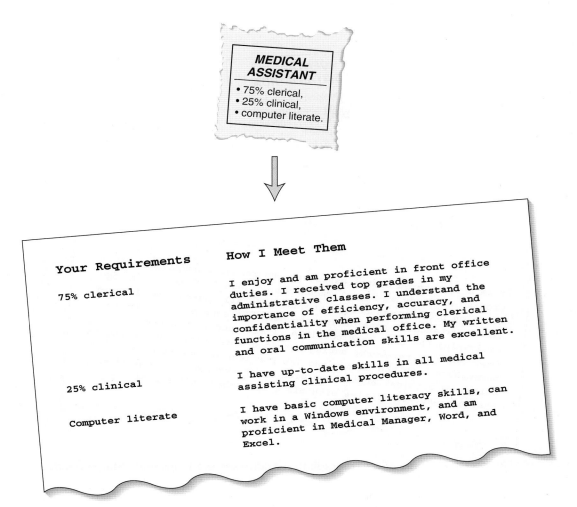

FIGURE 3-17 Example of a Direct, Point-By-Point Response to a Job Posting.

want to work there and what you have to offer. See Figure 3-19 for a sample letter of inquiry.

 WHAT IF?

You want to write cover letters but feel unsure about your grammar and spelling.

Applications

LEARNING OBJECTIVE 20: APPLICATIONS

- Explain the purpose of job applications.
- List ways to ensure that you fill out applications properly.

Most employers require applicants to fill out job applications, even if the individual has submitted a resume. Applications provide the employer with complete, standardized sources of information. Once you are hired, the application is placed in your personnel file and can serve as a legal document and record of information about you and your previous employment.

Some applications contain important statements you are required to read and sign. For example, employers of home health care workers may protect themselves from liability (i.e., responsibility) if employees have an accident when they are driving to and from job assignments. Read all statements carefully before signing. Applications and employment contracts may contain legal language and unfamiliar words. Don't hesitate to ask for an explanation of anything you don't understand.

After the work of constructing a resume, filling out an application may seem easy. But don't take it for granted. Take time to read the instructions and fill it out as accurately and neatly as possible. This is

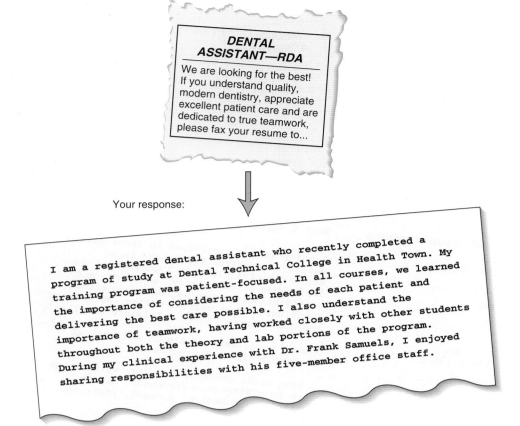

DENTAL ASSISTANT—RDA

We are looking for the best! If you understand quality, modern dentistry, appreciate excellent patient care and are dedicated to true teamwork, please fax your resume to...

Your response:

I am a registered dental assistant who recently completed a program of study at Dental Technical College in Health Town. My training program was patient-focused. In all courses, we learned the importance of considering the needs of each patient and delivering the best care possible. I also understand the importance of teamwork, having worked closely with other students throughout both the theory and lab portions of the program. During my clinical experience with Dr. Frank Samuels, I enjoyed sharing responsibilities with his five-member office staff.

FIGURE 3-18 Example of a Paragraph that Addresses the Employer's Stated Needs.

especially important when applying for health care positions because neatness and accuracy are job requirements. Use this opportunity to demonstrate that you meet these requirements.

Success Tips for Filling Out Job Applications

* Read the entire application before you begin to fill it in.
* Fill out all sections completely. Do not leave blanks or write in "See resume."
* Use black or blue pen, never pencil.
* Print neatly.
* Go to interviews prepared to fill out an application. Take complete information with you, including the following:
  * Social Security number
  * Education, including dates and locations
  * Work history, including names of employers and dates of employment
  * Military service
  * References

* Proofread what you have written before submitting it.
* Be honest when answering questions. Giving false information can be grounds for dismissal if you are hired.
* For questions that don't apply to you, write "N/A" instead of leaving them blank. This way it is clear that you saw the question and didn't accidentally skip over it.
* Many entry-level jobs have a set salary. If the one you are applying for does not, it is best to write "negotiable" in the space asking for your salary requirement.
* Be sure to sign and date the application.

Electronic Applications

Many employers now have application forms on their websites. When applying electronically, it is especially important to follow the directions and check your entries carefully before pushing the "send" button. Once you send the application, it is difficult to change incorrect information. In some cases, the online

10752 Learning Lane
Silver Stream, NY 10559
July 22, 2010

Ms. Sandra Walters, Manager
Caring Clinic
7992 Oates Road
Greenville, NY 10772

Dear Ms. Walters:

I am writing to inquire about job openings at Caring Clinic. My husband and I are relocating to Greenville in September and I am looking for a position in which I can apply my up-to-date skills as a phlebotomy technician. Caring Clinic has a reputation for excellent service to the health needs of the Greenville community and I would be proud to be a contributing member of your team.

As a recent graduate of Top Skill Institute, I had the opportunity to perform my internship at Goodwell Laboratory Services, an affiliate of Caring Clinic. I understand the importance of combining technical excellence with attention to customer service. While at Goodwell, my technical skills were highly praised by my supervisor, Mr. Jaime Gutierrez. In addition, I consistently received top ratings on patient satisfaction surveys.

My resume is enclosed for your review. I will call you in early September to see if I can set an appointment to meet with you. Thank you for your consideration.

Respectfully,

Carla Martinez
Carla Martinez

FIGURE 3-19 Example of a Cover Letter Used to Inquire About Possible Job Openings.

application takes the place of sending a resume. As with traditional written materials, what you submit is a reflection of you as a professional. In fact, some employers use electronic applications to test the computer skills of potential employees.

Keep a record of the electronic applications you send: your password (if any), and the specific information you have sent (for example, some applications ask for your salary requirements). Print your completed application and place it in your job search binder or files.

References

LEARNING OBJECTIVE 21: REFERENCES

- Give examples of credible references.
- List the characteristics of good references.

- List examples of people who might be good references.
- List the information that should be included on reference sheet.

Recall that references are people who will vouch for your qualifications and character. Good references can be a key factor in tipping the hiring scales in your favor. Give careful consideration about who you ask to be references. They must be considered credible (i.e., believable). Friends and relatives are not generally accepted as good work references, but they may be acceptable if you are asked to provide character references.

In addition to being credible, references must:
* Have the time and be willing to speak on your behalf to potential employers,
* Be able to speak positively about you, and
* Have the ability to speak clearly and in an organized way.

The following people are good candidates to be work references:
* Instructors
* Other school personnel
* Externship supervisor(s)
* Previous employers
* Supervisors at places where you've done volunteer work
* Professionals who you've worked with on committees or projects

Contact each person you want to serve as a reference. Do this before you begin your job search. Never give out a name and then ask the person for permission afterward. This can put the person on the spot and makes it difficult if he or she prefers not to be a reference. Inform your references about the types of jobs you are applying for and what qualifications are important. This will enable them to be prepared to answer the potential employer's questions.

Reference Sheet

Create a written list of at least three references. At a minimum, include their names, titles, telephone numbers, and email addresses. You may also want to include their addresses. Ask them if they can be contacted at work. If not, provide recommended times to call. It is essential that the telephone numbers be current and accurate. If you list a work number and the person is no longer employed there, your credibility may be questioned. Potential employers may not have time to call you back or make numerous calls

trying to locate your references. Make it easy for them. This makes it easier for them to hire you.

Organize your reference list in an easy-to-read format and print it on the same kind of paper as your resume. Write "References for (your name)" at the top of the page. The reference sheet should not be mailed with your resume unless it is specifically requested. Take copies with you to interviews to give to potential employers who ask for it. If you are visiting a Human Resources department, take a copy with you because many employment applications have a section for listing references.

Let your references know when you are hired. Thank them for their willingness to assist you. Keep them posted of your career progress. In the future, you may be in a position to help them, and that is what true networking is all about—mutual career support.

⭐ **EXPERIENTIAL EXERCISES**

1. Contact possible references.
2. Once you have their consent, gather the data you need about each person.
3. Prepare your reference sheet.

Letters of Recommendation

LEARNING OBJECTIVE 22: LETTERS OF RECOMMENDATION

- Explain who should write your letters of recommendation.
- Describe the proper etiquette when asking for letters of recommendation.

Another type of reference is provided through letters of recommendation. These letters are usually written by supervisors or people in authority, such as instructors, who write statements about your work record, skills, and personal qualities. It is a good idea to request reference letters from employers throughout your career because they can serve as a record of endorsements and achievements over the years. As you leave each job (on good terms, it is hoped!), ask for a letter of recommendation from your supervisor.

Make copies of your letters of recommendation to place in your portfolio and/or to give to potential employers who request them. It is appropriate at interviews to mention that you have them available.

As with other references, be considerate. Ask only those people who you believe can write a positive letter. Also, try to give people enough time to compose a letter. Avoid giving one day's notice. Finally, let your references know what kind of job you are seeking so they can phrase their letters appropriately.

The Portfolio: Supporting What You Say

LEARNING OBJECTIVE 23: THE PORTFOLIO: SUPPORTING WHAT YOU SAY

- Describe how the items in your portfolio should be organized.
- Describe the appropriate appearance of a portfolio.

Look over the items you have been collecting to put in your portfolio. Choose the ones that represent your best work and support the qualifications needed for your target jobs. Think about others you can include. For example, you might add a list of the courses you have taken if your educational program, including classes not commonly offered in your program of study.

Organize your materials in a logical order, grouping related items together in sections. Place them in a binder or presentation folder using plastic protection sheets. It is not necessary to go to a lot of expense, but the folder should be well made and in a plain, conservative color. Prepare a title page labeled "Professional Portfolio" and include your name, address, telephone number(s), and email address. If you have a large number of items, number the pages and prepare a table of contents.

You need to make only one portfolio if it is rather large; if it consists of only a few pages, make copies in case a potential employer asks you to leave it after the interview. Portfolios are not generally sent with your resume but are taken to interviews. You may mention to the interviewer that you have a portfolio. Don't simply hand it to the employer and expect him or her to read it. It is to be used during the interview to demonstrate your capabilities. For example, if you are asked about your knowledge of coding, you could show assignments in which you accurately coded a variety of diagnoses and procedures. The chapter on interviewing has a section on using your portfolio.

 EXPERIENTIAL EXERCISE

Put together your professional portfolio.

CASE STUDY 3-6

Cameron was getting increasingly nervous. He had almost completed his pharmacy technician program and was getting prepared for his externship. As he told his friend, Juan, "School has been okay, but going out after a job—I don't know. It's getting pretty nerve wracking."

Juan tried to reassure him. "You did okay in school. And you liked your classes, right?"

"Yeah," Cameron said. "Pharmacy is pretty interesting. But after working all those years in masonry, I feel like a fish out of water going in and asking for a job. And now I have to put together a resume for my job search class. I've been putting that off, too. What am I going to say that any employer would want? That I built walls and stuff for 20 years?"

"That does sound like a challenge. I guess I'm lucky I chose something less physical and can stay where I am," said Juan.

"The thing is, I really like masonry. Felt real creative sometimes, and I liked the physical part of it—kept me in shape!" explained Cameron.

"I understand. Too bad your back went out. That was a bummer," sympathized Juan.

"Well, I guess I'd better get myself together. I've got a job search class tomorrow, and the homework doesn't get done on its own," said Cameron.

The next day in class, the instructor, Mr. Harmond, asked the students how they were doing on their resumes. "Don't forget," he reminded them. "These are due next week so Ms. Garcia and I can look them over and give you comments."

Cameron spent the next few days worrying about this assignment. He just didn't know how he was going to fill a page when all he had done was graduate from high school, work for 20 years for Cedar Glen Tile and Masonry, and finish a pharmacy technician program. Not much to show for a guy 40 years old, he thought.

He finally sat down on Sunday night and put something together. It wasn't much, but he knew he had to have something to turn in on Monday. After class on Tuesday, Mr. Harmond asked Cameron to wait so they could talk.

"Cameron," said Mr. Harmond, "I reviewed your resume last night and was surprised by how little thought you put into it."

"Actually," Cameron replied, "I've put *days* of thought into that thing. Thought and worry. I just couldn't come up with anything."

"That really surprises me," said Mr. Harmond. "My impression is that you have a lot to offer an employer. You're dependable, never late for class, articulate, always ready to help a classmate. And I understand you have years of experience in masonry—worked for the same employer where you moved up into a supervisory position."

"Well," said Cameron. "I don't really understand what all that has to do with applying for a job as a pharmacy tech."

"It has everything to do with it." Mr. Harmond went on to explain how employers were looking for employees with more than just technical skills. "Think about it," he said to Cameron. "You didn't move up with Cedar Glen just because you had good technical skills. You also had good people skills, were dependable, and had a good attitude. These are all valuable. They're the transferable skills we talked about in class."

"I guess I missed the point," admitted Cameron.

"Well, let's do this," suggested Mr. Cameron. "Come by my office tomorrow after class and I'll help you come up with transferable skills you can put on your resume. Maybe we'll put together some categories that will supplement your job history section. We can also mention your achievements at Cedar Glen. It may have been a completely different field, but they show motivation and a good work ethic—all employers want to see those in their employees."

"I'll be there," said Cameron. "Thanks a lot, Mr. Harmond. I really appreciate the extra help."

QUESTIONS FOR THOUGHT AND CONSIDERATION

1. Why is it sometimes difficult for students to realize what they have to offer employers?
2. Why was it especially hard for Cameron to see what he could bring to a job as a pharmacy technician?
3. What other skills and characteristics might he have to offer other than those mentioned?
4. Do you think Cameron, along with Mr. Harmond's help, will be able to build a strong resume?

Down a Dark Road

Steve Bailey is another student in Mr. Harmond's class. He also came to pharmacy tech from another occupation—he was a dry waller. Like Cameron, he just couldn't continue with the physical aspects of the job. Unlike Cameron, he had never really liked his previous work. It was just something fairly easy he could get into after high school when a family friend offered him a job.

Steve didn't like the idea of a career where he would have to sit all day or be cooped up in an office, but pharmacy tech seemed okay. He could stand, walk around, be in an area that wasn't too closed in. He struggled with some with his courses, especially those that involved math, but got tutoring, passed his classes, and is now near graduation.

Again like Cameron, he is struggling with his resume. His spelling and grammar have never been very good and although he can use computers for data entry and work related to pharmacy tech, his word processing skills are weak. He doesn't understand why the career services department can't just take his information and put it together into a nice resume.

"After all," he tells his friend James, "they're the experts. Why should I be tearing what little hair I have left trying to figure out how to do this?"

"Didn't they give you any help in class?" asks James.

"Some, I guess," replied Steve. "But it seemed complicated. There's this kind of resume and that kind. How am I supposed to figure out which one to use? I'm working part-time. I don't have time to go to class, read the textbook, and do more research on top of that. I think it's unreasonable."

Steve decided he just wouldn't turn anything in on Monday. He'd passed the technical courses in his program and surely they're weren't going to do much about his not having a resume put together on time. At the class break on Tuesday morning, Mr. Harmond approached him.

"Steve, I noticed that you didn't turn in a draft of your resume," he said.

"You're right. I just didn't have time—and it's just not something I'm good at. I really think you people in career services should help me out. I'll give you the information about me—lots of it you already have from my school application—and you put it together. You must have some special software on the computers you have in your office."

Mr. Harmond paused. "Steve, that's not how we do it here. We give you the tools and guide you through the process, but we want our students to create their own resumes. It's like a portrait of *you*, not just a general picture."

"Great," muttered Steve. "I don't know. Maybe I'll find something online that I can get a friend to help me fill in."

QUESTIONS FOR THOUGHT AND CONSIDERATION

1. What is your opinion of Steve's attitude?
2. Why do you think Steve is so resistant about working on his resume?
3. How do you think his attitude will affect his prospects of getting a job?
4. Do you agree with Mr. Harmond that students should create their own resumes?

The Art of Interviewing

The Interview: Your Sales Opportunity

You don't have to be perfect. Just be the best for the job.

Rick Baird

LEARNING OBJECTIVE 24: THE INTERVIEW: YOUR SALES OPPORTUNITY

- Explain a positive way to approach interviewing for jobs.
- Understand the importance of preparing for job interviews.
- List sources of information about health care employers.
- Explain the importance of empathy when talking with interviewers.

Finally! The words you have been hoping to hear: "Let's set up a time for an interview." Your job search efforts are paying off. But wait a minute! You begin to worry: "What if I can't think of anything to say?" "What if I don't have the skills they are looking for?" "What if they ask me about ... ?"

The purpose of this chapter is to help you put the "what ifs" to rest and see the interviewing process as an opportunity to present yourself at your best. Many applicants view interviews as opportunities to be rejected. But you have another choice. You can view an interview as an opportunity to determine an employer's needs and show how you can meet them.

Employers are busy people who don't have time to conduct interviews with people who are unlikely job candidates. You obviously meet the minimum qualifications. The interviewer wants to see whether you are a person who can back up your qualifications, communicate well, and contribute to the organization.

By learning what will be expected of you at an interview and practicing your presentation skills, you can attend each interview with confidence. A common reason for not being hired is lack of preparation for the interview. And this is a factor over which you, not the interviewer, has control.

The Customer's Needs

Good sales presentations are based on showing customers—employers—how they can benefit by buying a product—in this case, by hiring you. You put yourself at a disadvantage if you attend an interview without knowing anything about what the employer needs. To interview successfully, complete the following in advance:

* Identify possible needs of the employer.
* Think of ways you might meet those needs as an employee.
* Anticipate what types of questions might be asked.
* Practice answering them.
* Create examples to demonstrate your qualifications.
* Prepare appropriate questions to ask.

All employers have general qualities they look for in applicants. Health care employers have expressed their needs through the National Healthcare Foundation Standards. Individual employers have specific requirements based on factors such as patient population, services offered, size of facility, budgets, and so on. Learn as much as possible before attending the interview. Here is a list of information sources:

* Direct contact by phone or in person: ask questions, request a job description, observe the facility
* Brochures produced by the organization
* People who work there, such as friends, classmates, or networking contacts
* The local newspaper: large facilities are sometimes the subject of news articles
* The employer's website
* Your school's career services department
* The local chamber of commerce and other organizations that have information about large employers
* The local chapter of your professional organization
* Information gathered at career fairs and employer orientation meetings
* Employment ad if the position was advertised

If the facility is small, such as a one-physician office, you should know, at a minimum, the type of specialty practiced and the patient population served. When you are unable to learn very much before the interview, it is especially important that you listen carefully to the employer and ask good questions. How to do this is discussed later in this chapter.

FIGURE 3-20 Understanding the needs and concerns of the interviewer helps an applicant navigate the interview process (Copyright © istock.com).

process. In reality, interviewers may be experiencing a number of pressures:

* Concern about finding the right candidate who can perform the job as needed
* An extremely busy schedule
* Lack of interviewing skills
* A demanding supervisor who will hold him or her responsible for the performance of the person who is hired
* Concern about finding the time and resources to orient and train a new employee

Understanding the interviewer's point of view requires empathy—attempting to see the world through the eyes of others (Figure 3-20). This may not seem easy in a job interview when you are nervous and concentrating on presenting yourself well. But it is this very shift of focus—from yourself to the interviewer—that leads to a more successful interviewing experience.

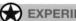 **EXPERIENTIAL EXERCISES**

1. Select a facilty where you might want to work.
2. Learn as much as possible about the facility: type of work they do, patient or client population, size of the staff, jobs for which you might qualify, mission of the organization.

The Interviewer Is Human, Too

Research into interviewing shows that the person conducting the interview is often more stressed than the candidate.

Allan-James Associates

Consider the personal situation of the interviewer. Many applicants view the interviewer as a person of great confidence who has all the power in the hiring

Knowing What to Expect

LEARNING OBJECTIVE 25: KNOWING WHAT TO EXPECT

■ Describe the different types of interviewing styles.
■ Describe the various types of interview questions, including traditional, behavioral, and situational. Give an example of each.
■ Understand how to use the STAR approach when answering behavioral questions.
■ Explain how to best answer questions in a personality test.
■ Describe the guidelines for answering computerized job interview questions.

Some interviews are highly structured, meaning that each candidate is asked the same set of prepared questions. Others are more like a conversation, with topics and questions generated freely. Most interviews fall somewhere between these patterns, with interviewers preparing at least a few questions in advance. The style of the interview and types of questions most likely depend on the size of the organization. Large health care systems, hospitals, and clinics usually have dedicated personnel to conduct initial interviews. As human resource professionals, they have the time and expertise to study the latest hiring practices and develop their interviewing skills. A physician who has a single practice is more likely to focus on what skills you have acquired through your education and experience—the specific skills he needs, for example, in a clinical medical assistant or receptionist.

Traditional Interview Questions

There are many "golden oldie" questions that interviewers have been using for years. Here are a few examples:

1. How would you describe yourself?
2. What are your long-range career objectives?
3. Why did you choose this career?
4. What makes you qualified for this position?
5. How well do you work with people?
6. What motivates you to go the extra mile on a job?
7. How do you define success?
8. Why should I hire you?

You can see that these questions are very open-ended. You can answer them in many ways, and this can present a problem if your answers are too vague or not related to the job under consideration. Employers want to know how your answer applies to *them*. For example, in explaining why you chose a career in health care, focus on what it is about you that relates to the job for which you are applying. Be specific. Saying, "I've always been a people person" doesn't give much information. Saying, "I've been interested in health care since I was 11 when I spent time playing chess with my grandfather after he had a stroke. I noticed how he really perked up when he played, and I became fascinated by how the brain works better when stimulated with an enjoyable activity. This led me to exploring a career in occupational therapy" is more specific and gives the interviewer more insight into who you are. When answering, "Why should I hire you?," mention specific skills and personal and professional qualities that will make a positive con-

tribution to the physician's practice, department's success, patient satisfaction, and so on.

 EXPERIENTIAL EXERCISES

1. Review your skills and qualities.
2. Create examples from your experience that demonstrate these.
3. Practice answering traditional interview questions using your examples.

Behavioral Interview Questions

Behavioral interviews have been part of the hiring process in many large organizations since the 1970s and are being increasingly used in the health care industry. In this type of interview, applicants are asked questions about their past performance: how they handled specific situations. Behavioral interviews are based on the premise that past performance is a good indicator of future performance.

Interviewers prepare in advance by listing the key qualifications for the jobs they post. Then they develop questions to help determine whether applicants possess the desired characteristics. Suppose that getting along with others is very important. A question might be "Describe a time when you had to work with someone who you felt was difficult to get along with." As you tell your story, the interviewer follows up with additional questions, such as "In what ways was this person difficult?" "What was it you needed to do together?" "What did you say to this person?" "Did you get the job done in spite of the difficulties?" "How did you feel about this situation?" "What did you learn from this?" There may be additional probing questions from the interviewer to get more detail as you tell your story and verify that this is an experience you really had. In the case of the difficult person, these might be "How did these difficulties affects others, such as co-workers and customers?" "Did your supervisor become involved?" Table 3-1 contains examples of behavioral interview questions.

This kind of questioning about real events can be more difficult for applicants to answer because they must be supported by facts. For this reason, behavioral interviewing has been found to be 55% predictive of future behavior on the job compared to traditional interviewing, which is 10% predictive (Hansen, 2009).

Preparing to answer behavioral questions usually takes more preparation than for traditional questions.

TABLE 3-1
Behavioral Interview Questions

Qualifications	Sample Questions
Interpersonal skills	Tell me about a time when someone disagreed with you about a major decision. What did you say or do? How was the decision ultimately made? Describe a situation in which you were able to use persuasion to successfully convince someone to consider your ideas.
Flexibility	Describe a situation in which you were required to conform to a work policy you really didn't agree with. What was the policy? Why didn't you agree? How did you feel about the situation? Give me an example of a job in which your working conditions frequently changed. How did you adapt to these changes? Tell me about a time when you had to reorganize your schedule in order to help a co-worker meet a deadline. How did you help? What was the result?
Communication	Give me a specific example that shows how you typically deal with conflict. Describe a time when you had to communicate something difficult to your supervisor. What was the situation? How did you plan your communication? What did you say? What was the result? Describe a situation in which you felt you didn't communicate well. How did you follow up? What did you learn?
Customer service skills	Tell me about a time when you had to deal with a very upset customer/patient? How did you handle the situation? What was the result? Give me a few examples of what you have said to customers/patients who have approached you for help. How did you decide the appropriate way to work with each one? Describe something you did to help another employer improve their customer service.
Stress management	Describe a stressful situation in which you applied your coping skills. What specifically caused the stress? How were you feeling at the time? What techniques did you use? How was the situation resolved?
Problem solving	Describe a time when you anticipated a potential problem(s) and developed preventive measures. How did you identify the problem? What were the signs? How did you determine ways to prevent it? How did others feel about your actions? What was the final result? Describe a time when you were asked or assigned to do a task you didn't feel qualified to handle. What did you do?
Integrity	Describe an incident in which you made a serious mistake. How did you handle this with your supervisor and/or co-workers? Tell me about a time when you had to make an unpopular decision. What were the circumstances? Why were others unhappy with the decision? Why did you believe you were making the right decision?

You are already preparing yourself if you have been collecting examples of your skills and qualifications. The key is to anticipate the kinds of qualifications an employer wants and then search your inventory—and memory—for experiences you've had that illustrate that qualification. Examples can come from any area of your life. You may never have worked in health care. In fact, you may have limited work experience of any kind. But perhaps you have raised children. That experience may help you answer questions about making unpopular decisions. These were likely based on good judgment, your values, even ethics and morality. In addition to family life, there are other experiences you can draw from:

* Externship
* Previous work

* School: classes, labs, extra activities
* Community and service work

In a behavioral interview, it is essential to *listen carefully.* Not only must you understand the question, but you need to understand *what it is the interviewer wants to know.* That is, what qualification is obviously important for this job, and how can you demonstrate that you have that qualification? Don't hesitate to ask for clarification if you don't understand the question.

It is totally acceptable to take a few moments to think about an answer. If the question asks about an experience you've never had—for example, "Tell me about a time when you had to fire a friend"—admit that this has never happened to you; don't try to make up a story. Some questions may even ask you to describe failures and how you've handled them, so you might think of some examples. Reflect on what you learned from experiences that didn't turn out as you hoped they would.

Many job search experts recommend using the **STAR** approach when answering a behaviorial question. It helps you organize your response and goes like this:

1. **S** and **T:** Choose and describe a **S**ituation or **T**ask that enables you to best demonstrate that you have the desired qualifications.
2. **A:** Explain the **A**ctions you took in dealing with the situation. Give enough details to show your skills, but take care not to ramble or give unnecessary information.
3. **R:** Describe the **R**esults. Explain what happened, what you learned, and how the results made a difference. Give numbers and percentages when possible.

Although it is advisable to have examples in mind and practice telling your "stories," take care not to try to memorize what to say. You need to think about what you are saying during the interview and not give a canned response that may not apply to the question.

Situational Questions

Situational questions present situations and problems you might encounter on the job. You are asked to explain how you would respond to and/or handle the problem. (See Box 3-19 for examples.) As with behavioral questions, you need to do some advance planning to be prepared to answer them:

* Learn as much as possible about the organization and the specific job. If possible, read the mission statement and goals of the organization.
* Recall your own values and mission statement. These may provide guidelines in anwering questions that don't have easy answers, but they can be based on your sense of right and wrong.
* Review your personal inventory of skills and qualifications.

EXPERIENTIAL EXERCISES

1. Review your skills and qualities.
2. Create examples from your experience that demonstrate these.
3. Practice answering behavioral interview questions using your examples.

EXPERIENTIAL EXERCISES

1. Review your skills and qualities.
2. Create examples from your experience that demonstrate these.
3. Practice answering situational interview questions using your examples.

Occupation-Specific Questions

Questions in this category explore your specific knowledge, skill mastery, willingness to learn new procedures, and the general content of your training. The type of question will vary:

* Describe how to perform a specific procedure.
* Explain how to operate certain equipment.
* Describe appropriate action to take in a given situation that directly relates to this job.
* Suggest how to solve a health care problem.
* Explain how you plan to keep your skills updated.
* What do you know about ... ? (a theory, new procedure, etc.)
* Why do you want to work in pediatrics/ dermatology/children's dentistry, etc.?

Some employers give practical skill tests or ask you to physically demonstrate your knowledge. Examples of these tests include a keyboarding speed test, filing or record-keeping exercise, spelling test, calculation of drug dosages, or demonstration of a procedure. If you are asked to perform a practical test that is appropriate for your level of training, do so willingly. Use the request to show that you have confidence in your abilities and can handle stress. If the task is something you have not been trained to do but is required for the job, tell the interviewer you would welcome the opportunity to learn.

Work Preference Questions

You may be asked about your job preferences. Be prepared to answer questions such as:

* Whether you want full-time or part-time work
* The hours you are willing to work
* The length of shift you prefer
* The days and time of day you can work

Remember to be realistic when applying for jobs. Don't waste employers' time—or your own—interviewing for jobs with conditions you already know are absolutely impossible for you to meet.

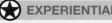 **EXPERIENTIAL EXERCISES**

1. Review your work preferences and needs.
2. Prepare to answer questions about your preferences and needs.

Personality Tests

You may be asked to take a personality test as part of the interviewing process. Personality assessment tests are increasingly being used, especially in larger organizations. As many as 30% of all companies now use personality tests (Cha, 2005). These tests involve answering a series of questions on paper or on the computer, and they measure qualities such as persistence and whether a person is an extrovert or introvert (highly social or more private). Studies claim that better matches are found when applicants take these tests. This is because certain jobs require specific characteristics and these are more reliably determined by tests than by interviews. Another claim is that the individuals hired tend to be happier with their jobs because of this matching process.

The best advice for taking a personality test is to answer the questions honestly. The tests contain a variety of questions to assess each trait. If you answer as you think you should or randomly select answers, this can show up negatively. If you do not "pass" such a test, it is very possible you would not have enjoyed either the work or the setting. This has been one of the reported benefits of personality assessments: less turnover among employees who, with traditional hiring methods, end up deciding the job just isn't for them.

Computerized Job Interviews

Some employers conduct interviews with the help of a computer. The advantage for the employer, in addition to saving time, is to prepare a set of questions, often up to 100, to ask of every applicant. Most interview programs consist of several answers from which the applicant must choose the correct one. This enables the employer to compare "apples with apples" when deciding whom to interview in person. The advantage for you is that you have more time to think about your answers and can, through the types of questions asked, learn a little about the organization before you have the face-to-face interview.

Answer the questions carefully and honestly. Computers report inconsistencies in your answers. Studies have shown that people are more likely to "tell" a computer information they would never tell a human being (Graber, 2000). If you are faced with a computerized interview, take care not to give unnecessary information that may harm your chance of getting hired. Also, be aware that most computer-assisted interviews must be completed in a certain length of time, so be sure you know how much time you have, and keep track of it as you move through the questions.

Another way computers are used in the hiring process involves presenting scenarios to applicants and asking them what they would do in that situation. Computers also administer skills tests, integrity tests, and personality tests. Some organizations administer computerized interviews and tests on their own computers at their facility; others make them available on the Internet and give applicants a password to gain access to testing websites.

Practice: Your Key to Success

Successful interviews usually depend on good preparation.

John D. Drake

LEARNING OBJECTIVE 26: PRACTICE: YOUR KEY TO SUCCESS

- List the skills a job applicant should be prepared to use at a job interview.
- Explain why it is important to practice interviewing skills.

Of course, you cannot anticipate the exact questions interviewers will ask. What you can do is prepare yourself to answer a variety of questions. Here are some actions you will use at an interview:

* Listening carefully
* Asking for clarification when necessary
* Thinking through your "inventory" of capabilities and characteristics that you can apply when answering questions
* Thinking of examples to back up your answers
* Projecting self-confidence

Preparation means practice—actually answering questions, aloud, under conditions as close to those of an actual interview as possible. The best way to practice is to role-play with someone who acts as the interviewer. This can be an instructor, classmate, mentor, networking contact, friend, or family member. Many schools require mock (pretend) interviews as part of professional development classes. Take advantage of these opportunities, and do your best to conduct yourself as if you were at a real interview. Videotaping or having an observer take notes can be helpful, even if it's a little nerve-wracking. It's better to make a few mistakes now so you can avoid them at interviews.

If you believe you might be asked to demonstrate skills or react to a scenario, include them in your practice sessions. The career services personnel at your school may be familiar with the interviewing practices of facilities in your area and can give you additional information about what to expect and how to best prepare.

The goal of "interview rehearsals" is not to memorize answers you can repeat. It is to develop a level of comfort about the interviewing process and have facts fresh in your mind so you can call on them as needed and respond to questions intelligently and confidently.

⭐ EXPERIENTIAL EXERCISES

1. Prepare a variety of interview questions.
2. Choose a partner who will read the questions for you to practice answering.

Be Prepared: What to Take Along

LEARNING OBJECTIVE 27: BE PREPARED: WHAT TO TAKE ALONG

- List the items the applicant should take to a job interview.
- Describe the best type of case or handbag for carrying these supplies.

Having everything you might need at the interview will help you feel organized and confident. It also demonstrates to employers that you are organized and think ahead—valuable qualities for health care professionals. Although your own list will be different, here are some suggestions for what to take along:

* Extra copies of your resume
* Your portfolio
* Copies of licenses, certifications, and other documentation
* Proof of immunizations and results of health tests
* Reference sheet
* Any documentation of skills and experience not included in your portfolio (or if you have chosen not to create a portfolio)
* Pens

* Small notepad
* Your list of questions (discussed later in this chapter)
* All information needed to fill out an application
* Appointment calendar/planner/electronic organizer/phone
* Anything you have been requested to bring
* For your eyes only: extra pantyhose, breath mints, other "emergency supplies"

A small case or large handbag is a convenient way to carry your papers and supplies. It can be inexpensive, but it should be a conservative color, in good repair, and neatly organized so you can quickly find what you need.

First Impressions: Make Them Count!

The way in which we think of ourselves has everything to do with how our world sees us.

Arlene Raven

LEARNING OBJECTIVE 28: FIRST IMPRESSIONS: MAKE THEM COUNT!

- Explain the importance of first impressions.
- Describe what a professional appearance communicates to an interviewer.
- List clothing that should not be worn to an interview.
- Give guidelines for appropriate dress and grooming for interviews.
- Explain steps to take to ensure you arrive to an interview on time.
- Describe appropriate posture and demeanor when meeting the interviewer.

Just 30 seconds! That's how long you have to make a lasting impression. The average person forms a strong opinion of another in less than 1 minute. This is why so much emphasis is placed on professional appearance both during the job search and on the job. While it is possible to eventually reverse a negative first impression, it's a lot easier to make a good one in the first place. At the interview, employers will be thinking, "If this is the best this person can do, what might I expect from him on the job?" Appropriate appearance tells the interviewer that you:

* Understand the impact of your appearance on others (patients, other professionals).
* Know what is appropriate for the job.

* Apply the principles of good hygiene.
* Respect both yourself and the interviewer.
* Take the interview seriously.

There is no universal agreement about the proper clothing to wear when applying for health care jobs. Some schools encourage their students to wear a clean, pressed uniform. Other schools advise them to wear neat, everyday clothing that is not too casual. It is important to pay attention to the professional advice of the staff at your school. The best choices for clothing are generally conservative colors and simple styles.

Appearance Do's and Don'ts

Never wear jeans or clothing that is revealing or intended for sports and outdoor activities. Don't wear a hat or sunglasses during the interview. If you're not sure about what to wear, ask your instructor or someone in your school's career service department for help. If money for buying interview clothes is a problem, ask if your school has a clothes-lending program. Many cities have excellent thrift shops that sell nice clothes at reasonable prices. Some even specialize in helping people dress for job interviews.

You may arrive at an interview and discover that most people at the facility are dressed very casually. Don't worry. It is better to be overdressed for a job interview than underdressed.

Here are some additional guidelines that apply to all health care job applicants:
* **Be squeaky clean.** Take a bath or shower, wash your hair, scrub your fingernails, and use a deodorant or antiperspirant.
* **Save the fashion trends for later.** Hair and nails should be natural colors, tattoos should be covered up, and visible rings and studs from piercings should be removed. Limit earrings to one set. Women should apply makeup lightly for a natural, not painted, look.
* **Show that you know what is acceptable for the health care professional.** Avoid long fingernails, free-flowing hair, and dangling accessories that can be grabbed by patients or caught in machinery. Wear closed-toe shoes. Strive to be odor-free. For example, don't smoke on the way to the interview. Even the fragrances in perfumes and other personal products, intended to be pleasant, should not be worn because many patients find them disagreeable or have allergic reactions.
* Men who wear facial hair should groom it neatly.

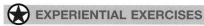

1. Select an appropriate outfit for interviewing, including shoes.
2. Make sure everything is clean and pressed.

Punctuality

Your appearance may be perfect, but if you arrive late for an interview, your appearance may not matter. Being late is a sure way to make a poor impression. Time management is an essential health care job skill, and you will have failed your first opportunity to demonstrate that you have mastered it. In addition, arriving late is a sign of rudeness and inconsideration for the interviewer's time. Make a few advance preparations to ensure that this doesn't happen to you:

* Write down the date and exact time of the appointment.
* Verify the address and ask for directions, if necessary.
* If the office is in a large building or complex, get additional instructions about how to find it.
* Inquire about parking, bus stops, or subway stops.
* If you are unsure of the location and it is not too far away, go there a couple of days before the interview to be sure you can find it.
* Allow extra time to arrive, and plan to be there about 10 minutes before the appointed time.

If there is an emergency that can't be avoided (a flat tire or unexpected snowstorm), call as soon as possible to offer an explanation and reschedule the interview.

First Contacts

Many job applicants don't realize that the interview actually starts before they sit down with the person asking the questions. From the first contact you made to inquire about a job opening or to schedule the appointment, you have been making an impression. If you arrive for the interview and are rude to the receptionist, you may have already failed in your bid for the job. You cannot know what information is shared with the hiring authority. Keep in mind, too, that these may be your future co-workers!

Learn the name of the person who will be conducting the interview. Be sure you have the correct spelling (for the thank-you letter, discussed later in this

BOX 3-20

Meeting the Interviewer

- Make and maintain eye contact.
- Give a healthy (not limp or hesitant) handshake.
- Express how glad you are to meet him or her and how much you appreciate the opportunity to be interviewed.
- Don't sit down until you are offered a chair or the other person is seated.

chapter) and pronunciation. See Box 3-20 for actions to express courtesy and self-confidence when meeting the interviewer.

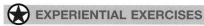

1. Practice your smile and posture in front of a mirror.
2. With a partner, practice your handshake.
3. Rehearse meeting an interviewer until you feel comfortable with these actions: approach, smile, handshake, sitting down, maintaining good posture.

Courtesy During the Interview

LEARNING OBJECTIVE 29: COURTESY DURING THE INTERVIEW

- List behaviors that should be avoided at interviews.
- Explain why it is important to act professionally.

Maintaining eye contact (without staring) while the other person is speaking indicates that you are interested in what he or she is saying. When you are speaking, it is natural to look away occasionally. Most of the time, however, you should look at the listener. This is a sign of openness and sincerity. The following is a summary of behaviors to definitely avoid (even if the interviewer engages in them):

* Interrupting
* Cursing
* Using poor grammar (such as the word "ain't") or slang

* Gossiping, such as commenting on the weaknesses of other facilities, professionals, or your previous employer
* Telling off-color jokes
* Putting yourself down
* Chewing gum
* Appearing to snoop by looking at papers or other materials on the interviewer's desk, shelves, and so forth
* Discussing personal problems

You don't want to come across as stiff or stuffy, but you do want to come across as professional. Try to be at ease and act natural, while maintaining your best "company manners."

Apply Your Communication Skills

- Explain the meaning and importance of active listening.
- Explain the role of active listening in the job interview.
- Define mirroring and explain its purpose in the job interview.
- Explain the purpose of feedback.
- Describe the three types of feedback.
- Define nonverbal communication (body language).
- Explain the importance of positive body language at the job interview.
- Give examples of positive body language.

A successful job interview depends on the effective use of communication. An interview is essentially a conversation between two people who are trying to determine whether they fit each other's employment needs. You have to express yourself clearly so the interviewer can understand you.

Active Listening

Understanding begins by listening actively. Active listening consists of paying attention, focusing on the speaker's words, and thinking about the meaning of what he or she says. This takes practice. During an interview, focus on listening carefully to the questions and then formulating an appropriate response. Pausing to think and compose a good answer will be appreciated by interviewers. You are more likely to be evaluated on the quality of your answer, not on how quickly you gave it.

The importance of listening carefully to the interviewer cannot be overemphasized. Often, we become so caught up in thinking about what we're going to say next that we fail to fully hear, let alone actively listen to, the other person. This is especially true in an interview when we are nervous and worried about whether we will say the right thing. This, however, is the very situation in which we can most benefit from listening carefully so we can base what we say on what we hear.

Mirroring

An effective communication technique for interviews is known as mirroring, which means observing the communication style of the interviewer and then matching it as closely as possible. This does not mean mimicking or appearing to make fun of the other person. It does mean adapting a style that will be most comfortable for the interviewer and help to build trust. Table 3-2 provides examples of mirroring.

TABLE 3-2
Examples of Mirroring at the Job Interview

If the Interviewer Is:	It Is Best to:
Very businesslike. Direct and to the point.	Answer questions concisely, quickly getting to the point. Avoid long introductions, wordiness, and unnecessary details.
Warm and friendly. Conversational tone.	Reflect the interviewer's warmth without becoming too casual. Include human interest and details, when appropriate, in your answers.
Seemingly unhurried. Spends time describing the job in detail.	Include details to support your answers without giving unnecessary or unrelated information.

Feedback

Whatever the style of the interviewer, use feedback when necessary to ensure that you understand the message. Feedback is a communication technique used to check your understanding of the speaker's intended message. It is not necessary—or even desirable—to repeat everything the speaker says, because this can be annoying to speakers. Used when needed, however, feedback can help you understand the other person so you can respond appropriately and intelligently. See Table 3-3 for examples.

Organization

When speaking, do your best to present your ideas in an organized manner so they are easy for the listener to follow. This can be difficult when you are nervous, so take your time to think before you speak. Recall the STAR technique described earlier in this chapter. Silence can feel uncomfortable, but taking a few moments to consider what you are going to say will result in better answers. Saying something meaningful after a pause is more important than simply responding quickly.

TABLE 3-3
Examples of Feedback

Paraphrasing
Saying what you heard the speaker say in your own words.

	What the Speaker Says	Feedback
Job Search	We really need employees we can rely on to be here on time every day. It's also essential they can get along with their co-workers.	It sounds like two of the most important characteristics you are looking for are punctuality and the ability to work well with others.
Career	It really hurts most when I get up in the mornings. I feel a little better as the day goes by.	It sounds like the pain is much worse when you first wake up in the morning but decreases during the day.

Reflecting
Repeating what the speaker said.

	What the Speaker Says	Feedback
Job Search	Here is a copy of the job description. It has most of the duties required for this position, although there are some others.	The job description has most of the duties required, but there are a few others. (The interviewer has given the impression that more may be expected than just what is listed on the job description.)
Career	I haven't lost any weight because the diet the doctor gave me isn't working.	You haven't lost any weight because the diet isn't working. (There may be other reasons, such as not following the diet exactly, lack of exercise, and so on.)

Clarifying
Asking the speaker to explain or give examples.

	What the Speaker Says	Feedback
Job Search	It's easy to find. We're really close to the Cross Town Shopping Center.	You said you are close to the Cross Town Shopping Center. Can you tell me about how many blocks that is?
Career	I give him the medication on schedule, but ever since he's been taking it, his behavior has been kind of strange.	Can you explain what you mean when you say your son has been acting "strangely" since he started taking the medication?

For the next week, take every opportunity to practice your communication skills: active listening, mirroring, and feedback.

Nonverbal Communication: It Can Make You or Break You

If you want a quality, act as if you already have it.

William James

You can speak smoothly and answer questions correctly and yet fail in your communication efforts. What has gone wrong? Your actions have betrayed you. What you *do* communicates as much as—or even more than—what you say. Up to half of the meaning of our messages is communicated nonverbally because our movements, posture, gestures, and facial expressions usually reveal our true feelings. You can enthusiastically claim that you would love the challenge of working in a fast-paced, think-on-your-feet clinical environment. But if your face and body language reflect fear, anxiety, or subtle expressions of "yuck!," your verbal message will not ring true. This is why videotaping yourself is very helpful when practicing interviewing skills. You can observe your nonverbal language and catch inappropriate facial expressions and other behaviors that might betray your words.

Developing a positive attitude about the interviewing process and having confidence in your own abilities will help ensure that your body language communicates appropriate positive messages. At the same time, developing the body language of a positive, confident person will help you become that person. Table 3-4 lists ways to communicate self-confidence and respect for the other person. Figure 3-21 illustrates positive body language.

1. Choose a day to observe other people as they communicate. Look for examples of body language. What do they communicate?
2. Describe actions you observe that communicate positive messages.
3. On another day, pay attention to your own body language. What do you think you are communicating to others?

TABLE 3-4
Positive Body Language

What You Do	The Message You Send
Stand up straight, with head held up and shoulders back	I am a candidate worthy of your consideration.
Maintain eye contact	I am sincere in what I am saying.
Avoid nervous action such as jiggling a leg	I want to be here.
Lean forward slightly toward the other person	I am interested in what you are saying.

FIGURE 3-21 Use body language that communicates respect for the interviewer and confidence in yourself (Copyright © istock.com).

Using Your Portfolio Wisely

LEARNING OBJECTIVE 31: USING YOUR PORTFOLIO WISELY

- Explain how to use the professional portfolio at the job interview.
- Give examples of questions or situations in which the portfolio could be used.

Portfolios are gaining popularity among job seekers, including those in the health care field. They can be a very effective way to support your claims of competence by providing evidence of your accomplishments and qualifications. The following interviewer questions and statements might be answered with material in your portfolio:

1. Asks a question about your skills and abilities
   "Can you ... ?"
   "Have you had experience ... ?"
   States what skills are needed or provides a job description
   "This job requires ..."
   "We need someone who can use medical terminology correctly and chart accurately."
2. Shares a problem or concern
   "One of our problems has been with ensuring accurate documentation ..."
   "We have difficulties with ..."
3. Isn't familiar with the contents of your training program
   "Did your program include ... ?"
   "What skills did you learn ... ?"
4. Asks for verification of licenses, certifications, and so on
   "Have you passed the _____ exam?"
   "Are you a certified medical assistant?"
   "Are you licensed in this state?"

If overused, a portfolio loses its effectiveness, and many questions are better answered with an oral explanation and/or example. Become very familiar with your portfolio's contents so you can find items quickly. If necessary, create an easy-to-read table of contents.

You might use your portfolio to give a brief summary presentation at the end of the interview. For example, the interviewer might say, "Tell me why I should hire you," or might ask, "What else should I know about you?" Use this presentation to quickly review your qualifications or to point out those you haven't yet mentioned.

You may attend interviews where you don't use your portfolio at all. This is okay. It is always better to be overprepared. This prevents you from missing opportunities when they do present themselves.

⭐ **EXPERIENTIAL EXERCISES**

1. Write five questions an interviewer might ask in which you could use your portfolio to support your answers.
2. Role-play with a partner. Have him or her play the part of the employer, choosing among your questions. Answer each question, using your portfolio.

Handling Sticky Interview Situations

LEARNING OBJECTIVE 32: HANDLING STICKY INTERVIEW SITUATIONS

- Give examples of difficult interviewer behaviors and how to best respond to each.
- List information that employers cannot legally use when making hiring decisions.
- Explain methods a job applicant can use when deciding how to respond to illegal questions.
- Explain how to address an employer's concerns without giving unnecessary information.

In spite of your best efforts, some interviews can be a little rocky. Table 3-5 contains difficult situations and suggestions for handling them gracefully. Keep in mind that the questions reveal something about the interviewer and possibly about the organization, so consider them when deciding if you would enjoy this job.

Illegal Questions

It is illegal for employers to discriminate against an applicant on the basis of any of the following factors:

* Age (as long as the applicant is old enough to work legally)
* Arrests (without a conviction—being proven guilty)
* Ethnic background
* Financial status
* Marital status and children
* Physical condition (as long as the applicant can perform the job tasks)
* Race
* Religion
* Sexual orientation

Although questions that require the applicant to reveal information about these factors are illegal, they are sometimes asked anyway. Some employers are ignorant of the laws, or sometimes the interview becomes friendly and conversational, and personal information is shared ("Oh, I went to Grady High School, too. What year did you graduate?"). Employers may take the chance that applicants won't know that the questions are illegal. Some will ask the questions because they know most applicants will not take the time to report them for discrimination. It may not

TABLE 3-5
Handling Difficult Interview Situations

If the Interviewer	What You Can Do
Keeps you waiting a long time	If you are interested in the job, do not show annoyance or anger. It is best not to schedule interviews when you have a very limited amount of time. Remember, this person may be overworked, and that's exactly why there is a potential position for you! Keep in mind that health care work does not always proceed at our convenience. A patient with an emergency, for example, will certainly have priority over an interviewee.
Allows constant interruptions with phone calls and/or people coming in	Again, do not show that you are irritated. This person may be very busy, disorganized, or simply having a difficult day. (This could be another good sign that this employer really needs your help.)
Does most of the talking and doesn't give you an opportunity to say much about yourself	Listen carefully, and try to determine how your qualifications relate to what you are hearing. Being a good listener in itself may be the most important quality you can demonstrate.
Seems to simply make conversation	Try to move the discussion to the job by asking questions: "Can you tell me about what you are looking for in a candidate?" "What are the principal duties that this person would perform?" It is possible that this is a test to see your reaction, so take care to be courteous.
Doesn't discuss the job or ask you questions	
Tries to engage you in gossip about school, personnel, and so on	Say you don't really know about the person or other professionals, facilities, or situations and cannot comment. Ask a question about the job to redirect the conversation.
Allows long periods of silence	This may be a test to see how you react under pressure. Don't feel that you have to speak, and do your best to remain comfortable. (Say to yourself, "This is just a test, and I'm doing fine.") If it goes on too long, you can ask, "Is there something you'd like me to tell you more about? Discuss further?"
Doesn't seem to understand your training or qualifications	Explain as clearly as possible. Use your portfolio, as appropriate, to illustrate your skills.
Makes inappropriate comments about your appearance, gender, ethnicity, and so on	Depending on the nature of the comment and your interpretation of the situation, it may be best to excuse yourself from the interview. For example, comments of a sexual nature or racial slurs should not be tolerated. You should discuss this situation with your instructor or career services department for device on how to proceed.
Is very friendly, chatty, and complimentary about you	Why in the world, you ask, is this a problem? It may not be. But be careful not to get so comfortable that you share personal problems and other information that may disqualify you for the job.

be obvious from the questions that answering them will, in fact, reveal information that cannot be considered when hiring. Table 3-6 contains examples.

Responding to Illegal Questions

Illegal questions put you in a difficult situation, and there are no easy formulas for handling them. In deciding what to do, you need to ask yourself several questions:

* Is the subject of the question of concern to me?
* Do I find the question offensive?
* Does the interviewer appear to be unaware that the question is illegal?

* What is my overall impression of the interviewer and the facility?
* Would I want to work here?
* How badly do I want this particular job?
* If this person is to be my immediate supervisor, is the question an indication that this is a person I don't really want to work with?
* What do I think the interviewer's real concern is? Is it valid?

Based on your answers, there are several ways you can respond to the interviewer:

1. Answer honestly.
2. Ask the interviewer to explain how the question relates to the job requirements.

3. Respond to the interviewer's apparent concern rather than to the question.
4. Ignore the question and talk about something else.
5. Refuse to answer.
6. Inform the interviewer that the question is illegal.
7. Excuse yourself from the interview and leave.
8. State that you plan to report the incident to the Civil Rights Commission or Equal Employment Opportunity Commission.

Legal Versus Illegal

Employers have the right—as well as the responsibility—to make sure that applicants can both physically and legally perform the job requirements. Sometimes there is only a small difference in wording between a legal and an illegal question, as in the following examples (Lock, 1996):

TABLE 3-6
Questions Requesting Information that Cannot Be Used for Hiring

Question	What It Can Reveal
What part of town do you live in?	Financial status
Do you own your home?	Financial status
Where are your parents from?	Ethnic background
Which holidays do you celebrate?	Religion
When did you graduate from high school?	Age

Illegal	Legal
How old are you?	Are you over 18?
Where were you born?	Do you have the legal right to work in the United States?
What is your maiden name?	Would your work records be listed under another name?
Have you ever been arrested?	Have you ever been convicted of a crime?

Are you beginning to understand how employers can get confused and ask illegal questions? It is possible to be an excellent dentist or physical therapist but not an expert in the details of employment law. However you choose to respond to questions you believe are illegal, it is best to remain calm and courteous. You may decide you don't want to work at that facility, but you should conduct yourself professionally at all times.

Responding to Employer Concerns

Many employment experts recommend that you respond to the employer's concerns rather than the questions. This requires that you determine what the concerns are. See Table 3-7 for examples.

One strategy for handling common employer concerns is to bring them up before the interviewer does. This gives you the opportunity to present them in a positive light. Employers may be uncomfortable addressing certain issues and will simply drop you from the "possible hire" list. By taking the initiative, you gain the opportunity to defend your position and

TABLE 3-7
Addressing Employer Concerns

Question	Possible Concern	Possible Responses
Do you have young children?	Your attendance and dependability	Explain your child care arrangements, good attendance in school and at other jobs, and your understanding of the importance of good attendance.
Where do you live?	Reliable transportation and punctuality	Describe your transportation and previous good attendance.
Which religious holidays are you unable to work?	Scheduling problems	Explain that you are a team player and understand that all workdays must be covered. You are willing to cover when co-workers have a holiday you do not observe.

TABLE 3-8
Point Out the Positives

The "Problem"	The Bright Side
You're young and have little work experience.	You are energetic, eager to learn, "trainable," and looking for long-term employment.
You have a criminal record.*	You have learned from your mistakes and are eager to have an opportunity to work and serve others.
You're over age 40.	You are experienced, have good work habits, and are patient.
You've had many jobs, none for very long.	You have a variety of experiences, are flexible, can adjust to the working environment, and have now found a career to which you want to dedicate your efforts.

*Some states do not allow individuals who have been convicted of specific crimes to work in certain health care occupations. In some cases, these individuals are not even allowed to take certification exams.

stay on the list. Table 3-8 contains suggestions for showing the employer the positive aspects of various employment "problems."

JOURNALING 3-14

Is there anything you think employers might see as an obstacle to hiring you? How can you turn the obstacle into a positive characteristic?

Stay Focused on the Positive

Employers are hiring based on attitude: "Give me a 'C' student with an 'A' attitude."

Melva Duran

LEARNING OBJECTIVE 33: STAY FOCUSED ON THE POSITIVE

■ Explain what you should emphasize to employers at interviews.

■ Explain why you should never criticize anyone or any organization at interviews.
■ Explain why you should not discuss your personal problems at interviews.
■ Give examples of questions you should not ask until you are offered a job.

Stay positive at interviews. They are not the place to bring up problems or what you believe you can't do or don't want to do. Be positive and future-oriented and prepared to emphasize the following:

* What you can do
* How you can help
* Ways you can apply what you've learned

Never criticize a previous employer, instructor, or anyone else. Potential employers realize they may someday be your previous employer and don't want to be the subject of your comments to others in the profession. It is also possible that the interviewer is a friend of the person you are criticizing!

Keep in mind that every interview is a sales presentation. Emphasize the positive aspects of your skills and character. However, if you sincerely feel that you are not qualified for a job (and this is an important consideration in health care), you should never pretend that you are. Lacking needed skills is not a negative reflection on you as a person. It simply means that this job is not appropriate for you. Other jobs will be. In fact, there may be many reasons why jobs and applicants do not match. After all, that's the whole purpose of job interviews: for you and the employer to make that determination. See Figure 3-22 for actions that demonstrate your positive qualities.

Subjects to Avoid

Don't mention your personal problems. You are there to help solve the employer's problems, not find solutions to your own. Employers are looking for independent problem solvers. There are exceptions. For example, if you are responsible for a disabled family member and need some consideration regarding your work schedule, it would be appropriate to mention this at the interview.

Giving the impression that you are more concerned with what you can get from the job than what you can give is a sure way to get nothing at all. The following questions send the message "What's in it for me?" and should be avoided until you know you are being considered for the job:

* How much does the job pay?
* What are the other benefits?

At the Interview: How To Show You've Got What It Takes	
Employers want to hire someone who is:	**How to show that you are that someone:**
Qualified to perform the job	1. Be familiar with and able to document all your skills 2. Create a portfolio that contains evidence of your qualifications
Reliable	1. Arrive on time to the interview 2. Send any requested follow-up materials
Trustworthy	1. Have a good handshake 2. Maintain appropriate eye contact 3. Include only accurate information on your resume and job application 4. Do not lie during your interview 5. Avoid saying anything negative about a previous employer 6. Do not engage in any type of gossip
Professional	1. Dress appropriately 2. Be clean and well-groomed 3. Bring needed materials to interview
Motivated and willing to learn	1. Know something about the facility and why you want to work there 2. Ask questions about the job 3. Inquire about learning opportunities on the job 4. Have a plan for professional development
A good communicator and able to work well with others	1. Show consideration for everyone at the interview site 2. Introduce yourself 3. Behave courteously 4. Listen actively throughout the interview 5. Use feedback appropriately to check your understanding of the speaker's message 6. Answer all questions completely but concisely 7. Speak clearly and with proper expression
Likable	1. Smile 2. Be enthusiastic 3. Have a sense of humor 4. Show interest in job 5. Express interest in employer's needs 6. Be comfortable with yourself 7. Show respect for interviewer 8. Avoid showing impatience, annoyance
A problem-solver	1. Describe examples of problems solved in the past 2. Be prepared and willing to participate in any problem-solving exercises given 3. Suggest specific ways you can help the employer

FIGURE 3-22 The interview is your sales opportunity.

* How many paid holidays will I get?
* Is Friday a casual day?
* Can I leave early if I finish my work?
* When will I get a raise?

It is acceptable to inquire about the work schedule, duties, and other expectations. The time to negotiate specific conditions, including your salary, is after you have been offered the job.

It's Your Interview, Too

LEARNING OBJECTIVE 34: IT'S YOUR INTERVIEW, TOO

■ Explain what you demonstrate to employers when you ask good questions about the organization and the job.

- Explain when it is appropriate to ask questions.
- Explain why you should prepare questions before the interview.
- Give examples of appropriate questions to ask.

You have the right—and the responsibility—to ask questions so you can evaluate the opportunities presented by the jobs for which you are applying. Well-stated questions about the job communicate motivation and interest.

When you are in class, it is generally true that "there are no stupid questions." However, at a job interview, the quality of your questions does count. There is a difference between questions that should be avoided and those that show you:

* Have a sincere interest in the job.
* Want to understand the employer's needs.
* Understand the nature of health care work.
* Have thought about your career goal.
* Want information that will enable you to do your best.

It is a good idea to prepare, in advance, a list of general questions, along with a few that are specific to the job and the facility. Not everyone is skilled at "thinking in the seat," especially when it feels like the hot seat!

Here are some questions to get you started:

1. How could I best contribute to the success of this facility?
2. What are the most important qualities needed to succeed in this position?
3. What is the mission of this organization/facility?
4. What are the major problems faced by this organization/facility?
5. How is the organization structured? Whom would I be reporting to?
6. What values are most important to the organization?
7. I want to continue learning and updating my skills. What opportunities would I have to do this?
8. How will I be evaluated and learn what I need to improve?
9. Are there opportunities for advancement for employees who work hard and perform well?

It is perfectly acceptable to ask questions throughout the interview where they are logical. This will be more natural and lead to a smoother interview than asking a long list at the end. You don't have to wait until you are invited to ask them.

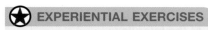 **EXPERIENTIAL EXERCISES**

Write at least five questions you could ask at an interview.

In addition to asking questions, observe the facility and the people who work there. Does this "feel" like a place you would want to work? Is it clean? Organized? Does it appear that safety precautions are followed? What is the pace? Are the people who work there courteous and helpful? How do they interact with patients and with one another? If your interview is with the person who would be your supervisor, do you think you would get along? Do you believe you would fit in?

It may not be possible for you to see anything other than the interviewer's office. In fact, at a large facility, your first interview may take place in the personnel office. You won't see the area where you would work. If this is the case, you will want to ask for a tour if you are offered a job.

Leaving Graciously

LEARNING OBJECTIVE 35: LEAVING GRACIOUSLY

- List the signs an interviewer gives to indicate that the interview is over.
- Explain the final steps you should take at the end of the interview.
- Describe the summary or wrap-up statement.
- Describe how to end the interview on a positive note.

The end of the interview provides you with an opportunity to make a final impression, so make it a good one. It is important to be sensitive to any signals the interviewer gives that it is time to wrap up. Failure to do so shows a lack of consideration for his or her time, and this is definitely not the parting message you want to leave. Some interviewers will make it obvious the interview is almost over by doing the following:

* Telling you directly
* Asking whether you have any "final" questions
* Telling you that everything has been covered

Less obvious signs include looking at their watch, clock, appointment book, or papers on their desk; pushing their chair back; or saying that they have "taken enough of your time." Show respect for their time by moving along with the final steps of the interview:

1. Ask any final questions (limit these to a couple of the most important ones that haven't been answered).
2. Make a brief wrap-up statement.
3. Thank them for their time.
4. Inquire about what comes next.

If you are interested in the job, say so in the wrap-up statement. Tell the interviewer why: you believe you can make a contribution, you are impressed with the organization, you believe your qualifications fit the position, and so on. Express your enthusiasm about working there, and state that you hope you are chosen for the position.

Whether you want the job or not, always thank the interviewer for his or her time. This applies even if the interview did not go well.

Finally, ask if there is anything you need to do to follow up. If requested, give the interviewer your reference sheet. Be sure to get the interviewer's last name and correct title. An easy way to do this is to ask for his or her business card. And be sure that he or she has your telephone number and any other information needed to contact you. Then smile, give a firm handshake, and leave as confidently as you entered.

⭐ EXPERIENTIAL EXERCISES

1. Create several short summaries that express your interest in various jobs.
2. Create statements about why you should be hired.
3. Practice your statements aloud until you are comfortable saying them. (Do not memorize.)

Some Final Thoughts

You wouldn't be nervous if you didn't care.

Robert Lock

LEARNING OBJECTIVE 36: SOME FINAL THOUGHTS

- Explain why it is natural to feel nervous and how this is viewed by employers.
- Explain why role playing is helpful in learning to interview.

You may be feeling a little (or very) overwhelmed at this point. "How can I remember all this and act natural and maintain eye contact and give good examples and ... ." It *is* a lot, and that's why it is so important to spend time learning about the interviewing process, preparing, and practicing. Take every opportunity to role-play. Make your practice sessions as realistic as possible.

When you inventoried your skills, were you surprised at how much you can do now that you would never have attempted before you started your educational program? You learned these skills by studying and practicing them—over and over. You are almost certainly more qualified for the job search than you realize.

It's okay to be nervous. It can even be a good thing, because it means you are taking the interview seriously. It tells interviewers that this job is important to you and that you care about the outcome. This is a positive message to communicate.

🕐 JOURNALING 3-15

What is my biggest concern about interviewing? What can I do to best prepare for interviews?

CASE STUDY 3-7

Emily, the medical administrative assistant student who interviewed Mr. Bard, the director of human resources at the clinic where she was doing her externship, felt she had learned a lot from the information he gave her about electronic applications and resumes. She shared what she learned with the class, and her instructor, Ms. Harris, wondered if Mr. Bard would be willing to come to BeWell and talk to the class about interviewing for jobs.

"You know," Ms. Harris told her husband that night, "I can give the students my best, but maybe if they hear it from people who do the actual hiring, they'll take it a little more seriously."

"I think you're on to something there. Interviewing for a job can be intimidating, especially for folks just starting a new career," her husband agreed.

Ms. Harris called St. Francis Clinic the next day. Mr. Bard said he was busy that week, but he could come on Tuesday of the following week. She had heard that a format in which students asked questions had worked well. It encouraged participation and enabled the guest speaker to address the immediate concerns of the students.

On Tuesday, Mr. Bard arrived, and the students asked their questions.

Student: What advice would you give applicants who are interviewing for a job at your clinic?

Mr. Bard: First, I would say they should use sound common sense. I might add here that common sense is not always so common! What I mean is, they need to think about the impression they are giving the employer. If applicants are not at their very best at an interview, what is the employer going to expect from them once they are on the job?

Student: Can you be more a little more specific?

Mr. Bard: Sure. Good candidates for jobs in health care are friendly, concerned, and respectful. They show this in the way they interact with the interviewer. For example, they are on time, showing they respect the other person's schedule. Health care today is a high-customer service environment, and we are looking for employees who take their work seriously. After all, we aren't selling shoes. Health *matters,* and that's what we're taking care of.

Student: You mentioned appearance. Have the standards changed in today's health care facilities?

Mr. Bard: To some degree, the answer is "yes." Social values drive business values, and as we all know, styles and trends have changed. What we're looking for are "reasonable standards." For example, piercings and tattoos used to be job-blockers. But now they're more accepted if they aren't excessive or too outlandish.

Related to appearance is language. Communication and the impressions given to patients are really important, so inappropriate language is really not okay. Anything off-color or offensive—that kind of thing.

Student: What kinds of questions should interviewees be prepared for?

Mr. Bard: Patients today are considered to be *customers,* so I'm interested in knowing what an applicant can do that will help us make our patients satisfied with our service. What will they do to make our patients feel important? Those are questions I would ask. The bottom line is that I'm looking for people who want to help make this place better. And I want to know how they're going to do it.

We sometimes give behavioral interviews. This means we give applicants scenarios of typical work situations and ask how they would handle them. What we are looking for is caring—respect for people—their general approach to work. Sometimes we require a demonstration of a skill related to the job.

QUESTIONS FOR THOUGHT AND REFLECTION

1. What does Mr. Bard mean by common sense?
2. Why are health providers today thinking of their patients as customers?
3. According to Mr. Bard, what are the most important personal characteristics employers want their employees to have?
4. What types of questions should applicants be prepared to answer?

Down a Dark Road

Abrianna has about had it with the job search. She graduated from her medical assisting program over two months ago and still isn't employed. She knows it's not her fault. After all, the career services people at her school just aren't giving her good leads. She's tried to tell them that the employers they've sent her to are really not interested in hiring a recent graduate, but they just keep encouraging her to keep the appointments.

As she told her friend Janice, "Last Thursday was a waste of time. I went to an interview, but how was I supposed to act enthusiastic about a job in a little office working with an older doctor? It didn't look like it would be a fun place to work. So I answered his questions, but I really couldn't pretend I was interested."

"So what did he say when you finished the interview?" asked Janice.

"He thanked me for coming in and said good-bye," answered Abrianna.

"That was all?" asked Janice.

"Yeah, imagine that," said Abrianna. "After I went to the trouble of getting dressed up and going in. Even if I didn't want the job, he could have said he would call me back or something."

Abrianna believes that she has bad luck with interviews. Sometimes she was late because "the office was hard to find, and they didn't give her good directions." Other times, career services called her at the last minute, and she didn't have time to get her clothes ready, her car gassed up, or her resume copied. As she told Janice, "What is that school thinking? That I'm just waiting around for them to call me about an interview?"

Yesterday, Mr. Craig called from her school. "Abrianna, I'd like you to come in so we can talk about your job search and the interviews you've been on."

Abrianna responded, "That sounds like a good idea, because I need to talk to *you* about these employers you've sent me to. What a waste of time."

Mr. Craig sighed. "Can you be here at 2:00?"

Abrianna arrived at Mr. Craig's office at 2:15. He looked at his watch. "Abrianna, our appointment was at 2:00. I want to help you, but this is one of the problems I'm hearing from the employers you've had interviews with."

"The babysitter arrived late, and I had to stop and get gas," explained Abrianna.

"Punctuality is very important to health care providers. They need their employees to be on time. And if you can't get to an interview on time, why would they think you will be on time for work?" Mr. Craig asked.

"Work is different. I can be on time. And even if I can't—you know, some kind of little emergency—there are co-workers who can cover for a few minutes. It won't kill them," said Abrianna.

"I must say that's a very unprofessional attitude, Abrianna. And it's not the only thing. You've had such a hard time becoming employed that I called a few of the employers who have interviewed you to see if there was something keeping you from receiving an offer," he said.

Abrianna was surprised but couldn't imagine any of them would have anything really negative to say about her.

Mr. Craig told her, "You seem to have a problem showing interest in the employers or their needs—or even showing respect for them. One employer told me you actually answered your cell phone during the interview! That is simply not done. It shows little regard for the employer and a lack of interest on your part in the interview or the job."

"Well," interrupted Abrianna. "That was an important call from a friend. I didn't think employers expected me to put my life on hold during an interview."

"The fact is, they want your full attention—just like they want it when you are working for them. The interview is like a test: are you the kind of person they want as an employee? And unfortunately, the behaviors you're demonstrating to me and to them are not going to get you employed."

QUESTIONS FOR THOUGHT AND REFLECTION

1. How is Abrianna's attitude affecting her job search?
2. What mistakes is she making at interviews?
3. How does she regard other people?
4. What advice would you give her?

After the Interview

Nothing is a waste of time if you use the experience wisely.

Auguste Rodin

LEARNING OBJECTIVE 37: AFTER THE INTERVIEW

- Explain why it is important to conduct a postinterview evaluation.
- List the contents of a postinterview evaluation.
- Explain the importance of sending thank-you letters.

- Describe a simple thank-you letter.
- Describe a thank-you-plus letter.
- Understand the importance of communicating with your references after each job interview.
- Describe the recommended strategy for contacting an employer after an interview.

Attending an interview is a success, whether or not you are hired for a particular job. You have qualifications that were worthy of the interviewer's time, you prepared well, and you met the challenge of presenting yourself one-on-one to a potential employer. Take a moment to reward yourself for completing this important step.

BOX 3-21

Postinterview Self-Evaluation

- Did I arrive on time?
- Did I use good communication skills?
- Did I present my qualifications effectively?
- Did I answer the interviewer's questions effectively?
- Did I ask good questions?
- What would I do differently if I could do it over?
- What did I learn from this experience?

Make the most of every interview by viewing each one as an opportunitiy to improve your presentation skills and learn more about the health care world. This knowledge can help you in future interviews and work-related situations such as performance evaluations. When you leave the interviewer's office, your reaction may be "Whew! That's over!" and the last thing you want to do is spend more time thinking about it. This is especially true if you feel the interview didn't go well. But this is precisely when you need to spend some time thinking about and evaluating the experience and your performance. Box 3-21 contains questions to ask yourself.

You might want to discuss your self-evaluation with someone you trust, such as your instructor, career services personnel, or mentor. You may have friends and family members who can provide insight and support. Create an improvement plan and practice so you'll feel more confident at the next interview.

When seeking help or discussing interviews with others, it is best not to make negative remarks about the interviewer or the facility. This serves no purpose, unless you are seeking advice about whether to accept a job you have doubts about. A friend may have a friend who works there, and your words, said "in confidence," may be passed along to the wrong party.

You may believe you will receive a job offer. You very well might. But don't cancel or turn down other interviews until you are formally hired. You may have done a superb job and the facility plans to hire you. Then the next day, your soon-to-be supervisor is informed of a facility-wide hiring freeze. You don't want to be left out in the cold with no other options. Stay actively involved in the search until you have a job.

Thank-You Letter

Whether the interview went like a dream or a nightmare, you should send a thank-you letter. Too many job seekers neglect this common courtesy, but it is a simple action that can set you apart from the others. Suppose the employer interviewed nine people in two days, in addition to carrying on a normal workload. Tired? Very likely. Able to remember each candidate clearly and recall who said what? Maybe. But why take the chance of being lost in the crowd?

Thank-you letters should be sent no later than the day after the interview. Consider keeping a box of cards in the car and writing the letter immediately after you leave the interview. Interviewers will be impressed when they receive your letter the very next day.

For some jobs, such as administrative positions, emailing a thank you may be acceptable because it demonstrates computer proficiency. Take the same care you would with a written letter: include a salutation, write complete sentences, use correct grammar, spell all words correctly, and use a proper closing. And regardless of how you send the thank you, be sure the name and title of the person who interviewed you are correct.

If you know for sure that you don't want the job, send a thank-you letter anyway. Keep it simple, say something positive about the interview, and express your appreciation for the time taken to meet with you. Do not say that you are not interested in the job. Figure 3-23 is an example of this kind of letter.

Why should you write if you don't want to work there? There are at least three good reasons:

1. The employer may know someone else who is hiring. Impressed by your follow-up, he or she recommends you.
2. An opening for a job that you do want becomes available at this facility. You are remembered for your thoughtfulness.
3. At this time, when courtesy and consideration for others are disappearing, it is the right thing to do.

WHAT IF?

You just left an interview for a job you now realize you would probably not accept. What would you say in your thank-you letter?

1642 Windhill Way
San Antonio, TX 78220
October 18, 2010

Nancy Henderson, Office Manager
Craigmore Pediatric Clinic
4979 Coffee Road
San Antonio, TX 78229

Dear Ms. Henderson:

Thank you so much for the time you spent with me yesterday. You have a busy schedule, and I appreciate the time you took to describe the opening for a medical assistant at Craigmore Pediatric. The Clinic enjoys a good reputation in San Antonio for the services it provides children in the community, and it was a pleasure to learn more about it.

Sincerely,

Karen Gonzalez

Karen Gonzalez

FIGURE 3-23 Simple Thank-You Letter.

Thank-You-Plus Letter

If you want the job, take the time to write a thank-you-plus letter. The "plus" refers to a paragraph or two in which you do at least one of the following:

* Briefly summarize your qualifications in relation to the job as it was discussed in the interview
* Point out specifically how you can make a positive contribution—again, based on details you learned

Let the employer know you want the job and hope to be the candidate selected. Include your full name and telephone number. Figure 3-24 shows an example of a thank-you-plus letter.

 WHAT IF?

You just left an interview for a job you want. What might you say in your thank-you letter?

1642 Windhill Way
San Antonio, TX 78220
October 18, 2010

Nancy Henderson, Office Manager
Craigmore Pediatric Clinic
4979 Coffee Road
San Antonio, TX 78229

Dear Ms. Henderson:

Thank you so much for the time you spent with me yesterday. You have a busy schedule, and I appreciate the time you took to describe the opening for a medical assistant at Craigmore Pediatric. The Clinic enjoys a good reputation in San Antonio for the services it provides children in the community, and it was a pleasure to learn more about it.

After visiting your facility and meeting the health professionals who work there, I sincerely believe I could make a positive contribution to your facility. My ability to communicate in both English and Spanish would allow me to work with patients from various cultural backgrounds. My previous experience working in a day care facility gave me a love for and understanding of children that enables me to work effectively with them. Finally, my organizational skills and knowledge of current insurance requirements would be of benefit in helping to develop the new billing system you described.

I am interested in this position and enthusiastic about working at Craigmore Pediatric. Please let me know if you need anything further from me. I can be reached at (210) 123-4567. I look forward to hearing from you.

Sincerely,

Karen Gonzalez

Karen Gonzalez

FIGURE 3-24 Thank-You-Plus Letter.

Alert Your References

If you left a reference sheet with the interviewer, call your references as soon as possible to tell them they may receive a call. Give them the job title, nature of the work, and type of facility. Add anything you learned about the type of candidate the employer is seeking. This gives your references an opportunity to stress those features that best support your bid for the job.

When to Call Back

Following up after an interview is a kind of balancing act: you don't want to be considered a pest by calling too soon and too frequently. On the other hand, you took the time to attend the interview and have a right to be informed when the hiring decision is made.

The best strategy is to wait until the day after you were told a decision would be made. Call or send an email and inquire about the decision. If none has been made, ask when you might expect to hear. Use your best manners. This is still part of the interview, and courtesy counts. Never express impatience about a delay. You want to show interest but not pressure the employer for a decision he or she is not ready to make. Sometimes the interviewer is deciding between two candidates and the decision may be influenced by your follow-up.

 EXPERIENTIAL EXERCISES

1. Read the following articles, available online:
   - "How to Follow Up After a Job Interview" http://jobsearch.about.com/od/interviewsnetworking/a/intfollowup.htm
   - "Job Interview Follow-Up Do's and Don'ts" www.quintcareers.com/interview_follow-up-dos-donts.html
   - "The Art of the Follow-Up After Job Interviews" www.quintcareers.com/job_interview_follow-up.html
2. List what you think are the five most important actions to take following an interview.

? WHAT IF?

What would you do if has been two weeks since you interviewed for a job you really want and you haven't heard anything?

Is This the Job for You?

LEARNING OBJECTIVE 38: IS THIS THE JOB FOR YOU?

- List the questions you should ask yourself when deciding whether to accept a job.
- Describe characteristics of jobs that are good for entry-level health care professionals.

Jobs are usually not offered on the spot during the first interview. If this does happen to you, it is a good idea to ask when a decision is needed and say that you are very interested (if you are) but need a little time to make a decision. There are exceptions, of course. You may have performed your externship at this site and know for sure that this is the place for you.

Interviewers will usually give you a time range during which a hiring decision will be made. You, too, need to make a decision: if this position is offered, will you accept it? Many factors will influence your decision. Box 3-22 contains questions to help you select an appropriate job.

BOX 3-22

Questions to Guide Your Job-Selection Process

Here are some questions to guide your thinking about the specific job and facility in which you will be working:

1. Do the job duties match my skills and interests?
2. How closely do the job and facility match my work preferences?
3. Does the facility appear to follow safe and ethical practices?
4. Do I agree with the mission and values of the organization?
5. Can I make a positive contribution?
6. Who are the clients/patients? Will I enjoy working with them?
7. How well do I think I would fit in?
8. Are there opportunities to learn?
9. Will there be opportunities for advancement?
10. Can I commit to the required schedule?
11. Is the management style compatible with my work style?
12. How did the facility "feel"?

Although you should consider these questions carefully, remember that the job that is "exactly what you want" probably doesn't exist. Finding the right job for you is a matter of finding a close match on the most important elements. You are starting a new career, and there are certain factors that will help your long-term success. Working with someone who is interested in teaching you, for example, may be a better choice than choosing a slightly higher-paying position that offers no opportunities for acquiring new skills. Many health care facilities make it a practice to promote from within. If there is a facility where you want to work, consider taking a job that gets you in the door.

Discussing Salary: When and How

- Explain when salary should be discussed with an employer.
- Explain why recent graduates may earn at the lower end of salary ranges.

Most career experts recommend that you not discuss salary with a potential employer until you have been offered the job. In many cases, this won't be an issue because salaries are predetermined and not negotiable. Some occupations, such as nursing, have labor unions, and the employer cannot change agreed-upon salaries for specific positions.

Doing your research before you attend an interview may provide you with this information. If a salary range for a position is given, the amount offered to you will most likely depend on the experience you bring to the job. Recent graduates tend to start at the low end of a range, earning more as they gain experience.

Considering an Offer

- List the information you should have when making a decision about accepting a job.
- Explain why you should state any special conditions you have before accepting a job offer.

A job offer may be extended in a telephone call, at a second or even third interview, or in a letter. Even if you feel quite sure that this is the right job, you still need to be sure that you have all the information needed to make a final decision. It is essential that you understand the following:

* The duties you will be required to perform. If you haven't seen a written job description, ask for it now. If there is no written description, ask for a detailed oral explanation if this wasn't done in the interview.
* The exact date and time you are to report for work.
* The days and hours you will work. Ask about the likelihood of required overtime and any change of hours or days that might take place in the future.
* Your salary. Earnings are expressed in various ways: hourly, weekly, biweekly, monthly, or annual rates. If you are quoted a rate that you aren't familiar with, you might want to convert it to one you know. For example, if you are accustomed to thinking in terms of amount per hour but are given a monthly salary, you may want to calculate the hourly equivalent.
* Orientation and/or training given. This is especially important for recent graduates. Learning the customs and practices of the facility can make a big difference in your success.

You may have received all this information in the interview(s). Don't hesitate, however, to ask about anything you don't fully understand. It is far better to take the time now rather than to discover later that the job or working conditions are not what you expected. If you didn't have an opportunity to see beyond the interviewer's office, ask for a tour of the facility before deciding whether to accept the job.

Understanding Benefits

- Explain why benefits are an important compensation consideration.
- List the types of benefits offered by some employers.
- Explain how to calculate the effect of benefits on your total compensation.

Benefits can represent a significant portion of your compensation. Health insurance, for example, can cost hundreds of dollars per month for a family of four. If full family coverage is offered by the employer, this may be worth thousands of dollars each year. Find out if you must pay part of the cost of the premiums and what type of coverage is provided. Health insurance for individuals (or families) is often more expensive than the group rates available through an employer. Health insurance is becoming an increasingly important benefit to consider when choosing where to work. There are other types of insurance, too, that can add value to the benefits package, including dental, vision, life, and disability.

If you are planning to continue your education, tuition benefits might be important to you. Some employers cover all or part of educational expenses if the studies are related to your work and you receive a grade of C or better. Time off to take classes and workshops is an additional advantage. This benefit is especially helpful for health care professionals who are required to earn continuing education units on a regular basis. Related professional expenses that some employers cover are the dues for professional organizations and required uniforms.

Other benefits to consider when calculating your overall compensation include the number of paid vacation, holiday, and personal days offered and whether there is a retirement plan such as a 401(k) plan. With this plan, you choose an amount to be deducted from your earnings each pay period. You pay no taxes on this money until you withdraw it anytime after you reach age 59½. The money is invested, often in mutual funds. Some employers match a certain percentage of the money you save, which is like giving you an additional, currently tax-free salary.

When considering the compensation offered by an employer, think in terms of the total package. One job may offer a higher hourly rate but require you to pay part of your health insurance premium. You may end up financially ahead by accepting the lower salary. On the other hand, if you are included on your spouse's group insurance plan, this might not be significant. Salary alone should not be the determining factor when deciding whether a job "pays enough."

Let's look at an example of an entry-level job. Suppose you are offered Job A, which pays $24,000 and includes medical insurance, for which the employer pays $2700. The total value of this package, then, is $26,700. Another employer offers you Job B at $27,000 in salary with no insurance benefits. You need insurance and plan to pay for it yourself with the extra

salary you will earn. Assuming that everything else about the two jobs is equal, which job would benefit you more financially? Surprisingly, it is Job A. Let's see why.

1. You will pay taxes on wages of $24,000 rather than $27,000. (Health insurance benefits are not taxed.)
2. The $2700 for medical insurance is the cost for a member of a group plan. If you buy insurance as an individual, it may cost you even more.

Job A

$24,000 − $7200 (standard tax deduction and single exemption)	= $16,800 (taxable income)
$16,800 × 15% tax rate	= $2520 (taxes)
$24,000 − $2520	= **$21,480** (amount of money you keep)

Job B

$27,000 − $7200	= $19,800 (taxable income)
$19,800 × 15%	= $2970 (taxes)
$27,000 − $2970	= $24,030
$24,030 − $2700 (amount spent on health insurance)	= **$21,330** (amount of money you keep)

Note: This is a simplified example. The numbers are not based on current tax rates and insurance costs. Also, because of the Affordable Care Act, there may be subsidies for privately purchased insurance.

The lesson here is to collect information and consider all aspects of the compensation plan. Although this is a simplified example and not based on current tax rates and insurance costs and subsidies, it shows how important it is to do the math. If you are unsure about how to do these calculations, ask for help.

Accepting an Offer

LEARNING OBJECTIVE 42: ACCEPTING AN OFFER

- Describe the ways in which a job offer may be accepted.
- Explain why it is important to write a letter of acceptance including the terms of employment.
- Understand the importance of disclosing future commitments when you accept a job.

When you accept a job, express your appreciation and enthusiasm. In addition to responding orally, write a letter of acceptance. The letter should include a summary of what you understand to be the terms of employment.

When speaking with the employer, inquire about any necessary follow-up activities. It is also a good idea to disclose any future commitments or other factors that will affect your work. For example, if your son is scheduled for surgery next month and you know you will need to take several days off to take care of him, let the employer know this during the hiring process. If the employer refuses to accommodate you, it is better to learn now that this job lacks flexibility regarding family needs. You may want to reconsider your acceptance. (Be aware, however, that employers cannot grant repeated requests for days off due to family responsibilities. Their first responsibility must be to the patients they serve.)

You may want this job but need to negotiate some conditions. For example, suppose the work hours are 8:00 a.m. to 5:00 p.m. You have a 3-year-old child who cannot be left at day care before 7:45 a.m., and it takes at least 25 minutes to drive to work. It is better to ask if you can work from 8:30 a.m. to 5:30 p.m. than to take the position and arrive late every day. Many problems on the job can be avoided by discussing them openly in advance. (Again, you must also consider the employer's needs. Accommodations like this are not always possible if they disrupt the facility's schedule and patient flow.) And sometimes, having a "Plan B" will save the day—in this case, having someone reliable who can take your child to day care.

What to Expect

> **LEARNING OBJECTIVE 43: WHAT TO EXPECT**

- List examples of information that employers may ask new hires to provide.
- Explain the types of tests and checks that may be required of new hires.

Once you are hired, employers can ask questions that were unacceptable during the hiring process. Information that cannot be used to make hiring decisions is often necessary to complete personnel requirements. Examples include the following:

1. Provide proof of your age (to ensure you are of legal age to work).
2. Provide verification that you can work legally in the United States.

3. Identify your race (for affirmative action statistics, if applicable in your state).
4. Supply a photograph (for identification).
5. State your marital status and number and ages of your children (for insurance).
6. Give the name and address of a relative (for notification in case of emergency).
7. Provide your Social Security number (for tax purposes).

There may be mandatory health tests and immunizations. In addition, some employers require drug tests and background checks for all employees.

If you are asked to sign an employment contract, read it carefully first. As with all other employment issues, ask about anything you don't understand. Ask for a copy of anything you sign.

Turning Down a Job Offer

After careful consideration, you may decide not to accept a job offer. It is not necessary to explain your reasons to the employer. Do express your appreciation and thanks for the opportunity, and do send a thank-you letter. In addition to being an expression of courtesy, this leaves a positive impression on all employers. You may want to work at this facility in the future.

If You Don't Get the Job

Failure is a delay, but not a defeat. It is a temporary detour, not a dead-end street.

William Arthur Ward

> **LEARNING OBJECTIVE 44: IF YOU DON'T GET THE JOB**

- Give examples of reasons for not being hired that are out of the control of the applicant.
- List common reasons for not being hired that are under the control of the applicant.

It can be difficult when you are not selected for a job you really want. There are many reasons why applicants don't get hired. Some you can't change and must simply accept, such as the following:

* Another applicant had more experience or skills that more closely met the employer's current needs.

* An employee in the organization decided to apply for the job.
* The employer believed that someone else was a better "match" for the organization in terms of work style, preferences, and so on.
* Budget cuts or other unexpected events prevented anyone from being hired at this time.

On the other hand, you may have lost this opportunity for reasons you can change. How do you know? First, do an honest review of your postinterview evaluation, school record, and resume. Are you presenting yourself in the best possible way? Second, look over the list in Box 3-23. Health care employers and career services personnel name these as major reasons why job applicants fail to get hired. Do you recognize anything that might apply to you?

You must be honest with yourself and commit to improving your attitude and/or job search skills. If necessary, seek advice from your instructor, career services personnel, or mentor. Work on adopting a winning attitude. Seek support from friends and family members if you are feeling down.

Although you may not feel enthusiastic about writing a letter to an employer who chooses another applicant, consider this: you may have come in a close second. The next opening may be yours! So take a few moments and demonstrate your high level of professionalism by thanking the employer and letting him or her know that you are still interested in working for the organization.

If you fail to get hired after attending an interview that you think went well, ask for assistance from an instructor or career services personnel. You may be

BOX 3-23

Why Job Applicants Fail to Get Hired

1. Failure to sell themselves by clearly presenting their skills and qualifications
2. Too much interest in what's in it for them rather than what they can give
3. Unprofessional behavior or lack of courtesy
4. Lack of enthusiasm and interest in the job
5. Poor appearance
6. Poor communication skills
7. Unrealistic job expectations
8. Negative or critical attitude
9. Arriving late, bringing children or the person who provided transportation, or other demonstrations of poor organizational skills

able to get good feedback. Or perhaps this person can call the employers on your behalf to find out how you might improve your presentation or to see if you appeared to lack needed skills. Employers are sometimes more willing to share reasons with school personnel so they can better assist their students. Be willing to listen to any constructive criticism offered and to make any needed changes.

 JOURNALING 3-16

If I don't get a job I want, what can I learn from the experience?

CASE STUDY 3-8

Jessica was really excited when she received the phone call yesterday from Blaine Clinic asking her to come in for an interview. This clinic had a reputation as a great place to work, and she had dropped off her resume there last week. She had learned through doing research on the clinic that it had several specialties and that there were advancement opportunities for employees who worked hard and showed promise.

She was surprised, then, by what happened at her interview. After arriving a few minutes early for her 10:30 appointment, she had to wait until almost 11:00 before Dr.

Spader, the director of the department that was looking to hire an administrative medical assistant, asked her into his office. As soon as she introduced herself and sat down, the phone rang. Dr. Spader took the call and was brief, but this was a sign of how the interview would be. The phone rang several times, staff members knocked on the door, and some employees just walked into Dr. Spader's office without knocking.

Jessica could see that Dr. Spader was stressed. He looked harried and apologized many times for the interruptions. Jessica tried her best to stay calm and answer his questions in ways that presented her as a good candidate for the job. Sometimes she lost her train of thought when an interruption occurred, but she would smile, take a breath, and continue. Dr. Spader seemed to understand that this was difficult for her.

That evening, Jessica thought about the interview and the clinic. It looked very busy with patients and personnel coming and going, especially in the department where she interviewed. She was still interested in working there, in spite of the interview that had seemed to go so wrong. She spent some time thinking about Dr. Spader and how stressed and apologetic he was. She didn't know whether to be annoyed or sympathetic and decided to think it over for a day or two.

The next day she remembered what she had learned in her job search class: focus on the employer's *needs*. Dr. Spader certainly had some needs. Obviously, there were problems in the department resulting in his not having the time to interview job candidates in a quiet environment. Jessica decided she really had nothing to lose and decided to write a thank-you letter that included her observations—and how she could help. She had always been an organized person, and she mentioned this in her letter. Of course, she didn't say she thought the department was disorganized, but she worded her letter carefully, mentioning how busy Dr. Spader seemed to be and how she knew her organizational skills could be a great help with his obviously heavy workload. She included a couple of specific suggestions based on what she saw and heard.

QUESTIONS FOR THOUGHT AND REFLECTION

1. What do you think of Jessica's strategy in writing a thank-you-plus letter?
2. Do you think Jessica got the job? Why or why not?
3. How would you have handled the situation?

Down a Dark Road

Sarah and Jessica were classmates and graduated together. Sarah did well in the administrative medical assistant program, and she prides herself on being punctual and organized. She and Jessica both received interviews with Dr. Spader at Blaine Clinic. Like Jessica's, Sarah's interview is sprinkled with phone calls and staff interruptions. She is finding it difficult to concentrate. She finally tells Dr. Spader that in spite of his apologies, she believes he is inconsiderate. Sarah says, "I took the time to come in for an interview. As a recent graduate, I'm still a little nervous about interviewing, and I expect to have your attention."

The situation doesn't improve, however, and by the time Sarah leaves, she is truly annoyed. "What a madhouse," she tells her boyfriend, Mike. "They could really use my organizational skills. Maybe Dr. Spader heard enough of what I said about myself to realize what a good employee I'd be."

"You're kidding, right?" asked Mike incredulously. "Why would you want to work in a place like that? Wouldn't it drive you crazy?"

"Probably. But that's only one department. The clinic has a good reputation, and they do pay well. I'm thinking if I just got my foot in the door, I could get to know people in the other departments and get a transfer as soon as possible," explained Sarah.

"That's my girl," said Mike. "Always thinking ahead. Are you going to drop him a note and thank him for the so-called interview?"

"That would be a waste of time. He'd probably just lose it!" she laughed.

QUESTIONS FOR THOUGHT AND REFLECTION

1. How was Sarah's reaction to Dr. Spader different from Jessica's?
2. What do you think of Sarah's reasons for wanting the job?
3. Do you think Sarah got the job? Why or why not?

References

Anderson R, Barbara A, Feldman S. (2009). *What patients want: A content analysis of key qualities that influence patient satisfaction.* Retrieved on July 28, 2015, from www.drscore.com/press/papers/whatpatientswant.pdf

Cha AE. Employers relying on personality tests to screen applicants. *Washington Post.* March 27, 2005. Page A01. http://www.washingtonpost.com/wp-dyn/content/article/2005/03/26/AR2005032605181.html (accessed July 28, 2015).

Dickel MR. (2004). Guide to Internet job searching 2004-2005, Columbus, OH: McGraw-Hill.

Ellis D, Lankowitz S, Stupka E, Toft D. (1997). Career planning (2nd ed.). New York, NY: Houghton Mifflin.

Graber S. (2000). The Everything online job search book. Holbrook, MA: Adams Media.

Hansen K. Behavioral interviewing strategies for job-seekers. www.quintcareers.com/behavioral_interviewing.html (accessed July 28, 2015).

Ireland S. (2014). Susan Ireland's Resume SiteI (website). Retrieved April 3, 2014, from susanireland.com

Lock RD. (1996). Job search: Career planning guide, book II (3rd ed.). Pacific Grove, CA: Brooks/Cole.

Lorenz Kate. Warning: Social networking can be hazardous to your job search. CareerBuilder.com Editor. Retrieved February 25, 2009, from http://www.careerbuilder.ca/blog/2006/07/12/cb-warning-social-networking-can-be-hazardous-to-your-job-search/

National Consortium on Health Science and Technology Education. *National Healthcare Foundation Standards and Accountability Criteria.* Retrieved on July 30, 2015, from http://www.healthscienceconsortium.org/docs/NCHSE_Standards_2015f.pdf.

CHAPTER 4

Ready for Work

- Act and look like a health care professional.
- Become someone other people look forward to seeing at work.
- Understand how your appearance affects your success.
- Fit in well with a variety of different people.
- Represent your employer to its customers.
- Develop self-reflection to change your habits and improve your performance.

Modeling Business Etiquette

Sticks and stones may break our bones, but words will break our hearts.

—Robert Fulghum

LEARNING OBJECTIVE 1: MODELING BUSINESS ETIQUETTE

- Understand your role in the support and success of the business where you work.
- Identify behavioral clues of your fellow workers.
- Make introductions easily and smoothly.
- Understand the importance of titles.
- Build your conversation skills.
- Learn to be on time and to be discreet.
- Practice the little courtesies that make a big difference.
- Create a positive reputation for yourself.

The Purposes of Business Etiquette

The first purpose of business etiquette is customer care. To each and every client or patient or family member with whom you interact, you *are* the facility you work for. Much of your customers' judgment about your employer will be based on their judgment of *you.*

⬅ JOURNALING 4-1

Recall the last time you sought health care, whether at a walk-in clinic, a dentist's office, or a physical therapy appointment. Describe your impression of the facility. Recall the workers you interacted with. How were you treated? How did these interactions contribute to the overall impression you have of the facility?

The second purpose of business etiquette is to do your part to make your facility a great place for you and your colleagues to work. A sense of business etiquette contributes to the smooth flow of operations in an environment that is often stressful and chaotic. Business etiquette contributes to clear communication, mutual support, and, ultimately, the delivery of quality health care. This requires flexibility and open-minded acceptance. For example, today's workplace is comprised of four generations (discussed more thoroughly in Chapter 9). You have to be able to step outside of your own generation and interact professionally with people of all ages. Aside from people of different ages, you will likely encounter clients and colleagues from dozens of different ethnic, national, and cultural backgrounds.

Regional Considerations

United States culture is well-blended. Few of us live more than a few miles from a national fast food restaurant or a gas station. Everyone is exposed to the same national news, sports, movies, and television programs, and local differences seem to be diminishing. Nevertheless, each region still retains some distinctive aspects of its own culture, and these aspects are sometimes reflected at work.

For instance, the degree of formality can vary from region to region. Regional differences at work can be very subtle, so you'll need to be sensitive to cultural variations such as formality, pace of action, small talk, and rules and regulations, and adapt your behavior accordingly.

Skills to Improve Your Business Etiquette

Conversation at Work

The "rules" of polite conversation are pretty much the same at work as anywhere else. In health care, where people work closely together, and the pace of work can vary, conversations about nonwork topics are not only common but also practical. Conversation builds relationships and makes work more enjoyable and rewarding. Much of the richness in life has to do with the quantity and quality of friendships you have in your life, and conversation is the fabric of friendship.

Unfortunately, many people don't have good conversation skills because they have never worked to develop them. Virtually anybody can become a better conversationalist by mindfully following a few strategies and techniques. For instance, paying someone a compliment is a great way to start a conversation. Then, ask questions and take a sincere interest in the answers. Ask "open-ended" questions that can't be answered with a simple, conversation-stalling *yes* or *no*. To ask open-ended questions, take Kipling's advice:

> I keep six honest serving-men
> (They taught me all I knew);
> Their names are What and Why and When
> and How and Where and Who.
>
> —Rudyard Kipling

Interestingly, people rate others who actually speak very little as good conversationalists. That means that good conversationalists are good listeners who ask a few good questions. People like to talk about themselves if they have an interested listener (Figure 4-1). It works the other way around, too. When you are asked an open-ended question, don't be afraid to reveal something about yourself. This "self-disclosure" is the kind of back-and-forth that creates friendships. When you open up, trust develops and friendships form.

If you have a sense of humor, use it. Sometimes it is hard to know whether it is appropriate to joke around, but you can always test the situation by using a little self-deprecating humor, which will never offend anyone. You should also reflect on topics you know about, so you always have something to talk about, and more importantly, to ask about. Common conversation topics include books, movies, sports, travel, food, music, and hobbies.

FIGURE 4-1 Support group members have a polite conversation (Copyright © istock.com).

At work, however, it is inappropriate to discuss controversial issues. Avoid topics such as politics, religion, immigration, abortion, or divorce.

Respecting Professional and Personal Titles

We may live in a free and equal society, but business etiquette demands that we honor each person's rank, status, and accomplishments. Nowhere is this more apparent than in the etiquette of introductions. In health care settings, where professionals work in teams and patients are usually new to the maze of professionals they encounter, it is important to know how to properly introduce people to one another. In fact, this is such a rarely seen skill that, if you can master it, your ability will mark you as a person of refinement and excellent manners.

Professional Titles

Physicians, of course, should always be addressed and introduced as *Doctor*. In our society, physicians and surgeons are always accorded the title of *Doctor*. Even if you are on a first-name basis with a physician, you should still refer to her and address her as *Doctor* at work.

In fact, any health professional who has earned a doctorate degree in his or her profession should be addressed as *Doctor*, unless he or she directs you otherwise. Thus, an audiologist with a PhD or AuD, a nurse with a PhD or DNSc, and a Respiratory Therapist with a PhD should each be called *Doctor*. You can always clarify the role of a doctorally prepared health professional to a patient by explaining the person's title or role. You can say, "Dr. Appleton is the Assistant Director of Nursing here." Or, "Dr. Loring is one of our Anesthesiologists." Or, "Dr. Harris manages the Speech Therapy Department."

Needless to say, when you are introduced to someone with a *Doctor* in their name, whether the person is a physician or any other doctorally prepared health professional, they may use their first name in their response, but that is not usually an invitation to call the doctor by his or her first name. If you are introduced like this:

"Dr. Tolland, this is Jim Holtz, the new Medical Assistant," and she says, "Hi Jim, I'm Monica Tolland. Welcome aboard," you should assume that she is just being friendly and is not inviting you to call her by her first name, unless she specifically says so. You should reply, "Thank you, Dr. Tolland. It's nice to meet you." If that is where it ends, then she is Dr.

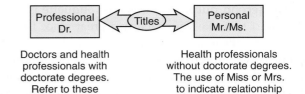

FIGURE 4-2 Professional and personal titles.

Tolland to you. See Figure 4-2 for a diagram on appropriate uses of titles.

Personal Titles

How do you know which feminine title to use when addressing women in the workplace? Women without doctoral degrees should be addressed as "Ms." unless you are specifically told otherwise. The use of "Miss" and "Mrs." to indicate whether a woman is married is outdated. The marital status of any man or woman is irrelevant at work and not something that needs to be disclosed or known for an effective working relationship to take place. Again, if the traditional titles of Miss or Mrs. are preferred, you will be informed. Otherwise, use Ms.

Making Introductions

The main rule about introductions is that you introduce the most important person, or the person with the most authority, first. Gender and age do not matter. However, you must remember this: The client or the patient is *always* the most important person. So when a client or patient is involved, you say:

"Mr. Adler, this is Dr. Berthold, the physician on duty today. Dr. Berthold, this is Saul Adler."

"Ms. Christy, this is Ms. Izzo, the Radiologic Technician. Ms. Izzo, this is Callie Christy."

When a patient is not involved, you revert back to the rule of the person with the highest title being introduced first, and say:

"Dr. Apollo, this is our new Surgical Technician, Sue Hale. Sue, Dr. Apollo is the Chief Resident."

Custom puts physicians and surgeons at the top of the status hierarchy, so introduce them first, even if the other person holds a doctoral degree, and say:

"Dr. Yang, this is Dr. Harold Reading, the new dentist for the clinic. Dr. Reading, Dr. Yang is a neurosurgeon here."

"Dr. Harvey, this is Dr. Bette Ringden, the Psychologist from the patient's school. Dr. Ringden, Dr. Harvey is our Psychiatrist-in-Chief."

Protocols for Introductions

- The most important person, or the person with the highest title, is introduced first.
- As the customer, the client or patient is *always* the most important person and should be introduced first, even to a physician or surgeon.
- Every doctorally prepared health professional should be introduced with the title *Doctor*.
- Physicians and surgeons should be introduced before other doctorally prepared health professionals.
- You can clarify the introduction by explaining the roles of the people you are introducing. This can be especially important in clarifying the role of a doctorally prepared health professional who is not a physician.
- Never address, refer to, or introduce a doctor by his or her first name, unless you are specifically told to do so.

This elegant way of introducing doctors enables the physician to choose whether to address the other person as *Doctor*, which gives the other person the opportunity to state their naming preference.

Very often, the circumstances will prevent you from making the full introduction. You may start out by saying:

"Dr. Hamid, this is Dr. Randall Whitaker, our new epidemiologist," and Dr. Hamid may jump in and say something like, "Hi, I'm Noori Hamid. It's nice to meet you, Dr. Whitaker." At that point, you have done your job, and you can let the newly introduced people settle on protocols for titles and first names.

When you introduce a patient to a doctor correctly, the rest of the introduction is out of your hands. If you say:

"Mr. Quirk, this is Dr. Clark, one of the Primary Care Physicians," and the Doctor interrupts to say, "Hi, Mr. Quirk. Bob Clark," and the patient says, "Nice to meet you, Bob," it is acceptable to move on.

Introductions can be confusing at times, mainly because most people are over-eager to make a good first impression. Protocols for making proper introductions are summarized in Box 4-1.

? WHAT IF?

1. What if you have to introduce someone, but you are not sure of their title or role?
2. What if you have to make an introduction, but you forgot the name of someone you are supposed to know?
3. What if a colleague's name is difficult?

Reliability in the Workplace

Can people count on you? Can you accomplish tasks on time and discreetly? For one thing, punctuality is absolutely essential in health care. The whole operation depends on getting things done on time. Health professionals and patients usually work on an appointment basis, and colleagues who have put in a full shift expect to be relieved on time. However, punctuality is not simply a matter of arriving on time. For example, many tasks have to be performed on a strict schedule. Vital signs may need to be taken at precise intervals. Input and output charts have to be maintained on a careful, timely basis. Meals are usually served at specific times. Breaks are scheduled to ensure a smooth workflow while giving every employee a break from their routine.

In addition to punctuality, discretion and confidentiality are essential to the practice of health care. The HIPAA law of 1996 requires that certain private medical information (PMI) be kept confidential, encoding in law what has always been an ethical responsibility for health care professionals. To protect your patients' medical information, file medical charts promptly and keep them away from anyone not directly involved in the patient's care. It is completely inappropriate to talk about a patient in a public place, inside or outside of your health facility. Whether in an elevator, walking down a corridor, or having lunch in the cafeteria, do not use the patient's name in conversation.

Little Courtesies

The simplest acts of courtesy can create a positive impression and attract people to you with very little effort. For example, a smile and a handshake are among the most open and welcoming gestures you can make (Figure 4-3). Similarly, saying *please* when you ask for something, whether it be information, some help with a task, advice, or some teaching, is all it usually takes to get positive results. Afterward, thanking people for their help makes them glad they gave it, solidifies relationships, and paves the way for future help.

FIGURE 4-3 A nurse greets a patient with a smile (Copyright © istock.com).

Another easy gesture of courtesy that can go a long way is that of addressing people by their name occasionally when you are speaking with them. Don't overdo it, but don't neglect names either. Dale Carnegie, who wrote *How to Make Friends and Influence People,* said that no sound is more pleasing to a person than the sound of his or her own name.

Next, you can earn a lot of respect by simply developing the habit of picking up after yourself and others. Health care facilities generate many little puddles of disorder, whether they are unfiled medical records, rain tracked in through the main entrance, or the leftovers from a medical procedure or treatment. You don't need to be the custodian, but everyone will appreciate your effort.

> *Practice random acts of kindness and senseless acts of beauty.*
>
> —Anne Herbert

Practicing random acts of kindness and paying it forward are two concepts from popular culture that express the idea that, if you do something nice for someone with no expectation of ever being repaid for it, two things will happen. First, the world will be a better place. Second, good things will come back to you. At work, your kindnesses will make your workplace a better place for everyone, and your reputation for kindness will repay you in ways unexpected and deeply rewarding.

When Someone Is Having a Bad Day

Let's face it. Some days will be tougher than others. It doesn't matter what is causing the bad day, whether it is a personal problem or a troubling issue at work. What matters is how you respond on these occasions.

> *Smooth seas do not make skillful sailors.*
>
> —African Proverb

Tackling Your Own Bad Days

If *you* are experiencing a bad day, you can try several strategies for maintaining a positive, professional approach at work:

* **Let work be therapeutic for you.** Even on the worst day, there are many positive aspects of work, such as the people you enjoy seeing, or specific activities you like tackling. Consider throwing yourself into your work as a means of shoving your other problems and concerns to the back of your mind.
* **Act "as if …"** Even if you don't feel like it, act the way you wish you felt. Act *as if* you are friendly. Act *as if* you are enthusiastic. Force yourself to smile. Chances are that your mood will get swept up in the act, and your day will go better.
* **Stop and reframe.** Cognitive psychologists urge people to reframe their outlook to gain a new perspective. Can you reframe your perspective on your problems by imagining how much worse they could be? Can you make a problem smaller in your mind by telling yourself that you will deal with it little by little until it's solved, just like the vast majority of problems you have ever encountered? Can you put the problem out of your mind by telling yourself that there is nothing you can do about it while you are at work, and you will confront the problem later at an appropriate time? If the problem is a work-related conflict, try simply resolving to take the high road rather than engage in disputes that are likely to be both petty and short-lived.
* **Practice mindfulness and relaxation techniques.** Every time you have a quiet moment, close your eyes and take some deep breaths to clear your mind. If you are feeling irritable, pause before you respond to someone and choose your responses thoughtfully. Without sharing too many details, explain to your co-workers that you are having a bad day and appreciate their understanding.

Finally, realize that bad times don't last forever and resolve to make the next day better.

Helping a Co-worker Experiencing a Bad Day

If one of your co-workers is having a bad day, try to be understanding and helpful by following these tips:

* **Make reasonable allowances.** Most people have good intentions, so a bad day can be tolerated now and then.
* **Be willing to listen.** If you are close to the person, you can offer to listen to them. Ask them if there is anything you can do to help.
* **Know when to step aside.** Naturally, if someone else's bad days are extensive enough to be chronic behavior problems, they are beyond your capacity to help. These are matters for supervisors and Human Resource professionals. If someone else's behavior becomes problematic for you, discuss the issue privately with your manager.

Social Networking and Business Etiquette

You probably have a work-related email account and are expected to communicate via email promptly and professionally. Your employer may even have a presence on such sites as LinkedIn, Facebook, and Twitter. In this age of hackers and security breaches, many companies find it necessary to employ filters and monitors that help to ensure responsible Internet use at work. Familiarize yourself with your company's written policies about Internet use, email, and professional social media. If no written policy exists, ask your supervisor what the acceptable practices are at your place of work.

In addition to security vulnerability, employers are as aware as the rest of us that the Internet can chew up a lot of time. Use your computer and Internet access at work only for business purposes. It might be permissible to check your personal email while on a break, but you should not be spending time on Facebook or other social networking sites. Using the Internet and social networking sites for your own interest while at work is contrary to the professionalism you are trying to build (Figure 4-4).

What You Can Expect From Your Workplace

What you can expect from your employer is usually codified by labor law. What you can expect from your colleagues is determined more by general behavior expectations. However, this distinction is not absolute.

Your employer must avoid all discrimination by either colleagues or supervisors. You cannot be sexually harassed or treated unfairly because of your gender, race, ethnicity, age, sexual orientation, disability, or religion and beliefs. You do not have to tolerate physical or verbal threats, coarse language, bullying, or gossip. Your employer must also provide fair compensation and adequate benefits, including time off. You have a right to a safe and drug-free work environment in which your personal information is confidential. Any criticism of you or your work must be delivered in a private and appropriate setting. Your employer's Human Resource professionals ensure compliance with occupational laws and can serve as mediators when disputes or conflicts arise in order to protect both you and your employer.

FIGURE 4-4 A distracted receptionist uses the company computer for her own interests (Copyright © istock.com).

CASE STUDY 4-1
Rookie

Stuart was the latest hire as a drug counselor in a drug treatment clinic in Madison, Wisconsin. He had been the first new hire for quite a long time and the rest of the staff had a strong bond with one another. Stuart learned all this on his first day, when everyone started calling him "Rookie."

The title was fine at first, but it began to annoy him. He actually had more education than many of the other counselors, and had worked with addiction cases for many years. He didn't see himself as a rookie.

After the first week, he found himself pacing around his living room as he talked to his wife. They had a good life in Milwaukee, with many friends and solid reputations at work. He agreed to the move to Madison because his wife, Antonia, a Master Teacher in Milwaukee, had been hired as a principal in Madison. And now, he was being called Rookie, and it looked as though it was going to stick. "I can't seem to connect with these people," he was saying. "They're nice enough to me, but I'm not part of the scene. It's like they speak in code about experiences they've all shared, and I'm on the outside." He shook his head.

"Who do you think should break the ice?" asked Antonia. "Who should take responsibility for it, you or them?"

"Oh, both of us. They have a responsibility too."

"Yes, they do. But you're not them. You can only do what you can do."

On Monday, Stuart decided to be more proactive. He picked up the staff room, which seemed to be in a perpetual state of disarray. He volunteered to run an activity group when one of the regulars became ill. A couple of people noticed the cleaned-up staff room. "It's good to have a rookie around," one person told him.

That night, Antonia asked who the leader was.

"The leader?"

"Yes, the person everyone else looks up to. The one whose opinion seems to matter more than others."

That would definitely be Schechter. She was quiet, but she commanded respect. The next day Stuart took an opportunity to sit down next to her while she was taking a break in the day room.

"What's up, Rookie," she said in her gruff way.

"Not much," said Stuart, "but I thought you could explain something to me."

She looked at him without responding, so he forged ahead.

"We have a lot of tough clients around here. Some are hard and kind of unapproachable, but you don't seem to care. You just go up to anybody and start talking, and pretty soon there's a good exchange going on. What is it about you?"

Schechter proved for the first time that she could actually smile. "I don't care how hard they are. They don't get to come here and be unapproachable. Neil Young said 'Every junkie is a setting sun.' These people don't have many of their nine lives left. They're not going to get much further down the road if they're just hard and unapproachable. That's not an option for me."

"For you?"

"Look Rookie, I lost my brother when I was fifteen. He was my only brother, and he was the only one who cared about me. He was hard and unapproachable. I knew him though. Underneath. I knew that's not the way he really was. But he didn't get any help, and he was dead before he was nineteen. I'm not giving these guys here a pass just because they're unapproachable."

Stuart told her he was sorry about her brother, and he wasn't giving any passes either, and he went back to work. Actually, Stuart felt the same way as Schechter did. He always had. He knew he was doing nobody a favor by letting them evade their issues. He was good at getting into people's faces. He could turn on an intensity that got people's attention, and he could use his body to maneuver a client into a suddenly serious conversation. Stuart had a cool, quiet voice that commanded attention, and he used his skills to get past a client's exterior and into the real issues. So he was on the same wavelength as Schechter, but he hadn't had to lose a brother to get there. He respected her for telling him that. And he was glad they had the same outlook in common.

Later that day, she called him "Rook."

On Wednesday evening Stuart came home to find Antonia collecting bags of flour and sugar on the kitchen counter, with bars of butter and unsweetened chocolate. She was going to make cupcakes for her faculty meeting the next day. Stuart said he would help her, because he wanted to make some extras for the gang at work.

At the staff meeting on Thursday afternoon, the cupcakes put everyone in a good mood. "Hey Rook," said Ted, "what are these sprinkles, Prozac?" Everybody laughed. Sarah said that a man's stomach is the shortest distance to his heart. "No," said Schechter. "It's his chest," and everyone roared. Stuart stayed afterward to pick up the staff room again, since he had made the mess today.

On Friday morning he found Schechter again on a break in the day room.

"Hey Schechter," he said, sitting down. "Do you actually have a first name?"

"Yeah," she said.

Stuart sat there in silence, gazing at the plaster swirls on the ceiling. He thought that if he could just stay silent for a few seconds, she might expand, but she didn't.

"That's OK," he said finally. "I'm sure that Bono and Moby have first names they wouldn't tell me either."

"My first name is Deborah," said Schechter. "But you can call me Shecky. That's what they called my brother. I can see you know what you're doing."

"Thanks, Shecky. You can call me Stuart."

"Not Stu?"

"No. When you call me *Stu*, you take the *art* out of *Stuart*."

Schechter rolled her eyes. "I was going to ask you if your wife made them cupcakes. Now I know she didn't."

"Actually, she did," said Stuart, and they had a good laugh.

At the staff meeting the following Wednesday, it was Stuart's turn to make his first case presentation. He had made these presentations hundreds of times before, and this one was no different, except at the end, he said, "I want to thank everybody for making me feel at home here. I feel like I was the first person that ever got the nickname *Rookie* here. I want to thank you for making me feel special. From now on, you can call me Stuart."

"With the *art*," chimed in Schechter.

"Sure, Rook," said Ted, and everyone laughed. But that was the last time anyone ever called Stuart "Rookie."

Except for Antonia.

QUESTIONS FOR THOUGHT AND REFLECTION

1. What would have happened to Stuart if he had not been proactive in changing the staff's initial perception of him?
2. What actions did Stuart take to establish himself as a member of the team?
3. Who helped Stuart?
4. In your opinion, what was more important: Stuart's ability as a drug counselor or Stuart's ability to fit in with the new team?

Down a Dark Road

Marianne Moscitello was having a bad day at work. First, her sister, who watched her young son during the day, was late. Then, the traffic was bad on her way to work. She arrived at the hospital 15 minutes late, and the administrative medical assistant who was waiting to be relieved yelled at Marianne, telling her she better "get it together," and "maybe you shouldn't be working at a place that expects you to be *on time!*"

Marianne's heart was pounding in her chest while she waited for her angry colleague to leave. "Give it a rest, Grandma," she said under her breath, while the nurses in the nursing station either looked down or made for the exit.

A little while later, one of the residents came in to enter some prescriptions and orders at the computer. All the terminals were busy, so he said brusquely to Marianne, "Do you mind?" She rolled her chair a minimal distance away and glared at him while he logged into his account.

After that, someone from Medical Records came up with an armload of files. "Give it to the new girl," said the charge nurse.

"I've got a name," said Marianne. Nobody asked her what it was.

The next day, Marianne was on time for work, but the person she relieved wasn't any friendlier. After she left, Marianne said in a loud voice, "I can see why she works nights." Everyone in the nursing station looked up. "She's not fit to be around in the daytime," she added. Again, everyone looked down, busied themselves with some work, or made their way toward the door.

That afternoon, after getting home from her shift, Marianne told her sister, "I don't think this job is working out. These people are jerks."

"The people are jerks? At a hospital?"

"Yeah, they're unfriendly. Like hostile. Nobody talks to you, except do this, do that."

"You're new, Marianne. You have to try harder."

"Yeah, you were no help. You made me late on my third day. How do you think *that* made me feel?"

Marianne's sister paused for a moment, trying to choose the best thing to say, and decided to say nothing. She just didn't want to get into it with Marianne.

QUESTIONS FOR THOUGHT AND REFLECTION

1. List the business etiquette mistakes that Marianne made.
2. What could she have done better to handle being late?
3. How would you characterize Marianne's personal style?
4. Is there anything Marianne can do to redeem herself?

⭐ EXPERIENTIAL EXERCISES

1. Practice introducing people.
2. Do something nice for someone today, but make sure they will never know who did it for them.
3. Initiate a conversation with a smile and a compliment. What response did you get?
4. Learn something new about a good friend today by asking her an open-ended question.
5. Create a LinkedIn site for yourself that reflects your professionalism.

↻ CROSS CURRENTS WITH OTHER SOFT SKILLS

LISTENING ACTIVELY: If you learn to listen actively, you will learn a lot and base your behavioral decisions on solid information. (pp. 263-269)

DRESSING FOR SUCCESS: Ralph Waldo Emerson once said to someone, "*Who* you are is speaking so loudly that I can't hear what you're saying." You should know what your appearance is saying about you, and make sure the message is what you want it to be. (pp. 178-183)

PROFESSIONAL PHONE TECHNIQUE: Speaking with customers and clients on the phone is a special case for business etiquette, with its own challenges. (pp. 257-261)

AIMING TO BE ADAPTABLE AND FLEXIBLE: It is hard to model proper business etiquette without a foundation of adaptability. (pp. 25-29)

MAINTAINING CONFIDENTIALITY AND DISCRETION: Every business benefits from discretion. Health care businesses demand it. (pp. 297-302)

Dressing for Success

What a strange power there is in clothing.

—Isaac Bashevis Singer

LEARNING OBJECTIVE 2: DRESSING FOR SUCCESS

- Review the written dress code of your employer.

- Familiarize yourself with Universal Precautions and wear protective garments when needed.
- Develop a strategy for what to wear on special occasions, like casual Fridays or holidays.
- Accept that visible tattoos and piercings are inappropriate in health care workplaces.
- Dress appropriately for your position in clean and pressed clothes.

Dressing well is one of the best things you can do to establish immediate credibility at work, whether in the eyes of your peers, your manager, or your clients and customers. Patients want to encounter health workers whose appearance reflects professionalism and competence.

❓ WHAT IF?

What if a friend or colleague of yours showed up for work in an inappropriate outfit? How would you bring this to his or her attention? What benefits would result from choosing a more appropriate outfit for work?

Everyday Professional Dress

In many health care facilities, employees are expected to wear scrubs or similar loose-fitting uniforms—sanitary garments that offer comfort while identifying you as a health professional. Scrubs are meant to be neutral and professional. They should not be tight, calling attention to your body. But they shouldn't be baggy either, causing safety and sanitation problems. Another alternative is lab coats worn over regular clothing (Figure 4-5). Scrubs and similar uniforms must always be freshly laundered and ironed, so change your scrubs or lab coat if they become soiled on the job. In addition to uniform policies, many facilities require badges for security purposes, identifying you as an employee with access to specific areas.

FIGURE 4-5 Work clothes should be conservative and tasteful.

When you are allowed to wear your own clothes at work, they should be conservative and tasteful. Clearly, there is nothing in these guidelines that says you can't be stylish, fashionable, or consistent with your gender, culture, or religion. Box 4-2 offers some considerations when choosing clothing appropriate for work.

Footwear

Health care professionals are typically on their feet for many hours during the work day. Comfort is certainly a primary consideration in choosing footwear. Other considerations include cleanliness, safety, and style. Many people don't realize that others, especially patients and clients, notice the state of our shoes—particularly whether or not they are clean.

Many workplaces encourage you to choose athletic-style shoes designed specifically for health professionals because they are comfortable, easy to clean, and have rubber soles and traction for safety. You may sometimes be required to wear shoe coverings such as surgical booties for sanitary purposes, although

BOX 4-2

Considerations for Buying and Wearing Work Clothes

- Choose fabrics that resist stains, shrinkage, fading, and wrinkling.
- Select colors and patterns that aren't distracting.
- For women, dresses and skirts should fall around the knee level. Pants or pantsuits may be appropriate.
- For men, trousers and shirts should be clean, pressed, and subdued in color.
- Avoid any clothes that are frayed, worn, ripped, or sloppy.
- Know the difference between your professional work clothes and your casual clothes.

this is becoming less common outside of surgical suites or settings with high risks for infectious diseases. Some traditional worksites encourage wearing white shoes, which require extra care to keep clean—shoelaces included.

Floors in health care workplaces can be slippery, and the pace is often hurried and hectic. If your employer allows ordinary street shoes, keep qualities such as comfort and traction at the top of your mind. Avoid open-toed shoes, high heels, straps, buckles, and ornaments that can be difficult to keep clean.

Jewelry and Body Adornments

Minimal jewelry such as a wedding band or a simple watch is fine, but most jewelry detracts from your professionalism and creates a safety or health hazard. Even tasteful jewelry can scratch, snag, or distract a client or patient. Agitated patients or small children have been known to snatch dangling earrings or necklaces. Jewelry can also collect harmful bacteria, a needless risk for a health professional.

Tattoos and body piercings, with the exception of pierced ears, might offend many of your patients. Make every effort to remove piercing jewelry and cover your tattoos at work.

Special Situations
Casual Fridays

Many workplaces have "casual Fridays" or may specify a preference for daily casual dress. However,

FIGURE 4-6 A, Proper business casual attire. **B,** Proper scrub attire.

an understanding of what constitutes casual work attire can be tricky. Should you play it safe and wear khakis and a polo shirt? Are denim skirts or blue jeans all right? Certainly, you should never wear shorts to work, unless they are specifically authorized. Even then, the health professional should be careful not to wear anything too revealing. No matter how casual the dress code, there is such a thing as *too* casual. Carefully investigate the guidelines where you work.

JOURNALING 4-4

Describe your style of dress. Differentiate between your weekend and the work week style. What influences have contributed to your style? Do you need to make any changes for work? How will you come to terms with these changes? Describe the role of dress at work.

Other Special Occasions

There may be other occasions during the course of a year that involve special considerations for dress. Some employers encourage employees to dress up for certain holidays, company photographs, or special visits from prominent local figures or the media. Finally, when representatives from accrediting organizations such as The Joint Commission arrive, your appearance and behavior should reflect positively on your employer.

The people depicted in Figure 4-6 display appropriate work attire.

JOURNALING 4-5

Record your thoughts about tattoos. Are some tasteful, while others are not? Why do people get tattoos? What messages are they trying to send? How might clients react to seeing a tattoo on their health care provider?

Special Attire to Reduce Risk of Infection

In treatment settings, patients with infectious diseases require the use of the most current Universal Precautions. These precautions affect the way you dress. You are likely to have to use gloves and even masks or surgical booties, which are often situated in the nurses' station or outside of a patient's room or a quarantined area. You may have to use a disposable paper gown to cover your uniform or clothing in such a situation. Your clothing choices should make it easy for you to put on these additional safety garments. The health care worker in Figure 4-7 is outfitted to protect himself and his patients from infections.

I base most of my fashion sense on what doesn't itch.

—Gilda Radner

FIGURE 4-7 A health care professional in a mask, disposable gown, and surgical booties. (From Proctor DB, Adams AP: *Kinn's the medical assistant: an applied learning approach*, ed 12, St Louis, 2014, Elsevier.)

First Impressions Last

On your first day at work, your peers and colleagues will formulate an impression of you in seven seconds. Every day, the process repeats as you meet clients or patients. Negative first impressions are difficult to overcome. Fortunately, dressing for a good first impression is something you can control.

> *Seldom do people discern eloquence under a threadbare cloak.*
>
> —Juvenal

CASE STUDY 4-2
A Difficult Conversation

Bill was very happy with Mary, the Medical Assistant he inherited from his predecessor. She was efficient and friendly. She answered his calls with professionalism and a cheerful note in her voice. One day, Bill stopped to talk with Helen, the vice president of Human Resources, in the hallway. She said, "Bill, did you see the announcement about the new dress code we're implementing?"

"Yes I did," he said, thinking privately to himself that he didn't care much for dress codes.

"What do you think of it?"

"It seems fine. But why do you think we need a dress code?

"Because of your assistant!" she almost snarled.

"Mary?"

"Yes! She wears those hip-hugger, capri things, and I've even seen her in a halter top!"

Bill knew that Mary's apparel was overly casual, but he hadn't given much thought to it. He wasn't really sure if he knew what a halter top was, and he had no idea what capris were. He felt somewhat annoyed to have been given this information. Perhaps he should have been more aware of the problem and done something about it already. Helen was always dressed appropriately in her gray pantsuit and sensible shoes.

Bill became concerned that Mary's style of dress could limit her opportunities. Apparently, it had already tarnished her reputation with some important people in the company. He decided to talk to Mary about her appearance.

"You know," he said to Mary in the privacy of a small conference room, "the way you dress is a problem."

"A problem?"

"Yes," he said. "For one thing, it's not in compliance with the new dress code. In fact, it's one of the reasons we have a new dress code."

Mary blushed with embarrassment and rising indignation. "Nobody's said anything to me before."

"Well, I'm saying it now."

"You know, I don't make much money here. I can't afford to buy fancy outfits." Mary was becoming defensive, probably without realizing it.

Bill decided to do a little reality testing with Mary. "You know," he said, "appropriate clothes don't cost any more than inappropriate clothes. It's all a matter of the choices you make when you shop. Your attire is certainly stylish—it's just not right for work."

At this point, Mary couldn't hide her anguish anymore, and she covered her face. Bill fell silent. He didn't know what to say and thought it might be best to let Mary have some privacy.

After a moment, he said, "Mary, you're excellent at your job and I'm very happy with your work. I'm having this conversation with you because I want you to succeed here and it would be unfortunate if your clothing were to interfere with your success. Will you give this some thought and consideration?"

Mary looked up and nodded.

The next day, Mary arrived wearing a white blouse and a pencil skirt. That afternoon, a young mother and her two small children were sitting in the waiting room. The mother's arm was in a sling and she seemed to be in pain. Mary introduced herself to the patient and asked her if she could take the children to the "playroom." The patient nodded, and Mary took the girls to a conference room with a big white board and lots of dry-erase markers. They played a few games of tic-tac-toe and then drew pictures. Mary transferred her calls to the phone in the conference room until the patient's appointment was over.

Shortly before the office closed, Bill called the medical assistants together and praised Mary for thinking on her feet and showing initiative in helping the patient and her family. A week later, Bill posted a handwritten letter from the mother, thanking his team for the caring and professionalism. There were also two crayon "portraits" of Mary enclosed in the envelope.

QUESTIONS FOR THOUGHT AND REFLECTION

1. Why do you think Mary might have had such little knowledge of what to wear in a professional health care setting?
2. Would you have handled this difficult conversation differently from the way Bill did?
3. If you were Mary, what would you have wanted Bill to do, under the circumstances?
4. What were the benefits of the caring that Mary demonstrated toward the patient's children?

Down a Dark Road

Lucy was a very competent member of the Emergency Department team at the hospital in her home town. She had special certification as an IV nurse, and she had a natural ability to perform such difficult skills as intubating patients. Her smile and a warm personality put patients at ease … once they got past her appearance!

One day she would wear a red skirt straight out of the 1940s, short in the front and long in the back. The next day she would wear a blouse with a shaggy fur collar. "Where do you get these things?" her friends would ask. "The Costumery?" Lucy would roll her eyes and brush off any discussion of her odd clothing style. But the physician in charge of the Emergency Department, Dr. Arthur, had lost patience with Lucy's strange appearance. "Do something about it," he told her supervisor. "It's an embarrassment." Natalie Palermo, the nursing supervisor, had tried to broach the topic with Lucy, but Lucy became sullen and refused to engage with Natalie. Lucy knew that everyone valued her clinical skills. But she didn't realize that, over time, she had become a "problem employee."

For one thing, everyone discussed the "Lucy problem" behind her back. Each day, Lucy's outlandish apparel became the subject of gossip. Natalie knew that this could not go on indefinitely. "What about an intervention?" suggested Mark, one of the EMTs. Natalie realized she had to do *something* so she arranged a meeting with Lucy for the next day. "I have to tell you," Natalie told her, "it's about your dress and professionalism." Lucy gave her the usual wordless scowl.

The next day, Lucy showed up in a pair of black slacks with a satin stripe down the sides, and a yellow cotton jersey with a smiley face pattern. Natalie got right to the point. "Lucy, you're a great clinician, but you dress like a clown."

"What?" said Lucy. "You can't talk to me like that!"

Ignoring her reaction, Natalie pressed on. "Your clothing contradicts the professionalism we're trying to convey in this department. Everyone likes and respects you, Lucy. But I'm not willing to tolerate it any longer. I need for you to take a clue from your colleagues here and dress in a professional, low-key manner that doesn't call negative attention to yourself and arouse concern in our patients. I'm telling you that you must improve your appearance to maintain your position here."

Lucy glanced over her shoulder at the closed office door, as if she wanted to escape this uncomfortable conversation, or at least ensure that nobody was within earshot.

"I've got a right to my personal style," she said. "I'm not some carbon copy of what you think I should be. I do my job very well, and that's all you should be concerned with. When you have a complaint about my clinical skills, let me know." With that, she got up and left the room, brushing past Dr. Arthur, who had just happened by.

As soon as Lucy turned the corner, Dr. Arthur shrugged his shoulders and opened his palms toward Natalie.

"I know, I know," she said. "She's just not willing to listen."

"Well, it's time to get HR involved," he said. "In the meantime, keep her out of the lobby and away from the patients' families as much as possible."

QUESTIONS FOR THOUGHT AND REFLECTION

1. Why do you think Lucy has chosen to respond to Natalie like this?
2. If you were Lucy's friend, what would you advise her?
3. If Lucy listened to your advice, what should her next move be?

⭐ EXPERIENTIAL EXERCISES

1. Spend a half-hour in a hospital lobby. It is easy to identify the staff? Are there staff members who, in your opinion, are particularly well dressed? Are there others who, in your perception, dress poorly or inappropriately?
2. Visit a local uniform store. Introduce yourself to the manager or owner, who can be a very knowledgeable resource to you, and discuss appropriate clothing options at health care facilities in your area. Examine the uniforms in the store and the various options. Learn about pricing, styles, colors, fabrics, and procedures for laundering and ironing.
3. What have you learned about professional attire while you have been a student? Are the school's dress code guidelines consistent with dress codes at local employers?
4. Prepare a checklist that details all the steps you should follow as you get dressed for work each day.

🔄 CROSS CURRENTS WITH OTHER SOFT SKILLS

ADOPTING A POSITIVE MENTAL ATTITUDE: Your clothing can reflect your attitude, positive or negative. (pp. 2-11)

DISPLAYING GOOD GROOMING, PERSONAL HYGIENE, AND CLEANLINESS: These are as important to your appearance and professionalism as *DRESSING FOR SUCCESS.* (pp. 183-189)

READING AND SPEAKING BODY LANGUAGE: Your dress is part of your body language, and your body language can dress up your clothing, appearance, and professionalism. (pp. 277-284)

FOLLOWING RULES AND REGULATIONS: You want your appearance to be within the range of appropriate guidelines at your place of employment. (pp. 291-297)

EXUDING OPTIMISM, ENTHUSIASM, AND POSITIVITY: Appropriate dress enhances your positivity; let your dress help your enthusiasm shine through! (pp. 380-384)

Displaying Good Grooming, Personal Hygiene, and Cleanliness

People often say that motivation doesn't last. Well, neither does bathing—that's why we recommend it daily.

—Zig Ziglar

LEARNING OBJECTIVE 3: DISPLAYING GOOD GROOMING, PERSONAL HYGIENE, AND CLEANLINESS

■ Review any written procedures pertaining to personal hygiene and grooming at your place of employment.

- Know what scents are appropriate for the workplace.
- Present yourself as a model of proper grooming for the workplace.
- List five solid strategies for maintaining sanitary hands.
- Explain ways in which pathogens can be spread at work.
- Explain how to change a habit.

Because there is a direct correlation between poor personal hygiene and transmissible illness, it is critical that health care workers understand and practice good basic hygiene habits, including proper hand washing, on a regular basis. Your healthy, vibrant appearance inspires confidence in people who have come to your facility to improve their own health, or visit family members and friends they care about. Some information in this section may not apply to you, but most professionals benefit from touching base now and then with a checklist of basic personal care.

The Health Care Professional's Checklist of Personal Work Hygiene

In our society, we face constant exposure to pollution, car exhaust, heat, and sweat. In addition, working in a health care facility will expose you to even more germs, odors, and dirt. Over the course of a day, your skin gets oily, your hair becomes drab, and bacteria accumulate on your skin. Practicing daily hygiene will ensure that you arrive at work looking clean and smelling fresh.

What separates two people most profoundly is a different sense and degree of cleanliness.

—Friedrich Nietzsche

JOURNALING 4-6

Talk with an elderly family member, friend, or client. Ask about hygiene practices from when they were young. What did they have to do to maintain proper personal hygiene? How much extra time and effort did it take? Write what you learned, and reflect on how much easier it is to maintain your personal hygiene in the 21st century.

The following checklist is a good basic guideline for daily personal hygiene for the health care professional:

- **Shower or bathe, and shampoo daily**—both before and after work if possible.
- **Use deodorant** after showering, especially unscented or lightly scented products.
- **Touch up your hair as needed** during the day; wear longer hair back or up so it does not hang in your face, impair your vision, or touch a patient in the course of your work.
- **Choose a hair style that does not call undue attention to itself.** In the health care setting, avoid hair that is dyed an unnatural color.
- **Apply makeup modestly.** If you wear makeup, use it sparingly. Although none of it is inappropriate, less is better.
- **Never wear fragrances at work.** Health facilities are loaded with people who are allergic to these products.
- **Cut your fingernails short,** straight across, and rounded at the corners. Keeping your nails trimmed will protect your nerve-rich fingertips, enable you to pick up small objects, and minimize the collection of disease-causing germs. Long, polished, and artificial fingernails are all germ hot spots.
- **Practice daily dental hygiene.** There are a host of benefits to good dental health. You should brush your teeth and floss at least twice daily. When brushing, remember to brush your gums as well. If you have cavities, tooth decay, gum disease, or teeth that are missing, chipped, or discolored, you should see a dentist. Box 4-3 lists tips on how to maintain oral hygiene.
- **Practice proper hand-washing technique all day.** A nail brush is one of the best small investments you can make in your arsenal of personal hygiene supplies. The stiff bristles whisk away dirt and germs. See Box 4-4 for a list of ways germs can be spread.

WHAT IF?

What if you had a friend who had a grooming problem? How would you try to help your friend?

Hand Washing

In the health care professions, special attention needs to be paid to hand-washing technique (Figure 4-8). Agents that cause disease (called *pathogens*) can be harbored in the hair, skin, nails, nose, eyes, blood, feces, mucus, saliva, lymph, and urine of an infected

Elements of a Good Personal Oral Hygiene Program

- Brush your teeth twice a day with toothpaste and a toothbrush bought within the last three months.
- Consider brushing your teeth after lunch, especially when you are working, since certain spices and foods can cause lasting bad breath.
- Brush for at least two minutes, paying attention to both the insides and outsides of your teeth, all four quarters of your mouth, and molars in the back, which can be hard to reach but are just as susceptible to decay as any other teeth.
- Use an antimicrobial mouthwash for good gum health and fresh breath.
- Floss your teeth twice a day. This is the only way to effectively clean between your teeth and under your gum line for good gum health.
- Scrape your tongue to remove bacteria that causes bad breath.
- Drink lots of water, and use it to flush food particles away from your teeth.

Common Ways Germs Spread

- Sick employees
- Unwashed hands or contaminated gloves
- Employees with open cuts and scrapes
- Employees who touch their faces and mouths with their hands
- Improperly disposed hygienic items (e.g., toilet paper, paper towels)
- Employees who do not wash their hands after using the restroom
- Unwashed and poorly sanitized preparation surfaces, utensils, and preparation areas
- Soiled wiping cloths and cleaning items

FIGURE 4-8 Thorough handwashing helps workers maintain a safe, sanitary health care environment (Copyright © istock.com).

Hands touch. They touch all the other bodily fluids and surfaces where pathogens live, and they touch your patients. Health care facilities are loaded with germs because the patients are sick and the environment is exposed to the bodily fluids where pathogens live. There is no question that the most important thing you can do to prevent the transmission of disease is to wash your hands frequently and properly. In fact, unless you are effective in your hand washing habits, you endanger your own health as much as that of your patients.

Therefore, you must establish sound, scientific hand-washing procedures right now and follow them throughout your career. Box 4-5 outlines the steps for properly washing your hands.

Much of the success of hand washing depends on the *frequency* and *timing* with which you wash your hands. First, you should recognize that your hands will accumulate dirt and germs over time even if you are not dressing a wound or collecting a urine specimen. Almost every surface or object you touch, whether a sink faucet or a computer keyboard, will transfer germs to your hands. Box 4-6 lists common places in the workplace where germs lurk. Develop the habit of washing your hands every hour or two at least, regardless of the type of work you are doing.

There are also many occasions when you *must* wash your hands (Box 4-7), sometimes *before* an activity (changing a dressing or administering care), and sometimes *after* (working with lab specimens or bodily fluids). Your workplace may even have specific rules about when to wash your hands. Ultimately, however, effective hand washing depends on your own good judgment, persistence, and personal commitment to the best possible sanitation you can bring to your work.

person, occurring in the form of some types of bacteria, viruses, toxins, parasites, chemicals, and even metals. The primary way that these pathogens are transmitted, however, is through contact with the hands.

BOX 4-5

Proper Hand-Washing Steps

1. Remove rings and bracelets except for plain wedding bands.
2. Use soap and warm running water. Heat offers a hostile environment for many pathogens.
3. Lather hands and arms up to elbows with soap, for 20 seconds. Silently, recite "Happy Birthday" twice.
4. Wash the backs of hands, wrists, between fingers, and under fingernails using a nailbrush.
5. Rinse hands and arms under running water.
6. Dry hands and arms with clean, disposable paper towels. Turn off running water with a paper towel, *not* with your bare hands.
7. If your place of employment has a hand sanitizer policy, this is the time to use hand sanitizer. Never use hand sanitizer to replace hand washing.

BOX 4-6

Common Sites for Germs in the Health Care Setting

- Floors and floor drains
- Cooling coils and cooling ducts
- Medical equipment
- Trash and medical waste receptacles
- Sinks, spigots, and handles
- Computer equipment, especially keyboards
- Examination tables and chairs

Disposable Gloves

Gloves do not replace proper hand washing. Disposable gloves become dirty, just like hands. Change your gloves every time you wash your hands, and wash your hands every time you change your gloves. However, using gloves properly and consistently helps establish a safe, sanitary environment for you and your patients. You should know how to don, remove, and dispose of gloves in a safe, effective manner.

BOX 4-7

When to Wash Your Hands

Before:
- Touching a patient
- Examining a patient
- Putting on new gloves
- Preparing food
- Consuming food
- Cleaning equipment and preparation surfaces

After:
- Visiting the restroom
- Touching any bare human body part, including skin, ears, nose, hair, or eyes
- Handling garbage, trash, or hazardous medical waste
- Smoking or doing other activities that soil your hands

Skin Wounds and Hand Sanitation

Working in health care, you will inevitably fall prey to cuts and burns on your hands. Every little incident, from a paper cut to a scrape against a rough surface, opens a new pathway to pathogens. A finger cot, a waterproof bandage, or gloving can minimize the dangers of cuts and open sores. You should treat even the most minor abrasion as a personal mini-emergency.

Hand Sanitizers

Alcohol-based hand sanitizers are now standard equipment at most health care facilities, sometimes with stations placed outside every patient or examination room. Research shows that hand sanitizers can be more effective than hand washing for removing germs from skin and nails, but they do not eliminate the need for effective hand washing. Instead, the increasing presence of hand sanitizer stations in your workplace should remind you to be vigilant and relentless in your efforts to keep your hands and nails as clean and virtually germ-free as possible at all times.

For Smokers

Any employer can refuse to let you smoke on company premises or on company time. The smell of smoke on your clothing, hair, or breath can be unpleasant for patients and clients. For that reason, you must make every effort to eliminate the smell of smoke and tobacco on your person if you do smoke. Even if you can't smell it, the odor of tobacco is likely to linger on your fingertips and elsewhere.

CASE STUDY 4-3
Twenty-One Days a Habit Makes

Elena Galindo grew up in a poor but loving family in California's Central Valley. She often says she didn't know she was poor until she got her first job as a licensed vocational nurse. Growing up, Elena and her two sisters moved constantly as her parents sought work.

Wherever they lived, the whole neighborhood became part of the family. At school, Elena was outgoing and a good student. Every time Elena moved, her friends would cry to see her go.

Most of the homes, apartments, and rooms they occupied were primitive. Still, Elena's mother always made sure her daughters were dressed in clean clothes, especially when they were in school. Elena's father was strict about homework, and he scrutinized the girls' friends, especially the boys, as they grew older. He wanted his children to escape from the life that he and Maria had lived. At her last high school, Elena enrolled in the LVN program at the adjoining Vo-Tech campus. She was good at science, and she was naturally warm and caring.

Elena passed her NCLEX-PN Exam on her first try and got a good job at a health clinic. Ultimately she wanted to be a public health nurse, but she was happy with her first job, where she vaccinated babies, took vital signs, and managed medical records. She was a good writer, and she was assigned to various writing jobs like revising the procedures manual and compiling an occasional internal newsletter.

One day she was working with Alberta, the community liaison manager, on a brochure they were writing together, to be distributed at area work sites and migrant camps. Suddenly Alberta stood up from her chair and said, "I gotta tell you, girl. You smell bad."

"It's hot. I've been working all day. Of course I do," she replied tentatively.

"No, I mean a lot. What do you do, take a shower every Saturday night?"

Elena was taken aback, but she didn't say anything.

"Listen, there are big things ahead for you, but you've got to get your act together," Alberta continued. "I'm going to put you on a program."

"A program?" Elena laughed nervously.

"A 21-day program to the rest of your life." Alberta went on to explain that it takes 21 days to form a new habit. "But you have to do the new thing every single day—no exceptions," she said.

Alberta took a fresh sheet of paper and drew a grid, 21 by 4. "Every day, for the next three weeks, you're going to report to me about four things," she told Elena. "Did you take a shower? Did you wash your hair? Did you use deodorant? Did you brush your teeth?"

"I always brush my teeth," said Elena.

"Good. Keep it up. If you do these four things for 21 days straight, with no exceptions—and I'm going to have to take your word for it on the weekends—then I'm going to take you to my spa for a massage, and makeover. I'm going to hold you accountable every day."

Elena nodded and quickly finished her work on the brochure. Her skin burned, but she was just stubborn enough to rise to this silly challenge. Anyway, she liked Alberta and it would be fun to spend a day in a spa.

The first several days were easy. Every day at work, Alberta would give her hair a sniff, and Elena could see the chart that Alberta had made was filling up.

"It takes 21 days to change a habit," Alberta kept saying. "Keep going."

On the tenth day, Elena overslept. She rushed through the bathroom and scrubbed the oil off her face, but she had no time for a shower, much less to wash her hair. She scrutinized her hair. After having washed it every day, she liked the luster her formerly drab hair had developed. Today it was drab and limp again. She shook some talcum powder into it, but that made it look worse. All day, she avoided Alberta at work, but it was awkward, and she noticed

Alberta looking at her occasionally. Alberta didn't ask to sniff her hair that day.

After work, Elena went home, but the lapse in her plan to form a new habit bothered her. The apartment building had a little workout room in the basement next to the laundry area, so she went down there and jogged on the treadmill for a half-hour. Then she went up to her apartment and took a shower. It was one of the best showers she had ever had.

Elena finished off the 21 days in a breeze. It worked! It seemed so natural to take a shower and wash her hair when she woke up. Alberta gave Elena her completed scorecard and they planned to spend the next Saturday at the spa.

QUESTIONS FOR THOUGHT AND REFLECTION

1. Now that you know it takes 21 days to change a habit, is there a habit you would like to establish in your life?
2. The trip to the spa was a reward that Elena found meaningful. What reward would you give yourself if you were going to change a habit?
3. Elena had a lot going for her because of her strong family background. What strengths do you carry from your background?
4. Did skipping a day discourage Elena?
5. How did Elena's personal goals help her make these changes?

 WHAT IF?

What if you saw a colleague biting his fingernails? How would you explain and illustrate the dangers of this habit?

 JOURNALING 4-7

Explain the importance of personal cleanliness to health care workers in a health care facility. Include your thoughts on why this skill is named *Displaying Good Grooming, Personal Hygiene, and Cleanliness.*

Down a Dark Road

THE TRUE STORY OF TYPHOID MARY

Mary Mallon was born in Ireland in 1869, and she immigrated to America when she was 15, settling in New York City. Like many Irish-Americans at the time, Mary found work as a domestic servant. Soon, her talent for cooking became apparent, so she sought better-paying positions as a cook.

In the summer of 1906, a wealthy New York banker, Charles Henry Warren, rented a house in Oyster Bay, Long Island, for a family vacation. He hired Mary Mallon as a cook. Within three weeks, six of the eleven members of Mr. Warren's family had come down with typhoid fever, a potentially serious bacterial illness spread by water and food. The owner of the summer rental, George Thompson, feared that he would never be able to rent his house again unless the cause of the outbreak was found, so he hired an investigator, George Soper, to get to the bottom of the puzzling case. Although typhoid fever was fairly common among poor people around 1900, especially those living in unsanitary conditions, it was a rare disease among the rich.

Soper discovered that, between 1900 and 1906, Mary Mallon had worked as a cook for seven families, and 22 cases of typhoid fever were reported shortly after her hiring, including one who died. Soper thought this was more than a coincidence, and he wanted to obtain blood, stool, and urine samples from Mary Mallon. This was when the trouble began.

Mary Mallon was not a person to mess with. She was big and strong. She had a terrible temper, and spoke coarsely. The Irish immigrants were commonly discriminated against at this time, and Mary was very touchy about being a victim of prejudice. She was healthy and had never had typhoid fever. She refused to provide samples of her bodily fluids to Mr. Soper.

Officials of the New York Board of Health arrived, and they received the same response from Mary. Finally, the police got involved, and it took five officers to wrestle Mary into an ambulance. Having obtained the desired samples by force, the health officials confirmed that she carried the *salmonella typhi* bacteria. In a case that was controversial even at that time, Miss Mallon, who had committed no crime, was remanded by the courts to a hospital island in the East River off the Bronx. Everyone else who was quarantined there was sick, but not Mary Mallon.

From Leavitt, Judith Walzer. *Typhoid Mary: Captive to the public's health*, Boston, 1996, Beacon Press, p. 180.

She sued the New York State Board of Health unsuccessfully but engaged a sympathetic public. "This contention that I am a perpetual menace in the spread of typhoid germs is not true," she said. "My own doctors say I have no typhoid germs. I am an innocent human being. I have committed no crime and I am treated like an outcast—a criminal. It is unjust, outrageous, uncivilized. It seems incredible that in a Christian community a defenseless woman can be treated in this manner." In 1910, a new Commissioner for the New York State Board of Public Health agreed to release Mary Mallon upon her promise and affidavit never to work as a cook again.

Grudgingly, Mary agreed, even though she never believed she was guilty of spreading typhoid fever. She worked in a laundry for some time, but the pay was low. Soon, there was an Irish-American cook, a "Mrs. Brown," who was hired to cook the staff's meals at the Sloan Maternity Hospital in Lower Manhattan. In 1915, 22 doctors and nurses at the hospital came down with typhoid, and two died. Mrs. Brown was soon unmasked as Mary Mallon, and she was returned to the quarantine island in the East River where she remained until her death at the age of 69 in 1938.

Mary had caused a total of 47 cases of typhoid fever, and three of those people died. Many other typhoid carriers caused many more cases and deaths, but none were quite so cantankerous as Miss Mallon. She never believed that she was a typhoid carrier, since she was healthy and had never had typhoid. It is likely that she contaminated so many people, though, because she didn't wash her hands as well and as frequently as she should have, especially after using the bathroom, when she worked as a cook.

Toward the end of her life, Mary Mallon was trained as a laboratory assistant and worked at the quarantine center and provided care to the sick people who were quarantined there. But the New York newspapers had long ago dubbed her "Typhoid Mary," a name she hated and no one would dare call her to her face. An autopsy revealed that the typhus bacteria were found in her gallbladder. Her mother had contracted typhoid fever back in Ireland, when she was pregnant with Mary.

Today, typhoid fever is rare. It is easily controlled by sanitary living conditions. Even carriers pose little risk, as long as they wash their hands carefully after using the bathroom.

QUESTIONS FOR THOUGHT AND REFLECTION

1. Was it fair that Mary Mallon was, in effect, incarcerated for much of her life? How would Mary Mallon's case be handled in today's society?
2. To what extent did Mary's personality contribute to her troubles?
3. What could Mary Mallon have done to reduce the risk of her spreading typhoid fever?
4. Why is typhoid fever so much less of a health problem today than it was just 100 years ago?

⭐ EXPERIENTIAL EXERCISES

1. Create a 21-day chart and record the successful completion of good grooming habits you want to maintain or create.
2. Use sticky notes to label places in your workplace where germs are likely to lurk.
3. What are the regulations in your workplace regarding smoking? Hand washing? Grooming and cleanliness?

Ⓢ CROSS CURRENTS WITH OTHER SOFT SKILLS

DRESSING FOR SUCCESS: So much of what you wear to work and at work has a direct bearing on your grooming, hygiene, and cleanliness. (pp. 178-183)
READING AND SPEAKING BODY LANGUAGE: Your personal hygiene is part of your body language. Poor personal hygiene *screams* in body language. (pp. 277-284)
FOLLOWING RULES AND REGULATIONS: Some aspects of your grooming and cleanliness are nonnegotiable. Whether they are Universal Precautions established by the CDC or rules in force at your workplace, your commitment must be to follow them without exception. (pp. 291-297)

CHAPTER 5

Gaining Energy and Reducing Stress

THEMES TO CONSIDER

- Build energy to support perseverance.
- Differentiate between short-term and long-term energy-building strategies.
- State why drug abuse and dependency are a special risk for health care professionals.
- Know what to do if a co-worker uses or diverts drugs.
- Gain insight into the physiological aspects of stress.
- Build a personal strategy for combating stress.

Gaining Energy, Persistence, and Perseverance

Nothing in the world can take the place of persistence. Talent will not; nothing is more common than unsuccessful men with talent. Genius will not; unrewarded genius is almost a proverb. Education will not; the world is full of educated derelicts. Persistence and determination alone are omnipotent.

—Calvin Coolidge

LEARNING OBJECTIVE 1: GAINING ENERGY, PERSISTENCE, AND PERSEVERANCE

- Name the basic elements of human energy.
- Know how to pace yourself.
- Apply strategies for boosting your energy when you need a lift.
- Know long-term strategies for developing higher energy.
- Understand why persistence works.

Health professions are physically and mentally demanding. The fast-paced environment is full of problems to solve and decisions to make. The work requires good judgment because answers are rarely black and white. A lot is at stake, including lives. It takes a lot of energy and persistence to be a health professional (Figure 5-1).

Think about the challenges a health professional faces on a typical day that take persistence to overcome. You might have to:

* Guide a confused and fragile patient
* Find an artery to take blood
* Keep a small child busy

FIGURE 5-1 With energy and persistence, a student can overcome obstacles and become a confident, competent medical professional (Copyright © istock.com).

* Communicate with someone who speaks little English or who is deaf
* Document a difficult incident
* Make sense of a cluster of lab results
* Mix dental cement perfectly
* Dispense medications correctly, determine blood gases, improve a client's range of motion, enter reimbursement codes for patients with multiple diagnoses and treatments

The list is virtually endless. You need strategies to build, maintain, and boost your energy.

Major Sources of Energy

How many times have you heard that your body needs fuel? While this is true, it's just one piece of the puzzle. Energy requires a balanced diet, physical activity, adequate sleep, satisfying work, and opportunities for positive interaction. A gap in any of these components can really sap your energy levels.

Get Enough to Eat and Drink, But Not Too Much

Let's start with nutrition, since food is the primary source of energy. Just eating is not enough. In order to function well on a daily basis, you need to choose food that produces stable blood sugar and provides vital nutrients throughout the day. Eating a healthy breakfast is important to your energy as well as keeping your weight in check. A mix of protein, healthy fats, and carbohydrates low on the glycemic scale will help you to start your day alert and will keep you energized until lunch. Hydration is also necessary in maintaining healthy circulation and normal brain function.

In many health care settings, there are days when you will have little or no time for lunch. A supply of low-glycemic snacks stashed away in your purse or backpack may come in handy on these days. Nuts, dried fruit, or energy bars are easy to store and eat whenever you have a spare moment or need to energize yourself.

Get Active

It may seem like a paradox, but exercise is energizing. Physical activity that gets you moving will increase your energy. Many people think exercise will tire them out, and it's true that *too much* exercise can tire you out. Many jobs require a person to sit all day, often staring at a computer screen. This will make anyone tired. If your job is sedentary, you should plan activity throughout the day. Maybe a trip to the gym before work is your style. Maybe walking works for you, whether it's a long walk or a few quick laps around the parking lot. Taking the stairs, volunteering for errands, or checking on patients will all keep you moving and keep your energy up.

Get Enough Sleep

Neuroscientists still have much to learn about sleep. It seems that the body uses sleep to repair cells, and the brain uses sleep to cement memories and integrate experience and learning in the form of building neural connections. Your body needs a minimum amount of sleep in order to perform these functions. The necessary amount varies, but it is usually between six and eight hours. Adolescents may need at least ten hours of sleep to thrive, and infants may need at least sixteen.

Who hasn't had the experience of going to bed so tired that you cannot imagine ever recovering, and then waking up eight hours later feeling refreshed? Clearly, something quite restorative happens during sleep.

By the same token, the consequences of too little sleep, especially on a prolonged basis, can be devastating to your state of mind and energy level (Figure 5-2). Your critical thinking skills deteriorate, leading to poor decisions and bad judgment. Your alertness is submerged, leading you to overlook important cues when communicating and treating patients. Your mood and emotions may be brittle, causing you to experience anger, depression, or frustration you

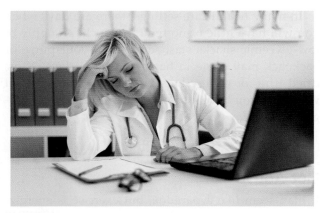

FIGURE 5-2 Sleep deprivation interferes with a health professional's ability to focus (Copyright © istock.com).

would normally move past. Somebody who is sleep-deprived is in no condition to be at work.

WHAT IF?

What if you didn't get enough sleep last night? What will you do to manage the work day ahead? What actions will you take to correct the lack of sleep you got?

Find Work You Love

As a health professional, you have chosen work that is meaningful and socially proactive, so you have already made a good choice in finding engaging work. Health professions are a unique blend of novel challenges such as physical activity, demanding thinking, social connection, and spiritual meaning. The more skilled and intuitive you become, the more engaged you can be as your interest and energy levels increase.

Still, even engaged professionals have to constantly renew their engagement at work. For one thing, even the most interesting work can lose its appeal if it becomes routine. To combat this tendency, you can reframe your view of your role. You can recognize that you are a big help to many people every day, even people you may not know such as family members of your patients. You may be an inspiration to others. Even if your job seems routine, take pride in the skills you worked so long to develop.

Besides adjusting your attitude, you can also adjust your routine. Introduce yourself to co-workers you don't know, or learn more about those you don't know well. Have lunch with different people. Learn a new skill. Research a health issue you encounter frequently. Drive to work by a different

route. Every novel change can renew interests you once treasured.

Connect With People

Human beings are wired to interact with other people, and health professionals have a particularly strong need to relate to people. Take advantage of this human need to create and build energy. A conversation, a discussion, a sharing of interests, the solving of a problem, a group decision, a feeling of connection in a crisis—these are all energy-building experiences because they fulfill our need for social connection.

Short-term Strategies for Boosting Energy

Everyone's energy fluctuates throughout the day because of our circadian rhythms, eating patterns, stress, emotional experiences, work load, and general health. So how do you boost energy when you really need it during those low-energy times? Plan ahead. Only *you* really know your individual energy pattern. Align the day's tasks to coincide with your own high-energy times as much as possible. If you have an energy dip after lunch, for instance, plan tasks that keep you moving around to restore your energy. Pick a time for your most mentally demanding tasks when you know you will be alert and able to concentrate. Let's examine some of the tools you have at your disposal to recharge your energy throughout the day.

JOURNALING 5-1

Outline your typical energy cycle throughout the day. Align your typical daily activities with your energy cycle.

Activity Tools

Use quick bursts of movement and activity to raise your energy (Figure 5-3). For instance, if you practice yoga, self-defense, aerobics, or dance, you can take a moment to perform a favorite exercise to increase your heart rate and circulation. Other activity tools include:

* Breathe deeply ten times, exhaling twice as long as you inhale. Concentrating on your breathing delivers oxygen to your brain and, more importantly, takes your mind off of everything else.
* Stretching or rolling your head around in a circle can also restore your equilibrium.

FIGURE 5-3 Taking a walk is a good way to reduce stress and regain energy (Copyright © istock.com).

* Accomplish small tasks leading up to larger projects.
* Plan bursts of activity. Spend 50 minutes on an important activity, followed by a preplanned 10-minute break doing something else you enjoy.
* If all else fails, get some fresh air by taking a walk outside.

Nutritional Tools

Fatigue is a symptom of dehydration. Your body is 60% to 70% water and water mediates virtually all of your bodily functions, including your brain function and energy systems, depending on your age, weight, and gender. You need water to keep you on the go all day long. Make plans to keep yourself well hydrated. Other nutritional tools include:

* Eat snacks that release energy slowly, like bananas, yogurt, trail mix, nuts, peanut butter on an apple, berries, or granola.
* Avoid sweets, junk food, and energy drinks that contain excessive sugar.
* Use caffeine sparingly but strategically. Try tea for its antioxidants. Or eat a small piece of chocolate for the caffeine and endorphin stimulation.
* Finally, take a daily multivitamin rich in vitamin C and B vitamins.

Refreshment Tools

Try the following strategies for an energy boost:
* Wash your face, hands, and wrists in cold water to stimulate circulation.
* Apply a cool, damp compress to hydrate and relieve the area around your eyes.

* Look on the bright side of a problem or tedious task. Can you learn something new? Can you remind yourself to see the value of what you are doing? This small attitude adjustment can restore interest and energy.
* If you are allowed to do so at work or on your breaks, listen to music.
* Close your eyes for a few minutes and let your cares draw away.
* If your energy depletion is severe, and if permitted, take a 20-minute nap—but no longer. You don't want to descend into deep sleep and wake up more groggy than refreshed.
* Avoid energy-sapping activities in the middle of a demanding routine, such as television, Internet, and email.

Other unconventional ideas are included in Box 5-1.

JOURNALING 5-2

List some of the boring things you have to do at work in one column. In another column, list the perks about these tasks that you may not have thought of before.

Socialization Tools

Few things restore energy faster than a good laugh, especially if you can share it with a co-worker. A short social conversation with a co-worker who's good at putting things in perspective will be a pick-me-up, especially if you do it while helping her in some way.

Finally, in your quest for an energy boost, take it easy on yourself so your stress doesn't act as a barrier to your refreshment.

Perfection is our goal; excellence will be tolerated.

—J. Yahl

Long-term Strategies for Gaining Energy

If you feel that you suffer chronically from low energy, plan to make some long-term changes. Many people can generate more energy by following healthy habits.

Lose Weight

If you suddenly had to carry around a 20-pound sack of flour strapped to your abdomen, you would definitely notice the load, and the energy that it took to carry it. If you are overweight, you probably put the weight on gradually. You adjusted to the stress it placed on your bones and muscles, so you hardly noticed the energy your excess weight robbed from you over time.

Almost without exception, people who lose significant weight are amazed at their newfound supply of energy. Losing weight is a difficult challenge requiring strong motivation and perseverance. Only you can motivate yourself to rise to the challenge, but regaining your lost energy might be part of that motivation. Even while you are losing weight, though, the exercise that is part of most weight-loss plans will begin restoring your energy right away. Try to include exercise as part of your weight-loss plan.

Evaluate Your Diet

If you are chronically tired, you may not be eating the right kind of diet. Heavy meals can make you feel lethargic as your blood is diverted from nourishing your brain to digesting your food. Foods high in sugar can spike your blood sugar, creating a short burst of energy followed by a long crash. Ideally, you want a consistent supply of nutrients that keeps your blood sugar steady and your brain supplied with glucose—the only substance it can burn—all day long.

Breakfast is an important part of such a program because it "breaks" the "fast" of sleeping all night, giving your body a much needed injection of blood sugar to start your day off right. After that, select protein, healthy fats, and carbohydrates that are low on the glycemic index and full of soluble and insoluble fiber (Box 5-2). Low-glycemic carbohydrates

BOX 5-2

Low-Glycemic Foods

- Most fruits, especially grapes, grapefruit, cantaloupe, raspberries, oranges, and avocados
- Most vegetables, especially broccoli, cauliflower, green beans, spinach, peppers, and squash
- Whole grains
- Fructose
- Most beans and legumes
- Most nuts

release sugars slowly and promote a feeling of fullness. Adding these foods to your diet will help to prevent blood sugar spikes and insulin surges that deplete sugars from the blood and prepare them for storage as fat.

Lower Stress

Providing health care is stressful work, and stress produces many negative effects besides lower energy. It can impair your judgment, reduce your happiness, and cause insomnia. In contrast, reduced stress leads to higher energy. Managing stress is discussed later in this chapter.

Sleep Well

If you don't sleep well, find out why and make adjustments. Most of the time, it is just a matter of going to bed earlier. In some cases, you may have to make a few more alterations such as cutting out late-night TV or eating earlier in the evening. Making your bedroom dark, quiet, and cool can help optimize the brain's ability to sleep. Develop a routine by waking up at the same time every day, going for a run, showering, and eating breakfast before going to work.

JOURNALING 5-3

Record your sleep pattern. Describe your bedroom, your bed, the darkness level, and any sounds or smells. How long does it take you to fall asleep? How deeply do you sleep? Do you remember your dreams? Do you have a routine before you retire or after you rise? What do you like best about your sleep-related behavior? What would you like to improve, and how would you do that?

If you snore, wake up with headaches, or feel exhausted despite sleeping all night, you might have sleep apnea. People who suffer from sleep apnea frequently stop breathing during the night, which deprives the brain of oxygen and stresses the heart. Seek help at a sleep clinic, where the clinician may recommend a polysomnograph (sleep study) and possibly prescribe a continuous positive airway pressure (CPAP) device. In rare cases, you may have a thyroid test to make sure you don't have hypothyroidism, which can cause fatigue.

Finally, if stress and anxiety are giving you insomnia, pursue some of the remedies discussed later in this chapter.

Seek Happiness

A final long-term strategy for increasing energy in your life is to make time to engage in activities that make you happy (Figure 5-4). Happiness is a natural energy boost. This can be as simple as spending more time socializing with friends, co-workers, or family. Maybe activities that feed your spirituality bring you a great deal of joy. Perhaps you are engrossed in a hobby such as swimming, pottery, or playing a musical instrument. Pursuing activities improves your brain waves and makes problems more manageable so they don't sap your energy.

Persistence and Perseverance

Now that we've examined ways to boost and maintain your energy levels, keep in mind that the health

FIGURE 5-4 Establishing a healthy work-life balance improves individual happiness. Boost your energy by engaging in the activities you enjoy (Copyright © istock.com).

care environment requires you to know how to be persistent. During stressful times, your perseverance will make a big difference.

Many problems yield to a solution only after attempting a number of approaches. For example, the needle will not always find the artery the first time. The first medication may prove ineffective. The patient may not become a regular until after a number of cancellations. These situations can be frustrating, but don't think about quitting. When you dwell on the various pros and cons of a tough job, you will eventually rationalize reasons to quit. Instead, turn your attention to the next most important task, and then the next. If you practice this approach, the work eventually disappears one small task at a time.

CASE STUDY 5-1
Picker-Upper

Penelope Traktakis added a lot of fun to the hospital pharmacy where she worked as a pharmacy technician. She had a big personality, a big family, and a big social life. She was high energy and never had any trouble getting her work done. In fact, she eagerly volunteered to help when others felt overwhelmed, making medication deliveries to the units, working overtime to fill prescriptions, and starting new lines of customers to get everything moving faster.

One Monday morning, Penny wasn't herself. Her father, Gus, was a roofer and had fallen off a ladder. Fortunately, he only broke his leg, but it still put him out of work. With a heavy sigh, Penny started filling prescriptions at half of her usual pace.

Later that day, an irritated customer started speaking harshly to Penny. "If you can read, Penelope," he said, reading her name tag, "the doctor wants me to take 40 milligrams now, not 20." Penny calmly apologized to the man, but Lane, the pharmacy manager, noticed that Penny was breathing deeply. After a few minutes, he said, "Penny, could you come with me? The new epidemiologist needs some help."

Lane took Penny to the conference room and introduced her to George Papa, a dark-haired young man hovering over a keyboard. "I don't know how to do this," he told Penny. "I'm studying off-label uses of atypical antipsychotics, and I can't figure out how to access the data." Penny sat down as George explained the criteria he was searching for. "Actually, that's pretty easy," she said. "You use cross tabs. Here, let me show you."

After an hour, George had what he needed. "Penny, I think I'm going to need your expertise with SAS. How can I reach you?"

Penny returned to the pharmacy with a familiar pep in her step.

QUESTIONS FOR THOUGHT AND REFLECTION

1. What effects did Penny's down mood have on her performance of her job?
2. Why was Lane's intervention effective?
3. Why do you think Penny hit it off with the epidemiologist?
4. Can you see the pattern of Penny's energy?

Down a Dark Road

Anthony had spent practically the whole night at the Italian Festival, and he was dazed when he arrived for his 7:00 shift on Sunday morning. As a patient services clerk, he never knew how busy his days were going to be at the public hospital he worked at downtown. Sundays were usually slower, but that wasn't always true. As he took his seat in his cubicle, he felt like he could sleep sitting up, right there.

But there was no time for that. Somebody sat down at his station, and he drearily started collecting the information. It was middle-aged man, but Anthony barely acknowledged him until the man said he forgot his insurance card. Anthony made eye contact with the man. "How are we supposed to treat you, sir, if you can't give us your insurance information?

"I know it's Aetna," said the man. "I'm a regular patient here. Do you think you have the number on file?"

"Sir, do you think I should know your policy number, if you have one? Do I look like a Rolodex to you?" The volume of his voice started to rise.

"I've been a patient here before," the man said again.

"Then you should know to bring your insurance card with you!" said Anthony, almost shouting.

"Is there a problem here?" asked Ranni, who came over when she heard Anthony's angry voice.

"Oh, just a little one," said Anthony, sprawled in his chair and jerking his thumb toward the man. "Vincent here wants to know if I have his insurance number."

"Excuse me, sir," she said to the man. "I can have you helped over here." She took the man by his hand and inserted him in Karla's line, apologizing to the woman who would have been next for Karla. "This gentleman needs your assistance, Karla," said Ranni.

"I know," said Karla with a knowing glance at Ranni. "How can I help you, sir?

Ranni returned immediately to Anthony's station, before another patient could be called. "You look like a street urchin," she told him. "You haven't even combed your hair, and your shirt is wrinkled.

"We don't have street urchins in this country, Ranni," he said with a sneer.

"You are not presentable for work. You were rude to that man. I am sending you home today, Anthony. You will be lucky if I let you come back."

QUESTIONS FOR THOUGHT AND REFLECTION

1. How did Anthony's lack of sleep affect his behavior?
2. Did you sense that Anthony's manner of speaking might have not been his usual way? Is there any indication that others disapproved of his behavior?
3. How did Ranni handle the situation? Would you have done anything differently?
4. What should Anthony do when he returns to work on Monday?

1. Create a "to stop" list of activities that deplete your energy.
2. Plan a brief exercise routine or dance you can do almost anywhere to boost your energy.
3. Prepare a list of snacks that you like, that you can carry with you, that would boost your energy without spoiling your appetite and adding weight. Look up their calories and nutritional value.
4. Collect 10 jokes that you find funny. Write them down and memorize them. Try them out on your friends. Use them at strategic times to raise somebody's spirits through laughter.
5. Perform a fine motor skill, like writing or eating, with your nondominant hand. Persist until you find the activity just a little bit easier.

CROSS CURRENTS WITH OTHER SOFT SKILLS

PRACTICING PATIENCE: Persistence takes energy, and also patience. (pp. 361-364)

STRENGTHENING RESILIENCE: You need resilience to overcome the obstacles that make persistence difficult. (pp. 364-368)

MANAGING YOUR TIME AND ORGANIZING YOUR LIFE: If you can take care of all the little distractions by planning your time and being organized, you can devote your energy to the challenges of your work and your life. (pp. 11-18)

EXUDING OPTIMISM, ENTHUSIASM, AND POSITIVITY: These traits will support your perseverance. (pp. 380-384)

Vowing to Be Drug-Free and Unimpaired

I did it to myself. It wasn't society... it wasn't a pusher, it wasn't being blind or being black or being poor. It was all my doing.

—Ray Charles

LEARNING OBJECTIVE 2: VOWING TO BE DRUG-FREE AND UNIMPAIRED

- Understand why drug abuse and dependency are issues for health care professionals.
- Describe the role of law enforcement in preventing drug abuse, particularly in the health industry.
- Describe the role and responsibilities of the Drug Enforcement Administration (DEA).
- Explain how drugs can be diverted in a health care facility, and the systems in place to prevent this.
- Know what three factors are necessary for someone to abuse or become dependent on drugs.
- Know what to do if you encounter an impaired co-worker or a co-worker who is stealing drugs.
- Describe two requirements necessary for recovery from drug dependency.

Working in a health care environment demands a lot of energy, which can lead to stress. If you combine this setting with the increased availability—both legal and illegal—of drugs, it is easy to see why the industry that prescribes and dispenses drugs poses a special risk to its workers.

Any substance, legal or illegal, that impairs performance is a drug. It doesn't matter whether the use of the drug is an addiction, a habit, or a recreational use. These substances can be obtained legally or illegally, but a health care professional is impaired if he or she is under the influence of a drug at work.

Drug abuse by a health professional is unacceptable. Professionals owe it to their clients and co-workers to be in a clear state of mind, to make the best decisions possible, to be observant and aware, to solve problems, and to maintain a high standard of conduct, empathy, and care. None of this is possible when workers are impaired by drugs or alcohol. Unfortunately, drug abuse exists among health professionals at every level.

The Basics of Drug Abuse Laws, Regulations, and Enforcement

Legal and illegal drugs are an enormous enterprise in the United States. The pharmaceutical industry develops and manufactures prescription and over-the-counter drugs, while the illegal drug industry manufactures and distributes drugs for addicts or recreational drug users. Drug addiction generates crime and can ruin the lives of its users.

Law Enforcement

Combating criminal activities generated by the demand for drugs requires a massive federal, state, and local effort. The Controlled Substance Act, a federal law enacted in 1970, regulates drug handling and distribution. It created five drug classifications (see Table 5-1) and ordered the Food and Drug Administration (FDA) and the Drug Enforcement Administration (DEA) to regulate and enforce the act. These agencies update the drugs, and Congress occasionally updates the law. In addition, numerous federal agencies have a role in regulating and enforcing drug laws, from the Department of Justice to the Department of Health and Human Resources to the Department of Agriculture. As explained by the variety of commonly abused drugs in Box 5-3, the "war on drugs" is a massive undertaking. Although penalties vary from state to state, the penalty for possessing drugs illegally can be up to seven years in prison, and penalties for trafficking drugs can be as long as life in prison.

The Drug Enforcement Administration (DEA) issues DEA numbers to physicians and others entitled to prescribe drugs. Physicians, pharmacists, dentists, veterinarians, and nurse practitioners have to apply to the DEA to get their number and their authorization, and the DEA conducts an investigation of these applicants before issuing a DEA number. Any medication that requires a prescription is controlled because it is not available over the counter. There are five classifications of controlled substances that are defined as having the potential for abuse and dependency (Table 5-1).

Within the Drug Enforcement Administration of the Department of Justice, the Office of Diversion Control determines how to dispose of expired, unused, or unwanted drugs. It also solicits reports of illicit pharmaceutical activities and seeks to keep illegal pharmaceuticals off the street and Internet. It also investigates health professionals accused of improper use or diversion of drugs and makes rulings on their future ability to prescribe drugs. It makes rulings about which drugs are classified as controlled substances, and it determines the levels of these classifications. It also tries to combat illegal drug manufacturing and importing. For instance, to help stem the epidemic of methamphetamine production, the Office of Diversion Control made some of the drug's key ingredients, such as pseudoephedrine,

BOX 5-3

Top 20 Most Abused Drugs

1. Cocaine
2. Marijuana
3. Heroin
4. Unspecified benzodiazepine
5. Alprazolam (Xanax)
6. Clonazepam (Klonopin)
7. Hydrocodone (Vicodin, Lorcet, Lortab)
8. Amphetamine
9. Diazepam (Valium)
10. Lorazepam (Ativan)
11. Methamphetamine (speed)
12. Trazodone (Desyrel)
13. Fluoxetine (Prozac)
14. Carisoprodol
15. Oxycodone (Percocet 5, Perdocan, Tylox, OxyContin)
16. Valproic acid
17. d-Propoxyphene (Darvocet N, Darvon)
18. Amitriptyline (Elavil)
19. Methadone
20. LSD

Source: Drug Abuse Warning Network (DAWN), operated by the Substance Abuse and Mental Health Services Administration (SAMHSA), an agency of the Department of Health and Human Services. The data comes from surveys of medical examiners and data that emergency rooms are required to report.

TABLE 5-1
Federal Schedules for Controlled Substances

Schedule	Definition	Examples
I	Substances that have no known current or approved medical use, but a high potential for abuse	Marijuana, LSD, Peyote, Ecstasy
II	Substances that can be prescribed but lend themselves to abuse and dependency	Cocaine, opiates, morphine, amphetamines, Ritalin, Adderol
III	Substances with less potential for abuse but still carry the risk of dependency	Codeine, anabolic steroids
IV	Mild narcotics and substances with less potential for abuse	Darvon, Valium, Prozac, Xanax, Ativan
V	Combination drugs with only a small amount of narcotics	Robitussin, Lomotil

controlled substances, which require a doctor's prescription.

Drug Diversion

Legal pharmaceutical agents—drugs—are said to be diverted when they are stolen or diverted away from their intended legal use. Drugs—or their key ingredients—can be diverted in innumerable ways. They can be stolen, transported, and sold illegally. Perhaps less obviously, patients who received a drug legitimately can become addicted to it and seek it illegally. Many addicts and drug abusers "doctor shop," seeking prescriptions from one practitioner and emergency room to another, using some of what they get and selling the rest. The effects of addiction are so powerful that addicts will pursue them relentlessly and even engage in criminal behavior to obtain drugs.

Characteristics of Drug Abusers and Addicts

Three factors are necessary for a person to develop an addiction to a drug. First, the person must experience the intense relief or pleasurable "high" that a drug supplies. Second, the person must be motivated to keep using the drug, either to pursue the pleasure or mask pain. The pain can be physical pain or emotional pain such as depression or loneliness. Usually, as the motivation drives more frequent use, the dosage must rise to keep producing the high, a factor that can lead to overdosing and prompt criminal activity necessary to finance the addiction. Third, the person must be susceptible to addiction. Many of the genetic and neurochemical intricacies of addiction are not yet known, but it is clear that different people have different vulnerabilities to addiction, and these susceptibility levels vary from substance to substance.

> *Drugs are a waste of time. They destroy your memory and your self-respect and everything that goes along with your self-esteem.*
>
> —Kurt Cobain

When Health Professionals Abuse Drugs

Because of a defense mechanism called denial, the impaired or addicted person is often the last to realize the problem. Everyone else, particularly their family and co-workers, can see that they are impaired. However, most impaired people try to deny or minimize their behavior when confronted. Being impaired is unacceptable and the incident cannot be ignored. Work as a team to address the matter.

Responding to an Impaired Colleague

If you detect or suspect that a co-worker is impaired at work, you must report your concern to a supervisor. The impaired worker may be reprimanded and sent home, or be given a second chance. Other consequences will be more serious. The impaired worker will almost certainly lose trust. They may be mandated to take an education or treatment program. They may be subjected to a formal monitoring program, such as random drug screenings.

Even more seriously, the person's career and personal life could both be in jeopardy. They may be subject to arrest, or their behavior could be reported to their licensing or certification bodies, where their certification could be suspended or revoked. Certainly, these are not outcomes anyone should ever want to risk.

 WHAT IF?

What if you smell alcohol on a co-worker's breath, and they tell you it is from drinking the previous night? Should the co-worker be considered impaired? What would you do?

Responding to a Colleague Who Diverts Drugs

In most states, if you see a drug theft or suspect a colleague of diverting drugs, you are required by law to report it. Large employers will have reporting procedures in place. In other instances, you may have to seek hotlines set up by state and federal drug enforcement agencies. If you ever have to report your suspicions that a colleague may be diverting drugs, you are not having the person arrested; rather, your report will initiate an investigation, which may or may not include law enforcement officials initially.

It may be very difficult to detect drug diversion (Figure 5-5). You may feel that the colleague is not acting like her usual self. There may be discrepancies

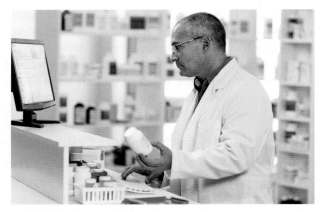

FIGURE 5-5 A pharmacy worker checks records for accuracy (Copyright © istock.com).

in drug inventories, or changes in the documentation supporting them. The worker engaged in drug diversion may seek extraordinary privacy by locking herself inside med rooms, handling runs to the pharmacy, working nights or weekends, or seeking other opportunities when surveillance or general precautions may not be as rigorous.

Most sinister of all is the health professional who removes liquid drugs from vials and replaces them with saline solutions. This kind of diversion is very hard to detect, but it almost always means that a patient who needs that pain medication will not experience any relief. Certainly, a pattern of ineffective medications should alert workers of the possibility that drugs are being diverted.

JOURNALING 5-4

Imagine that a family member being treated in a hospital were the victim of drug diversion. How would that make you feel?

It is hard to imagine a greater breach of faith than a health professional withholding medication from patients for personal gain. Even so, it is easy to see why reporting these co-workers is a difficult responsibility. The proper path is not always clear. How *sure* do you have to be to subject a co-worker to such a serious charge? A frivolous and false charge could still be devastating to the person falsely accused. On the other hand, patient safety is at stake. If you are uncertain about what to do, you should discuss your concerns with your supervisor.

Treatment Options for Impaired Workers

Fortunately, many programs treat impaired and addicted health professionals by addressing their problems and providing opportunities to save their career and their right to practice. These programs are generically called *impaired professionals* programs. Most treat any health professional and may also treat other professionals as well. Recently, employers, regulators, and professional associations have concluded that it is cost effective and morally just to assist an impaired colleague. If addiction is a disease, then don't these health professionals deserve an opportunity for treatment?

A seminal study out of the University of Pittsburgh (Baldisseri, 2007) showed that 10% to 15% of all health professionals will abuse drugs or alcohol at some point in their career. Although this rate of abuse is about the same as the general population, the recovery rate has been shown to be much higher than that of the general population. This rate is attributed to the availability of structured treatment programs, which often include a reentry to practice component. However, it has also been shown that laws and policies force intervention, so these impaired professionals are usually identified at the beginning of their substance abuse. Once they have recovered, their clear thinking returns, enabling them to make good decisions about their careers and their commitments.

Two conditions must be met for recovery to succeed. First, the individual must admit that he or she has a drug or alcohol problem. Second, the individual must be willing to change. The motivation for health professionals to change is usually high. Their right to practice is in jeopardy. Fortunately, recovering health professionals usually receive the support of their colleagues.

A Final Word

Working in an impaired state can lead down a dark road. Always seek positive solutions to problems you encounter at work. Drugs are never a solution. If one of your colleagues starts abusing drugs, use the tools discussed in this chapter to help them.

Every junkie's like a setting sun.

—Neil Young

Old Friends

Pritha Verma worked nights as an LPN at the County Nursing Home in Charleston so she could be home with her young children during the day while her husband worked. Despite working during the nighttime hours, her shifts were surprisingly busy. Patients could be disoriented and wander out of their rooms. Bed linens would need changing. Bathroom trips were scheduled for some patients. Others needed PRN sleeping medication and tranquilizers. Pritha was used to the pace, though, and all of the activity made the time pass quickly. She worked with the same nurse and nursing assistants most of the time, and they were her friends. Whenever she had a spare moment, she would check supplies and reorder when necessary, or complete other tasks that were difficult to accomplish during the day.

The night nurse, Margaret Woods, was Pritha's neighbor and they usually carpooled. They had worked together for more than three years, and Pritha always felt energized by Margaret's high spirits and sense of humor whenever things became chaotic. Perhaps that's why she didn't notice the signs of Margaret's drug diversions immediately.

At first, there were some minor discrepancies in the narcotic counts. Margaret would claim that some pills fell into the sink, but Margaret would dutifully document the loss. Other times, Margaret would say she dropped some tablets and asked Pritha to help her look for them, but they could never be found. Then, Margaret's behavior became more jittery than energetic. Margaret monopolized Pritha and prevented her from getting her work done. Pritha spoke to Margaret about it, but Margaret got agitated in a way that Pritha had never seen her before. One night when they were pouring the meds together, Pritha thought she saw Margaret slipping a pair of pills into her pocket. She didn't say anything that time, but she started to observe Margaret more closely.

When she saw Margaret do it again, Pritha confronted her immediately. Hesitantly, Margaret produced a Halcion pill from her pocket. "I just can't seem to sleep anymore when I get home," she explained to Pritha. "I should just get a prescription." She put the Halcion tablet back in the jar, but Pritha was pretty sure she saw her take two.

After the two friends drove home together that morning, Pritha went back to work. Walter, the nursing supervisor, was surprised to see her and immediately ushered her into his office when she asked to speak with him.

"I can't believe this," he said, "but I know it must be true. I trust you, and I've been concerned about the inventory discrepancies myself. Unfortunately, Pritha, an investigation is in order. Until this matter is resolved, I am going to ask you to pour the meds at night and keep the med closet locked. I'm going to have to ask Margaret for her keys." Later that morning, Walter alerted the County Health Commissioner and asked Gino, the pharmacy manager, to start an audit. He collected the bottle of aspirin labeled OxyContin from the meds room.

That night, neither Margaret nor Pritha were in top form. Pritha had not been able to sleep and Margaret seemed angry. They had both driven to work separately. Pritha poured the meds and kept the med room locked.

The following night, Margaret was too angry to keep silent. "I can't believe you would do such a thing to me, Pritha. We're supposed to be friends. Now I have to give blood for a drug screening, because of you. As if I don't have enough stress in my life already. Now I could lose my license, because of you. I'd just quit, but that would be admitting guilt, and I'd lose my license for sure, and so I have to go to work and be with *you*," she finished with a sneer.

"None of this is because of me," Pritha said quietly, and Margaret strode off toward the sitting area. Pritha thought she saw Margaret sleeping around 4:00 a.m.

After the weekend, Walter announced to the staff that Margaret would be away on administrative leave to deal with some personal problems. He asked the evening nurses to rotate through the night shifts to cover for Margaret. It turned out that many of the nurses had shared Pritha's concerns and praised her professionalism.

Six weeks later, Pritha saw Margaret and her husband drive their car up their driveway. She had not seen Margaret all this time and assumed she was away, although she didn't know where. She kept telling her husband she hoped she wouldn't run into Margaret in the neighborhood, but her husband said it would happen eventually. Now she saw Margaret walking up the sidewalk and turning up Pritha's front walk. When Pritha opened her door, Margaret was holding back tears.

"Pritha," she said. "Thank you. I—" she stopped, and shook her head. "You are a wonderful friend." They hugged.

QUESTIONS FOR THOUGHT AND REFLECTION

1. What were the early signs of Margaret's drug problem? If you were Pritha, would you have ignored them too?

2. Why did Pritha report her friend to Walter? Should she had done anything differently?

3. How did Margaret deny or minimize her drug dependency?

4. Were you surprised to learn that so many other people were suspicious of Margaret's drug diversions?

5. Why did Margaret call Pritha a friend?

Down a Dark Road

Corrina was a pleasant young woman who enjoyed her first job as a Medical Assistant. She was introverted and had trouble making eye contact with patients who approached the reception desk, but she felt that the job was helping her overcome her shyness. After her mother went to bed each night, Corrina retreated to the little "getaway" she had created for herself in the house's half-finished attic. There was a comfortable old chair, a footstool and side table, a small TV, and a big window with a fan in it. She always made a snack, lit some incense, turned on the television, and measured a few pinches of marijuana in an old Plexi-glas pipe. She exhaled the smoke into the fan in the window and carefully hid her stash. She imagined what her first apartment would be like, what she would buy for it, what kind of a kitchen it would have, and what friends she would have over for dinner. At the end of the night, she returned to her bedroom and woke up refreshed for work.

This particular day was the most chaotic, stressed-out day she had worked so far, and it made Corrina feel jittery. First, there was the really angry guy who hadn't shown up for his appointment the day before and then blew up when she told him that he missed his appointment. It was nice of Dr. Adelman to work him in, but he just glared at her in the waiting room the whole time, as if it were *her* fault that he wrote the appointment down on the wrong day. By the time lunch rolled around, she felt as if she had already done a whole day's work, and the afternoon didn't look any easier.

Returning from lunch, though, Corrina felt calm. Taking some deep breaths, she opened the door and strode through the lobby, nodding and smiling at everyone she saw, and took up her post behind the desk. Three patients approached at once, and that confused her for a moment. "Who's first?" she called out cheerily, surprised at the volume of her own voice. The patients looked quizzically at one another, a little annoyed. "I'll take you left to right," she said. "My left, your right," she laughed. Then she couldn't

get the spelling right for the first man. Brisinsky, or something. "Corrina," said Dr. Ollinger.

Where did *she* come from?

"Corrina, do you have Mrs. Summers yet?"

"Do I have Mrs. Summers yet?" mimicked Corrina, looking at the faces in front of her. One of them identified herself as Mrs. Summers, but Corrina just couldn't think of what to do next. Dr. Ollinger eventually grabbed the patient's chart herself.

At the end of the day, Dr. Ollinger and Corrina's supervisor, Imogene, asked to speak with Corrina in private.

"Were you smoking marijuana during your lunch, Corrina?"

"What? What? Whoa, no way."

"Because you were behaving very strangely when you got back," Dr. Ollinger went on, "and I'm sure I smelled it in your hair."

"No, no," was all that Corrina could think of to say.

"Corrina, we would like to help you, but you have to want the help," said Imogene.

"Yeah, sure, I mean, you guys have been very helpful to me. Thank you. Thank you *soooo* much."

"I want you to think this over during the weekend, Corrina, and we'll revisit this conversation on Monday. Deal?"

"Sure. Deal. Yeah."

On Monday, Corrina slept in late. Her cell phone rang several times, but she could see it was from the clinic, so she let the messages go to her voice mail. "I'm going to look for a different job when my vacation is over," she told her mother.

"Oh why, Corrina? I thought you liked that job."

"It was fine," said Corrina. "The people were nice. But I think I can do better."

That afternoon, she deleted the phone messages without listening to them.

1. How did Corrina's marijuana use influence her personality?
2. What can you say about Corrina's confidence and self-esteem?
3. Did the clinic staff respond appropriately to Corrina's behavior?
4. Were the clinic staff willing to give Corrina a second chance?
5. What could Corrina have done to give herself a more positive outcome?

⭐ EXPERIENTIAL EXERCISES

1. Watch an episode of the series "Nurse Jackie." How does the character played by Edie Falco behave when she is impaired at work?
2. Spend some time on the site of the Drug Enforcement Administration (www.dea.gov) to familiarize yourself with the scope of America's drug problem and the government's law enforcement effort and other services to health professionals.
3. Volunteer at a drug treatment center to learn more about addiction.
4. Familiarize yourself with your employer's policies on reporting drug diversion and impaired employees.
5. Write a promise to yourself in your journal that you will never work while you are impaired.

🔄 CROSS CURRENTS WITH OTHER SOFT SKILLS

ACHIEVING HONESTY AND INTEGRITY: Being impaired is living a lie built on denial. (pp. 18-25)

MANAGING AND RESOLVING CONFLICT: Working with an impaired or drug-diverting co-worker is a recipe for conflict. (pp. 224-231)

FOLLOWING RULES AND REGULATIONS: There is no place in health care for drug abuse and dependency. In most states, you are required to report colleagues who are impaired or divert drugs. (pp. 291-297)

CONTROLLING ANXIETY: Anxiety is part of life. You need a solid approach to managing anxiety that doesn't involve drugs or alcohol. (pp. 356-361)

Managing Stress

Instead of thoughtful lives they savor, people are in danger of living superficial, sound-bite lives they barely notice.

—Edward M. Hallowell

LEARNING OBJECTIVE 3: MANAGING STRESS

- Describe the stress response.
- Explain the causes of chronic stress.
- List six strategies for managing stress that might work for you.
- Describe the role of control in causing and managing stress.
- Describe the effect of human connection on the management of stress.

The Stress Response

As we have reviewed, stress is a continuous energy drain. So how do we manage our stress?

The human stress response evolved ages ago to help us effectively respond to physical danger. Danger triggers a flood of hormones to our muscles to enable us to fight or flee. These hormones—namely, adrenaline and cortisol—enhance our natural strength and stamina. Bodily functions unrelated to fighting or fleeing, like digestion, shut down as all resources are diverted to responding to the immediate danger. Triggers might include an interaction with a difficult co-worker, a chaotic work environment, or being late for an appointment.

Of course, a certain amount of stress is necessary for effective functioning. Stress that makes us alert, energized, and focused is necessary to accomplish our work every day. Once stress exceeds optimal effectiveness, however, it becomes negative energy and must be controlled. The Yerkes-Dodson graph, in Figure 5-6, developed early in the 20th century, shows how stress can be suboptimal, optimal, or out of control.

The psychological demands of modern life frequently leave people in a permanent stress response, which produces terrible consequences for our physical and mental health. All those danger hormones that

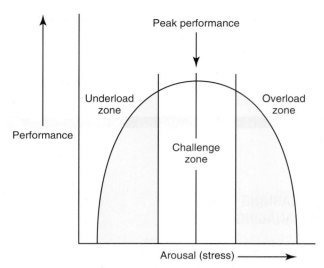

FIGURE 5-6 The Yerkes-Dodson graph shows the effects of stress on performance.

flood your bloodstream and muscles but are never expended in physical activity produce lethargy and fatigue. Glucose enters your bloodstream to prepare your body for physical action, but raises your blood sugar if it is not released. Unexpended energy also leads to high blood pressure.

Chronic stress exposure can also contribute to health complications, including immune dysfunction, cardiovascular disease, suppressed growth, erratic menstrual cycles, erectile dysfunction, and digestive disorders.

Ultimately, stress can damage your quality of life and shorten your lifespan. Stress affects our mental health by causing anxiety. It causes us to express negative emotions inappropriately and without good judgment. This establishes a negative feedback loop in which these same outbursts create new problems that compound stress. Box 5-4 contains additional negative health outcomes related to stress.

Sources of Stress

The rate of change and the resulting demands placed on you are increasing at an unprecedented pace. Stress is coming at you from virtually all directions.

Technology, Addictions, and Productivity Demands

Technology makes our lives easier, faster, more fun, and more immediate, but the pace of technological change can also be stressful. Most people in the 21st century are continually managing multiple modes of technology-mediated communication. You follow people on Twitter, Facebook, and LinkedIn. You are reachable 24/7 on your cell phone, mobile device, and email. You text, and friends send you links to videos, photos, and web sites.

Although new devices and software enhance our lives, change requires constantly learning how to operate and optimize new technology. Moreover, face-to-face human connections decrease as communication is more mediated by technology, depriving us of a proven stress remedy. As productivity demands increase at work and at home, we often turn to television, video games, the Internet, and social media to escape from the world around us.

You can't have everything. Where would you put it?

—Stephen Wright

JOURNALING 5-5

Make a list of the technology you use every day. Consider how these devices actually add to your stress. Brainstorm ideas to lower technology's impact on your stress.

Multitasking

Many people respond to these demands by resorting to multitasking, but this can be a deceptive strategy because it doesn't always work. Computers can execute multiple tasks without stress, but your brain doesn't operate the same way. Although you may be able to manage habitual tasks while giving your attention to something else, you can only concentrate on one thing that demands your attention at time (Figure 5-7). For instance, you may be able to sign routine documents while talking on the phone. If you try to process your email while you talk on the phone, you might miss subtle details in an email or have to ask

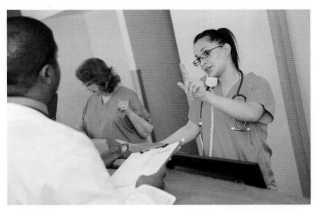

FIGURE 5-7 Responding to multiple demands can be overwhelming. When you cannot effectively multitask, it is best to prioritize your work and concentrate on one issue at a time (Copyright © istock.com).

your caller to repeat herself. When multitasking, make sure all of the tasks are manageable. If not, tackle them individually.

? WHAT IF?

What if you are called upon to perform two tasks at once, both of which require your attention? What happens to your attention? What happens to your performance on each task?

Worry

Unlike other animals, which respond only to immediate dangers and then return to normal, humans can generate the stress response about events that haven't even occurred, maintaining a constant stress level. In fact, comedian and stress expert Loretta LaRoche describes severe worrying as "catastrophizing," fixating on the absolute worst thing that could possibly happen. Do you occasionally catastrophize, or know people who do?

> *I am an old man and have known a great many troubles, but most of them never happened.*
>
> —Mark Twain

In fact, approximately 90% of the outcomes that people worry about never come to pass. Worrying about the future will not make it better, but it can damage your well-being.

Managing Stress

When stress becomes severe enough to be a medical condition, many effective treatments are available. Unfortunately, these treatments are beyond the scope of this book. However, let's consider stress-busting measures within our control such as laughter, meditation, exercise, nature, sleep, and positive social interaction.

Laughter

The old expression that laughter is the best medicine is true. Laughter is an antidote to stress. Laughing releases endorphins, pleasure hormones in your brain, that bash the hormonal effects of stress. If you have a great sense of humor, or work around people who do, you have a powerful weapon against stress. In *Anatomy of an Illness* by Norman Cousins, he describes how he responded when his doctors told him he had weeks to live. He watched Marx Brothers and other funny movies, training himself to laugh. He lived another ten highly productive and active years.

Meditation and Relaxation

A couple of basic meditation techniques such as deep breathing and visualization can help quell your stress. To practice deep breathing, simply breathe from your diaphragm. You know you are breathing deeply enough to get the benefits of stress relief if, when you place your hand just below your rib cage and above your stomach, it moves up and down as you breathe. This simple deep breathing exercise is meditation at its simplest: concentrating on the rhythm of your breath.

Deep breathing lowers your heart rate and your blood pressure, sending oxygen into your blood and brain. It makes you feel calm and anchors you in the present. What's not to like? Moreover, you can practice deep breathing virtually any time you like, and it is not apparent to anyone else.

Another basic form of meditation is visualization. You may be able to intensify the benefits of your deep breathing by closing your eyes and visualizing a sensory-rich environment. It's best to have this destination at your disposal so start imagining it now. Visualization can also be a focused tensing and relaxing of the muscles of your body, in sequence from head to toe.

Dr. Herbert Benson, a Harvard-trained cardiologist and founder of the Mind/Body Institute at Massachusetts General Hospital, calls the result of meditation the "relaxation response." This relaxation response involves a number of physiological changes, including the release of nitric oxide in the blood, which dilates blood vessels. Box 5-5 offers some steps in pursuing the relaxation response.

FIGURE 5-8 Taking a yoga class is a positive way to manage stress (Copyright © istock.com).

Regardless of the meditation method you choose, the objective is to become acutely aware of your body, your mind, and your present. You should find meditation stimulating, grounding, and refreshing.

Exercise

Exercise relieves stress. For one thing, it uses up the stress hormones and glucose that stress has poured into your blood system and muscles. Left unburned and unused, these chemicals will cause fatigue. That is why you frequently feel more energetic after exercise, particularly if you are stressed out.

Exercise, movement, and fun also release endorphins, hormones that make us feel good. When you see children running around a playground, you will also see smiles on their faces. So, consider play if you don't like exercise. You can pursue lots of fun activities which provide therapeutic exercise. Seek fun activities that you can fit into your lifestyle. You are only limited by your imagination. You could shoot baskets, run, dance, swim, cycle, shadow-box, garden, or shovel snow. Better yet, seek activities that you can enjoy with a friend. You can hike, play tennis, play handball, or play catch. Finally, you can even join a team and play softball, field hockey, flag football, or soccer. Yoga is also an appealing activity to combat stress because it combines exercise with meditation in a group setting (Figure 5-8).

Eliminate Worry

Bobby McFerrin's hit song says "Don't Worry, Be Happy," but that is easier said than done. The solution to worry is to take action to prevent the worry from surfacing. If you are in a situation where you cannot take the appropriate action, acknowledge how useless it is to worry and let go. Box 5-6 offers a recipe to reduce or eliminate worry.

Action is the antidote to despair.

—Joan Baez

Sleep

If you don't get at least six hours of sound sleep every night, you are contributing to your stress level. The effects of insufficient sleep are well documented and discussed earlier in this chapter under "Gaining Energy, Persistence, and Perseverance."

Sleep knits up the ravell'd sleeve of care.

—William Shakespeare

Control

There are many things you have no control over: the weather; your supervisor's personality; your physical limitations; the number of patients and calls you get on any given day, and the severity of their problems. Accept this. Identify the areas in your life where you *do* have control, and concentrate on them. You may not be able to control everything, but you *can* choose to control your response to them.

FIGURE 5-9 Coworkers take a break and laugh together (Copyright © istock.com).

Connect

The most important thing you can do in your life to manage and minimize stress is to connect with other people, nature, work, and your spiritual self (Figure 5-9). We are in fact neurologically wired to find peace in our connections, especially with the important people in our lives. We are energized by these interactions and feel support, empathy, and relief in communicating our stress with others. Even interacting with strangers can be strangely relieving. Connecting with people is completely under our control as a means of controlling stress.

Your work, as odd as it sounds, can be a fortification against stress. If you love your work, excel in and find meaning in it, you can often lose yourself in the flow of your work. This experience of "flow" liberates you from the stress your work might otherwise cause you, and enables you to focus intently on getting your work done well.

Finally, connect with your spiritual self. You don't have to be religious to feel that you are connected with something much bigger and more powerful than yourself. This is a perspective that many people find liberating and energizing as an antidote to stress.

Specific religious beliefs, prayer, or meditation can be a source of personal strength against what Shakespeare called "the slings and arrows of outrageous fortune."

Additional Stress Management Strategies

Put yourself in the present moment to the best of your ability. Be on time and be dependable. If you eliminate the anxiety of being late or distracted, you have significantly reduced the stress in your life.

Choose to be positive. Many people think that positive circumstances will produce a positive outlook. In reality, though, a positive perspective produces positive circumstances. If you have close family, friends, and co-workers, you have many of the qualities that lead to happiness and the ability to handle the stress in your life. Additionally, if you tend toward hope instead of worry and maintain a sense of humor when dealing with setbacks, you will find meaning in everything you do. You will have everything you need to conquer stressful experiences.

Finally, go slow. This may seem paradoxical in our fast-paced world, but choosing your own pace allows you to control the situation. If you are caring for an anxious patient with puzzling symptoms, slow down when addressing his or her needs.

Got a problem that's stressing you out? Trade it for a bigger problem. Volunteer for a charity such as a children's hospital or a disease foundation. This experience will put your problems in perspective. In addition, altruism—working on the behalf of others—will reduce your stress.

Box 5-7 suggests additional unconventional strategies that may work for you in your quest to control your stress.

CASE STUDY 5-3

Skittles and Bits

Karalee had a pounding headache by the time she got to work at Pediatric Associates and the parking lot was full of patients waiting for the clinic to open. The doctors wouldn't even be there for another half hour. She unlocked the doors and let the patients fill the waiting room. When she went in the back room to put on her lab coat, the other medical assistants, Mindy and Carlos, were already there, drinking coffee. "Why didn't you guys open up?" she said.

They just looked at her as though no reply was necessary.

Karalee was pretty new compared to them, so she just took some ibuprofen for her headache and put a smile on her face as she headed out to the reception desk, followed by Mindy and Carlos. As if in a wave, the patients rose from their seats and approached the reception desk. Karalee took a deep breath and greeted the mom and her two children who were first in line. Karalee couldn't help but notice that she was processing patients in at about the same rate as her two colleagues put together, but she just assumed their patients had more complex issues.

Once the patients were checked in, Karalee pulled all the charts for the day's appointments. Pretty soon, Dr. Agawam came out and demanded to know who pulled the charts. Karalee stepped up. "Well, this is the wrong 'Murphy,' Karalee. Please try to be more careful."

Her ears burned as she overheard Carlos referring to her as "Karaless." But she closed her eyes for a moment and took some deep breaths. Everybody makes mistakes, she told herself. I will be more careful next time.

Then she approached her co-workers. "Wow," she said, "that was crazy. In this city, *everybody's* name is Murphy. I gotta be more careful."

"It's just a mistake," said Mindy.

"I know. Hey, what did you guys do over the weekend?"

Just then, there was a commotion in the waiting room. "Allie, Allie!" screamed a woman's voice. Karalee looked up and saw little Allison Sallah with a surprised look on her little face, which had started to turn blue, especially around her lips. Her mother was kneeling in front of her, shouting her name. The three medical assistants rushed to the waiting room. "She's choking on a Skittle," the mother said.

"Go get one of the doctors," Karalee ordered Mindy, who ran off. "Carlos, get everybody back. We need some room here." She gently turned Allison around and placed the heel of her hand on Allison's sternum, being careful it was in the right spot. She gave her a Heimlich maneuver, a rather gentle one, but nothing happened. Carlos had created some space around the scene, gesturing people back and moving some chairs out of the way. Karalee gave the toddler another Heimlich, hard this time, but no response. She could hear that Allison wasn't breathing, nor gasping for air. Just as Dr. Levin and Mindy rushed in the room together, Karalee gave it another try, and out flew the Skittle. Allison sucked in a deep breath and let it out with the loudest, best-sounding cry Karalee had ever heard.

The mother swept up Allison into the waiting arms of Dr. Levin. Everybody crowded around Karalee as Allison's wailing retreated into the back.

"I could use some air," she said good-naturedly.

Everybody stood back. "What if you didn't get it out?" said another mother.

"Well, it did come out, so let's not make it worse than it was," said Karalee. "I'd like to recompose myself. How about you guys?" she said, and everyone took a seat as if by cue.

Later on, Dr. Levin pulled Karalee into an office with Dr. Agawam. "I talked to Mrs. Sallah, and I asked around," Dr. Levin told her. "You showed great skill today, Karalee, and even greater leadership. You really took command of a very serious situation. How did you do that?"

"For one thing, I took some very deep breaths," said Karalee. "It calmed me down, and it helped me understand how little Allison must have felt, not being able to breathe at all."

That evening, Karalee finally got a chance to reflect on the day. It was stressful, but she managed it well. She loved that Dr. Levin said she showed leadership. From now on, she was going to think of herself as a leader too.

QUESTIONS FOR THOUGHT AND REFLECTION

1. What little, almost automatic, actions did Karalee take to keep her stress in check?
2. Underline all the actions that Karalee took to manage her stress.
3. Was Karalee offended by any unkindness shown to her by her co-workers?
4. Things seemed to go better when Karalee connected with her patients and co-workers. What did she do to initiate these connections?
5. Is Karalee a natural leader? Why or why not?

Down a Dark Road

Brinna was in a foul mood. She had just learned that her sister got engaged to be married.

"And you're not happy for her?" asked Nick, one of the other pharm techs. "You don't like the guy?"

"The guy's fine. For her. I wouldn't marry him. So I'm happy enough for her. It's just that she's younger than me, and I'm the pretty one. I should be the one getting married."

"She has a boyfriend, and you don't," said Eleanor, the other pharm tech.

Brinna gave her a baleful look. "I have plenty of boyfriends. I just wouldn't marry any of them, that's all."

"Have any asked?" said Eleanor.

Brinna gave Eleanor another withering look. She didn't like that girl.

Ralph, one of the pharmacists, stuck his head in. "Brinna, is that Hobson script ready yet?"

"You made me lose count!" she shouted, forgetting whom she was speaking to. "Oh, sorry. What?"

"The Hobson script. I told you to get it out here right away. Where is it?"

Brinna looked blank. "The Hobson script?"

"Come on, Brinna. If you didn't talk so much, I wouldn't have to tell you twice."

She found the script and started filling it. "Like he doesn't talk too much," she muttered, counting out the 200 mg pills.

He stuck his head back in. "Those are 200s," he shouted, startling Brinna, who knocked over the big jug and dumped 200s everywhere. "100s, 100s," he shouted. "And I want you to count every one of these 200s when you pick them up and sign off on them." Brinna immediately stooped down and started scooping up the 200s. "I said after, *after*," shouted Ralph. Brinna stood, but she was immobilized. Ralph threw up his hands and left. She could hear Ralph apologizing to Mrs. Hobson.

"She'll get her script," Brinna muttered to herself and looked up to see Eleanor and Nick watching her. "I could use some help here," she snapped, but they both wandered away.

Brinna's cell phone rang. "Oh hi," she said. "OK. I'm working with idiots, that's all." She saw Eleanor pass by and roll her eyes just as she said that. "Look, I can't talk. Wait till you hear the news, though. I'll call you back." She could see Ralph trolling. "Let's see, 100s, 100s." She stepped on more 200s as she finally delivered the script to Ralph.

"This is 90?" he said.

"Oh boy, she wants 90?"

"No," said Ralph. "The doctor who ordered the medication for Mrs. Hobson wants 90. That's why he wrote '90' on the script. Eleanor, would you please fill this script for Mrs. Hobson. And recount these, to make sure you have 30 to start with."

QUESTIONS FOR THOUGHT AND REFLECTION

1. In what ways is Brinna contributing to her own stress?
2. Can Brinna count on solid relationships with her co-workers to help her out in a jam?
3. What can you say about Brinna's center of attention?
4. If you were Brinna, what would you do in response to Ralph telling Eleanor to fill the prescription?

1. Don't buy anything for a week. What did you really miss having?
2. Keep track of everything you do for 24 hours. Do you have any regrets about how you spent your time? Is there something else you wish you had done, or done more of?
3. Take a yoga class. Go ahead. See if you like it!
4. Pick a pleasurable, relaxing place you have been in the past. Visualize it intensely, using the senses of sight, sound, smell, taste, and touch. Visualize the colors. Recall the feelings you experienced when you were in this place. Visualize your chosen relaxing place so intensely that you can call upon it at will when the need to relax arises.
5. Start a collection of videos you find hilarious, and remember to use them in times of acute stress.
6. Catch yourself breathing. When you do, deepen and lengthen your breaths. See if you can feel the sense of calm this gives you. Do this repeatedly until you make deep breathing a habit and always have it as a remedy in times of stress and anxiety.

CROSS CURRENTS WITH OTHER SOFT SKILLS

BEING DEPENDABLE: If you are dependable, you have removed many stressors, like being late, from your life. (pp. 35-38)

MANAGING AND RESOLVING CONFLICT: You cannot eliminate conflict from your life, but you can manage it effectively to minimize the stress associated with it. (pp. 224-231)

CONTROLLING ANXIETY: Anxiety is caused by stress; if you can combat anxiety, you can combat stress. (pp. 356-361)

EXUDING OPTIMISM, ENTHUSIASM, AND POSITIVITY: These traits can be effective in shielding you from the ravages of stress. (pp. 380-384)

Bibliography

Baldisseri MR. Impaired healthcare professional. *Crit Care Med* 35(2 suppl):S106-S116, 2007.

Griffin RA, Polit DF, Byrne MW. Stereotyping and nurses' recommendations for treating pain in hospitalized children. *Res Nurs Health* 30(6):655-666, 2007. DOI: 10.1002/nur.20209.

INTERPERSONAL SKILLS

CHAPTER 6

Being Easy to Deal With

THEMES TO CONSIDER	
	■ Know how important trust is to your success in the health professions.
	■ Have a strategy to earn and keep trust in your new job.
	■ Understand why empathy is a necessary trait in the health professions.
	■ Explain the neurologic basis for empathy.
	■ Describe an empathic organization.

Building Trust

The best way to find out if you can trust somebody is to trust them.

—Ernest Hemingway

LEARNING OBJECTIVE 1: BUILDING TRUST

■ Learn to trust yourself.
■ Understand how people learn to trust others.
■ Know how to build trust in yourself among your co-workers.
■ State the benefits of a trusting organization.
■ Consider the advantages of forgiveness.
■ Gain insight into how broken trust can be rebuilt.

As soon as you trust yourself, you will know how to live.

—Goethe

Ever heard of a New Year's resolution? Ever make a promise to yourself (e.g., "Someday I'm going to...")? Ever break those promises?

Trust must start from within and *only then* radiate outward to the rest of the world. To become trustworthy, you must first be able to trust yourself, so keep promises you make to yourself. Then you can begin to build trust with others—a process comprised of respect, empathy, and listening skills, which requires time and practice.

⬅ JOURNALING 6-1

Because likability counts in building trust, list the characteristics that make you likable. Explain how you can make these traits more obvious to people you meet.

The Building Blocks of Trust

Listening

Let's start with the skill of listening. A trusting work relationship begins like any other—through conversation. Questions drive conversations; statements stop them. Ask more questions. Make fewer statements.

In baseball, no matter how well you play defense, you cannot score runs while you are in the field. Listening works the same way. You can only learn by listening, no matter how good of a speaker you are. See Chapter 7 for strategies on becoming a good listener.

Cultivating Respect

The next component of trust is respect. Everyone deserves to be treated with respect and equality. To treat others equally, you must forget your ego. Humility generates trust; arrogance destroys it.

So how do you demonstrate respect? First, remember that small efforts make a big difference: use names, ask about family or experiences, offer to help, pay sincere compliments. When you demonstrate this kind of interest and acceptance, people perceive you as accepting, reasonable, and intelligent. They will know that you respect them. Figure 6-1 shows a health professional expressing genuine interest in her patients. This interaction displays the trust that you should work to achieve with every patient.

Empathy

The final building block of trust is empathy, also explored later in this chapter. Others will care for you if you exhibit caring for others. *You get what you want*

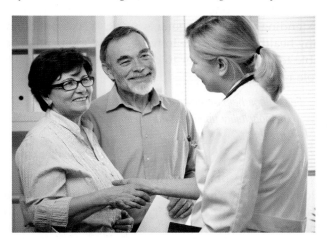

FIGURE 6-1 Health professionals can show interest in patients through interaction (Copyright © istock.com).

when you help others get what they want. When you listen to others, they will listen to you. When you accept others, they will accept you. When you trust others, they will trust you.

And in the end, the love you take is equal to the love you make.

—**Paul McCartney & John Lennon**

How to Instill Trust in Others

Ronald Reagan said, "Trust, but verify." He knew that earning trust takes a long time. Trust requires honesty *and* competence. You will have to demonstrate both of these qualities repeatedly before your co-workers will be able to trust you. You must be honest and you must contribute to the fullest of your capacity, day after day. People want to achieve mutual trust, but we still have to earn it in the long run. Trust will develop only after you have demonstrated that you deserve it.

If you want to start building trust right away, follow the tips in Box 6-1.

BOX 6-1

Basic Behaviors that Build Trust

- Be on time all the time. No exceptions!
- Be friendly. Greet people you encounter. Make eye contact.
- Remember the names of the people you are introduced to.
- Ask for help and advice.
- Have your standard, short, and interesting introduction at the tip of your tongue.
- Dress professionally and be well groomed at all times.
- Observe business etiquette and culture so that you will be in sync at your workplace.
- Complete all your tasks professionally.
- Pitch in when there is work to be done.
- Show kindness toward patients and clients at all times.
- Display a positive attitude.

FIGURE 6-2 New employees can learn about job duties and build positive work relationships by communicating with coworkers (Copyright © istock.com).

Communicate

Communicate clearly. Speak loud enough for others to hear you. Ask and answer questions. Asking for help is one of the strongest relationship builders you can employ (Figure 6-2). Most new co-workers will be happy to help you, and the time you spend with them contributes to relationship building. At first, observe, help, and focus on executing your job correctly. As a new team member, you are just beginning to comprehend your new role and are interacting with a lot of new people, so refrain from offering strong opinions until you have formed relationships with your new co-workers.

Always clarify expectations. Never make assumptions or walk away from a conversation with only a vague understanding of your expectations. Communicate clearly to avoid misunderstanding.

 WHAT IF?

What if someone doesn't remember your name? How will you be able to tell? How can you tactfully remind them of your name?

Show Transparency

Demonstrating your skills will prove that you are reliable. Carefully document your work in patients' charts. Over time, as you become more familiar with routines and procedures, you will overcome the "learning curve" that accompanies being new. You will find yourself improving and developing a sense of where your skills are most needed. As your

performance naturally evolves, you can start to contribute your own ideas and experiences.

Next, demonstrate loyalty. Say positive things about your co-workers, knowing that your comments could get back to them. By the same token, if you speak negatively about someone, your co-workers will be wondering what you say about *them* when they're not around.

Achieve Results

Patients and co-workers alike award their trust to employees who tackle problems and address difficult issues when they arise. Failure to hold yourself and others accountable destroys trust. Practicing accountability can be similar to setting limits with children: it may be difficult to do consistently, but it creates productive adults. Accountability establishes expectations, boundaries, safety, and—yes—trust. Finally, demonstrate your own accountability by making commitments and consistently keeping them. Over time, your impeccable track record will inspire trust.

WHAT IF?

What if you are called upon to demonstrate your clinical skills? What skills have you mastered?

Organizational Trust

Sometimes health care professionals who receive promotions have a difficult time giving up their duties, because they trust their capabilities and are hesitant to trust someone else's standards. Even though extending trust to someone is a risk, it is essential for any health care practice to work. Co-workers must be able to trust each other to do their jobs because each role is interrelated.

Few things help an individual more than to place responsibility upon him and to let him know that you trust him.

—Booker T. Washington

In an atmosphere of trust, people share information and tolerate mistakes because they acknowledge that mistakes are necessary steps on the path to excellence. People are loyal and support one another. The environment fosters creativity, innovation, and workflow improvements. Co-workers regularly

FIGURE 6-3 Important aspects of trust.

TABLE 6-1
Characteristics of Organizations that Trust and Those that Don't Trust

Trusting Organizations	Organizations Without Trust
Information is shared	Information is withheld
People support one another	People look out for themselves
Teams	Cliques
Communication	Gossip
Autonomy	Micromanagement
Innovation	Bureaucracy
Fun place to work	Low morale
Longevity, experience	Turnover
Satisfied customers	Customer turnover

demonstrate a high degree of productivity and good morale. Figure 6-3 shows important aspects of trust.

In contrast, a distrustful environment is divisive. Morale suffers, turnover increases, and patients leave after acknowledging this dynamic. Table 6-1 compares characteristics of trusting organizations and organizations where trust is lacking.

Trust is the lubrication that makes it possible for organizations to work.

—Warren Bennis

When Trust Is Broken

Our distrust is very expensive.

—Ralph Waldo Emerson

Trust is fragile. It takes a long time to build it, but it can be broken in a heartbeat. Even when trust is sustained, it takes a lot of work to keep it going day after day.

If you break someone's trust, there are only two things you can do to repair the damage. First, you must apologize. Then, you will have to start all over to slowly rebuild trust one act at a time. You will be able to redeem yourself eventually.

◄ JOURNALING 6-3

Reflect on a time when you betrayed someone's trust. Imagine how the other person felt. Did they forgive you? Did you redeem yourself? Where does the relationship stand today, and why it is the way it is?

What if a co-worker betrays your trust? It is tempting to lash out emotionally, but it is best to restrain this urge.

Saying nothing is sometimes the wisest course. After all, everyone slips up now and then, and we usually feel bad enough without being reminded of our errors. However, if the error is significant and you feel it is more constructive to say something, it might be appropriate to calmly address your co-worker. Make your feedback easier to deliver by first calling attention to your co-worker's strengths: "You're usually such a great team player, Anna. That kind of behavior was the last thing I would have expected from you."

Whether you address the situation or not, give yourself a little time to heal before attempting to mend the relationship.

It's best to forgive a co-worker even if they don't ask for your forgiveness. When you forgive someone, you feel better. We all make mistakes. Forgive, move on, and leave the door open to repair the relationship. After all, you have to work with this person, and it's difficult to work effectively without trust. Forgiveness means letting go of resentment and bitterness, not forgetting. Although you may remember the incident, you are no longer emotionally affected by it.

The weak can never forgive.
Forgiveness is the attribute of the strong.

—Mahatma Gandhi

Like a broken bone that has healed, trust that is rebuilt can be stronger than it was before it was broken. Once everyone involved forgives, the relationship can become stronger than it was before the incident. Your perception changes when you strive for forgiveness because you gain understanding of how the incident happened in the first place, and learn how to avoid similar instances in the future.

CASE STUDY 6-1
Trust Me

Richard Fecht wasn't even born when his father was killed in Vietnam. He had two older brothers, but they weren't close. Richard struggled through high school and worked a series of odd jobs since graduating.

After several years stuck in a rut, Richard decided he needed to start over. He packed up the Jeep and drove to Flagstaff because he heard they needed EMTs. The training was even subsidized by the county. Richard signed on and worked at a nursing home to make ends meet.

Richard's EMT-Basic class was a diverse group. At 40, Richard wasn't among the youngest in his class. Most of the people were young, just beginning careers that many of them had been committed to pursuing for a long time. Once the training began, Richard started to think that being an EMT could be the solution to his lack of direction.

Richard was hired once he completed his training. The company put Richard with a different crew every few days, so he could get to know the other employees. He asked everyone he met the same questions. How long would it take to feel comfortable with the job? What did they like about the company? What was their background? He heard about memorable runs and imagined what he might have done if he was faced with the same situations.

One day, the company installed new defibrillators on each unit. Everybody received training, but some of the EMTs complained about always having to get used to new equipment. Rather than complaining, Richard picked up a copy of the training manual and familiarized himself with all of the defibrillator's functions.

A few days later, Richard's efforts paid off. His unit got a call from a hysterical mother. Her infant son wasn't breathing and was turning blue. His crew started performing heart compressions as they carried the infant to the ambulance. The team wasn't able to find a heartbeat, so Richard prepared the defibrillator. "Here," said Richard. "We need to turn the infant key."

"Are we ready?" one of Richard's teammates, Rachel, asked as she grabbed the paddles.

Richard nodded. "Clear!" yelled Rachel. She shocked the infant twice and was able to detect a feeble heartbeat. The heartbeat continued all the way to the Medical Center, but it was erratic. Richard located a cable to attach his iPhone to the strip stored in the HeartStart's memory. As soon as they got the infant into the ER, he worked with one of the emergency department technicians to download the strip from his iPhone to their main system.

Back in the unit, Richard explained the infant key to the rest of his team and explained how he downloaded the sinus rhythm strip.

"Lucky to have you aboard," said Art, the crew chief.

Mr. Carmichael, the vice president of operations, asked Richard to develop a more in-depth training course for the defibrillator.

QUESTIONS FOR THOUGHT AND REFLECTION
1. What was missing from Richard's life before he arrived in Flagstaff?
2. What listening skills did Richard demonstrate?
3. Even though he was new to the profession and the company, how did Richard manage to demonstrate his clinical skill competency?
4. List the trust-building efforts that Richard made throughout this story.

Down a Dark Road

Willie Davis had been working at the Arcadia State Hospital for more than 40 years. He had seen huge changes in the care of the mentally ill, but he thought his job as a mental health worker was more dangerous now than it had ever been. Long ago, patients had few rights. Many were committed by courts. Restraints and seclusion rooms were common responses to patients who were aggressive or suicidal. Now, the least dangerous patients have been moved out of the state hospitals and into the community, in halfway houses and group homes. Many are cared for by their families, but a large percentage of the homeless population is now made up of mentally ill people who used to receive treatment in state-supported psychiatric hospitals.

Now, Willie thought that only the most dangerous patients remained. Mental health workers have to think on their feet to manage patients and assaults are common. "A lot of people I've worked with over the years live on disability," he told a group of new employees. He was teaching a class on restraints and self-defense, and he wanted them to understand how important these skills would be to them.

One of the six new employees, Keith Cummings, was assigned to the unit where Willie worked. Willie was paying special attention to him because he had a few concerns. For one thing, Keith wasn't maintaining eye contact with Willie.

"You have to be on the same exact team as your fellow staff members at all times," Willie barked at the newbies. Willie demonstrated all the physical techniques, having the new staff members stand in as patients. They learned how to protect against assaults. They learned how to safely restrain a patient, getting him to the floor and immobilizing all the limbs. "It takes four to carry a patient so nobody gets hurt," he explained. "You carry him face down," he said as he demonstrated the skill. "He won't be as strong, and he won't be as panicked." Keith seemed tentative, even when Willie showed him the techniques. "Grab the wrist and put your other hand on his shoulder. If he's still fighting you, twist the wrist a little." Willie told them that if they worked as a team, built their skills, and learned to trust one another, they could minimize the chances of getting hurt or injuring a patient. "Everything we do here," he declared, "is in the interest of the patient."

One week after orientation, Keith showed up for his first shift with Willie. Fortunately, the unit was going through a quiet time. The mix of patients did not seem too combustible, and the staff seemed to have developed strong relationships even with the more dangerous patients. Keith had majored in psychology at Bates College, and he hoped to become a psychologist eventually. This looked like a difficult job, but he wanted to get some exposure to people who had severe mental illnesses, and he hoped the experience would help him get accepted to graduate school in a year or two.

He introduced himself to the psychiatrists and residents and tried to draw them into conversations about the patients. He wanted to understand the etiology of their illnesses, the dysfunctional parts of their brains, the treatment and prognosis.

At the end of the first week, there was a minor scuffle involving a new patient, Larry M., which was quickly defused. Willie, Keith, and two other experienced staff members were on the scene. They lowered the patient to the carpet, keeping his arms and legs immobilized until he calmed down. Keith was confused about his responsibility as he moved around the scene. By the time he regained control, the patient was ready to be escorted to the day room.

Keith's poor performance confirmed Willie's worries. He took Keith out to the side yard to practice some of the moves. He was trying to be patient, but got frustrated when he realized that Keith wasn't even trying. "I don't think I like this part of the job," he told Willie. "Nobody does," said Willie, "but it's not optional."

Everything stayed quiet for the next few weeks until a serious incident occurred. Willie was by himself with Lou, a burly patient with a persecution complex. Without warning, he attacked Willie, who shouted "Help" as the two crashed to the floor. Willie had to cover himself from the blows. He thought he saw Keith walk by and then retreat around the corner. Help arrived after several seconds, but Keith wasn't among them.

"Where'd that kid go?" said one of them, after Lou had been subdued.

"He called for help, but that's the last we saw of him."

QUESTIONS FOR THOUGHT AND REFLECTION

1. What cues should Keith have taken from Willie to help gain Willie's confidence?
2. What interest did Keith show in learning his new job?
3. Do you think Keith's behavior was normal during the first physical scuffle?
4. Do you think Keith will be able to keep his job?

 EXPERIENTIAL EXERCISES

1. Ask an acquaintance to do a favor for you today.
2. Ask a friend for some advice on a problem you are having.
3. Make a trust chart. Using graph paper, list the important people in your life across the top. Color in the squares of the graph paper below each name to show your level of trust in each of the people.
4. Forgive somebody today, and really mean it.

 CROSS CURRENTS WITH OTHER SOFT SKILLS

ADOPTING A POSITIVE ATTITUDE: A positive attitude is basic to forming trust. (pp. 2-11)

ACHIEVING HONESTY AND INTEGRITY: Building trust is all about consistently honest behavior. (pp. 18-25)

STRIVING FOR TOLERANCE: Building trust means being open minded. If you are tolerant and open minded, you will be amazed and delighted by what you will learn. (pp. 29-35)

LISTENING ACTIVELY: This is a key skill for building trust. (pp. 263-269)
CONTRIBUTING AS A MEMBER OF THE TEAM: Trust is a social enterprise. (pp. 336-346)

Showing Empathy, Sensitivity, and Caring

How far you go in life depends on you being tender with the young, compassionate with the aged, sympathetic with the striving and tolerant of the weak and the strong.
Because someday in life you will have been all of these.

—George Washington Carver

LEARNING OBJECTIVE 2: SHOWING EMPATHY, SENSITIVITY, AND CARING

- Define empathy.
- Describe the limbic system of the brain and its relationship to empathy.
- Explain the importance of intuition for health care professionals.
- Identify multiple ways of increasing and deepening your empathy.
- Explain mirroring and its effect on empathy.
- Describe the empathic organization.

Empathy is the capacity to understand the emotions of another person. It makes us feel connected to others. Without empathy, we would be isolated, lonely, and misunderstood.

When you start to develop your powers of empathy and imagination, the whole world opens up to you.

—Susan Sarandon

Health care professionals must have empathy. We are in the business of helping others alleviate worry and suffering, helping them to heal, and maximizing their wellness. These outcomes are difficult to achieve without empathy.

Research shows that it is easier to experience empathy with people who are like us than with people who are from different cultural backgrounds. Health care professionals are required to develop empathy for all kinds of people. Curiosity is the first step in achieving this empathy.

People, people who need people,
are the luckiest people in the world.

—Bob Merrill

Wired to Care: The Neuroscience of Empathy

The Primitive Brain

To understand how we develop empathy for others, let's examine the neuroscience of empathy. In broad terms, humans have developed three brains, starting with the medulla, which sits at the top of the spinal column at the core of the brain. This "reptilian" brain controls involuntary physical actions such as breathing and heart rate, and primitive responses such as sex drive and the "fight or flee" stress response (see Chapter 5).

The Highly Evolved Brain

The neocortex makes up about 80% of the total mass of the human brain. This recently evolved outer layer of the brain controls thinking, imagination, logic, symbolism, and language.

The Limbic System, the Seat of Memory and Emotion

The limbic system controls memory and emotions. In the limbic system, two structures are especially important, the amygdala, which is the emotional processing control center of the brain, and the hippocampus, which manages memory functions. Their communication circuits are highly interrelated. As a result, events with strong emotional content tend to survive vividly in our memories for a long time.

The limbic system also enables us to interpret emotions and body language, which aids our capability to empathize with others. The amygdala and the hippocampus enable us to form relationships, passionate values and beliefs, and commitments to the most important people in our lives.

Interesting phenomena emerge from the limbic system. For one thing, all the information we have learned from relationships forms an emotional context that is unique in each individual. This limbic context helps us evaluate new people and experiences by making us naturally more or less trusting, more suspicious or more accepting, more introverted or more extroverted, more distant or more empathetic. It's difficult to remove genetic components that help determine these traits, but our "nature" is definitely modified by the "nurture" of our experiences, and the way we process them emotionally in the limbic structures.

A person is a person because he recognizes others as persons.

—Bishop Desmond Tutu

What we know as a result of our limbic brain makes us curious about the new people we meet. How do they fit into our personal context? What is the first impression we form? Do we see similarities and contrasts with other people we know? Is our first impulse to like or dislike the new person? Health professionals tend to have a highly developed sense of empathy, and our limbic brains help us help people.

The capabilities of the human brain are beyond imagination. Scientists are only beginning to understand its workings. One such capability is intuition. Somehow, we gather information, filter it through our context, power it with our curiosity, interpret subtle body language, and find unspoken meanings. Intuition can manifest as an instant feeling of deep understanding and connection, or as a hunch that something "doesn't feel right." It is an advanced sense of empathy, resulting from rich limbic context.

The great gift of human beings is that we have the power of empathy,
we can all sense a mysterious connection to each other.

—Meryl Streep

Ways to Discover, Enhance, and Deepen Your Empathy

Since empathy is a natural state of being, you already have it. But by understanding the way we are wired to be empathetic, there are a number of strategies you can pursue to become even more acutely empathetic and thus improve your emotional intelligence—the kind of intelligence needed most in health care facilities (Box 6-2).

Social Intelligence

Examining the context of your social intelligence can be helpful in deepening your sense of empathy. Social intelligence itself has five components: situational awareness, presence, authenticity, clarity, and empathy (Figure 6-4).

Situational awareness involves knowing how to act appropriately in a situation. People who lack

---

BOX 6-2

Strategies for Becoming More Emotionally Attuned

- Develop a plan to improve your active listening skills and practice this plan.
- Consciously search for the emotional content expressed by others.
- Reflect upon your own emotions in a quiet place.
- Make eye contact and observe body language.
- Allow pauses and silences in conversations.
- Confirm your observation of others' emotions by using statements such as, "You seem disappointed" and "How did that make you feel?"
- See other people as puzzles that you want to solve.

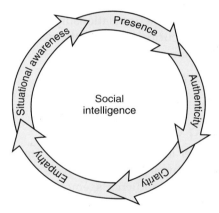

FIGURE 6-4 Components of social intelligence.

situational awareness might have poor manners, for example. Presence is also referred to as your overall "bearing" or total impression you make on people through your behavior, body language, and charisma. Authenticity is a question of how deeply your ethics influence your behavior. It involves the honesty of your reactions. Some people have a difficult time expressing their ideas coherently, while others are plainspoken. People with good clarity will use colorful language and express ideas dramatically. Moreover, people who possess clarity will use their verbal ability to cater to their audience and build empathy.

Empathy, as we have seen, is more than just identifying with others. It involves building connections with others so that you understand how they feel. Developing a sense of empathy will help create a smooth work environment. Patients are admitted and cared for, and they leave satisfied. Treatments are conducted expeditiously, with the patient's cooperation. Unexpected problems are solved quickly.

The cost of operating without empathy is significant. If someone is demeaning, argumentative, hostile, or unaware of the needs of others around him, he will not generate the empathy and cooperation he needs from others to achieve his objectives.

Questioning and Listening

Ask perceptive questions, and then listen actively. This is the way to build empathy. Listening actively (see Chapter 9) involves a lot more than hearing and understanding words. While you are listening, notice the paracommunication that accompanies the speaker's words, such as their gestures, facial expressions, pauses, and tone. What can you tell about their emotions? How do they *feel* about what they are saying? What are they conveying that you want to ask about next? Showing interest in people is the first step in forming an empathetic relationship, followed up by your genuine curiosity about them as individuals. Withhold judgment; just learn.

Compassion begins with attention.

—Daniel Goleman

Imagining Others

Have you ever identified with a character in a movie or a book? Of course, films and novels are constructed to maximize the audience's emotional response as they imagine what it must be like to be in a character's shoes. Use your empathetic skills to try to relate to a patient or a colleague as if they were a character you are curious about, reflecting on what they are saying and paying attention to their emotional content (Figure 6-5).

JOURNALING 6-4

List three of your behaviors you would like to change. Record when these negative behaviors occur, and consider how you can become more aware of them so you can change them more effectively.

Mirroring

One way we can connect with others is to mirror their behavior. All of us can practice empathy by picking

FIGURE 6-5 A counselor and group members console a distraught man (Copyright © istock.com).

up on facial expressions, tone, gestures, or posture. It seems we even have mirror neurons in the premotor cortex of our brains, the area responsible for planning actions. These cells fire automatically, helping us mirror each other's actions almost automatically. We see this when babies mimic their parents' facial expressions, for example. These neurons also help us learn by watching someone perform a skill. They help us "read" each other, laughing when others laugh, and wincing when we see violence.

The existence and role of mirror neurons suggest that human beings are wired for social interaction, and that empathy is a natural state of being.

Organizational Empathy

WHAT IF?

What if you became ill or needed treatment? Would you choose to seek it at your place of employment? Why or why not? Is your decision influenced by the amount of empathy you would receive?

Every patient or client is looking for empathy as a large part of their experience when they come to your facility. Knowing that, you can either meet this need or not. If you are empathetic toward everyone who comes to your facility, you are supporting the mission of your health care organization and meeting your needs for emotional connection. If you are not empathetic, even if it is just because you are having a bad day, you are detracting from the organization's mission. Empathy only delivers its benefits when it is given consistently and genuinely. The organization suffers when even one employee lacks empathy.

WHAT IF?

What if you are ordering toilet tissue for the restrooms? You are about to select the least expensive brand when a co-worker says she hates cheap toilet tissue and would prefer to have better quality tissue. What would you do?

JOURNALING 6-5

Record an experience where you experienced the "golden rule" in a health care facility, where you were treated exactly how you would have wanted to be treated. What did the providers do to create this experience for you? How did it make you feel?

Service providers sometimes lose contact with their customers. Fortunately, health care providers meet face to face with customers. Health care will never be mass produced. Therapists will deliver massages to one customer at a time. Physician assistants will address all of a patient's injuries before moving on to the next person in line. The ability to provide this level of attention for each patient is part of what makes working in health care so rewarding. However, empathy is essential in delivering services in this one-on-one model.

Never forget to put yourself in your patient's shoes. What's worrying her? Is she feeling any pain or anxiety? What kind of care is she expecting from you? You will become a great health care professional when you can understand where your patients are coming from, and can respond to their needs with those insights.

CASE STUDY 6-2
Sister Act

Simone had already had a long work day as a Home Health Aide before heading back to the office to complete her paperwork. The agency manager, Iris, was speaking with two middle-aged sisters and their elderly mother who was in a wheelchair.

Simone listened as the sisters, Ella and Diane, spoke "It's become unmanageable," Diane said. "Mother is going downhill fast, but she insists on staying in her house."

"Mrs. Carter," Iris said, speaking directly to the mother, "what kind of help do you need in order to stay in your home?"

"She's incontinent and she forgets to take her medicine," Ella said. "She needs a cane and she can't cook anything for herself. She could fall or starve. I don't think she would be able to use the phone to call for an emergency. It's just so exasperating!"

"Can you walk without a wheelchair, Mrs. Carter?" asked Iris.

"Yes, but it would take a year," said Diane. "We only brought her because we thought you would want to see her. If a home aide doesn't work, a nursing home is the next stop."

"Yes, well I am very glad you came, Mrs. Carter. I think we should give home health a try," said Iris.

Two days later, Simone arrived at Mrs. Carter's home. Although it took a long time for Mrs. Carter to answer the door, Simone was surprised to see how clean the house was.

"Do your daughters help you with the housework?" Simone asked.

"I do it myself, just when they're not here," Mrs. Carter said. "They don't think I can do it. Diane thinks Ella picks up and Ella thinks Diane does it. I'm sure they think it doesn't need much cleaning, with me just sitting in a chair all day."

Over tea, Simone asked Mrs. Carter about what she needed help with. "A hot lunch," she said immediately. "And a light snack for later. I left the gas on once, which frightened me and upset my daughters. I am becoming forgetful. It worries me. Can you cook, dear?"

"Oh yes, Mrs. Carter. You will be very happy with my cooking." Working from a checklist, Simone spoke with Mrs. Carter about her finances, her daily routine, her ambulatory ability, her general health and her medication. They agreed that Simone would come from 10:00 to 12:00 every weekday. She would buy groceries before she arrived on Monday, from a list Mrs. Carter would give her on Friday. She would make sure that Mrs. Carter took her medication correctly. She offered to help Mrs. Carter with the housework, and she said she would conduct regular assessments to review her functioning and also drive her to doctor appointments.

On Friday morning, Ella and Diane were there when Simone arrived. Simone offered to cut them some of the blueberry pie she made for Mrs. Carter the day before. Both accepted as the four of them sat around the kitchen table.

"Mother is so happy with your cooking, Simone," Diane said. "It's such a load off of our minds, to know that you are taking care of her."

"Does she take her medicine?" Ella asked Simone.

"Have you noticed how forgetful she can be?" added Diane.

"Mrs. Carter, would you mind if I spoke privately with your daughters?"

"Of course she doesn't mind," said Diane.

"I don't mind," said Mrs. Carter.

As they walked out to the backyard, Simone welcomed the sisters to share their worries about their mother.

"Oh, she's just going downhill so fast," Ella said.

"What makes you say that?" Simone said.

"Did you hear about how she left the gas on?" Ella said.

"She told me about that," Simone said. "It frightened her too, but it's good that she could remember and agree that it's a problem."

"And we just can't spend all our time over here anymore," said Diane. "We have our own families to consider."

"Well, ladies," said Simone. "I feel very confident that the ten hours I spend with your mother every week will assure her care and her ability to live here in her own home." The sisters nodded. Before heading back inside, Simone shared one last tip. "Speak directly to her. Engage her in your concerns. That will help her feel that she is actively involved in her own self care. Allow her to do as much as she can for herself. It may take her a little longer than if you did things for her, but she seems to take pride in her abilities."

Ella and Diane kept nodding.

"My ears were burning," said Mrs. Carter, "but I'm pretty sure it didn't have anything to do with the stove." The sisters laughed and Simone could tell their discussion helped to relieve their worries.

QUESTIONS FOR THOUGHT AND REFLECTION

1. Did Simone judge the sisters and let them know what she thought of them?
2. What information about Mrs. Carter's functioning became clearer as Simone talked to her?
3. What do you think the sisters' true concerns were?
4. Although Mrs. Carter needed some help, what made Simone think she could function in her own home?

Down a Dark Road

Miranda was the new administrative medical assistant at the practice of Drs. Shaw, Sybil, Martinez, and Rao. The practice manager, Candice Yang, hired Miranda based on the reputation of the school she went to, her grades, and her portfolio. Miranda was to welcome patients, confirm their appointments, and pull charts. If she worked out, Candice would give her additional responsibilities.

Candice handled the administrative responsibilities for the first two days, so Miranda could shadow her. Candice introduced her to the rest of the staff, explained the medical records system, and gave her the insurance and intake forms to review. "Are you sure you don't have any questions?" asked Candice.

"Nope," said Miranda.

On Wednesday, Candice turned the receptionist desk over to Miranda. "Are you sure you feel comfortable with everything?" Candice asked her.

"Yup."

That afternoon, Candice started receiving complaints about Miranda. "I told her my name twice," said Andy, the lab tech, "and she still can't remember." Leslie, one of the LPNs, was miffed when her greeting to Miranda went unanswered. "Friendly, the new girl," she told Candice. "Can't wait to hear her voice."

"Give her a chance," said Candice nervously. "I'm sure she's feeling a little overwhelmed." Then Dr. Shaw stuck his head in her office. "I had to fish my 2:30 appointment out of the lobby. She hadn't even been greeted. Can you do something about this?"

Candice confronted Miranda.

"I didn't even see her come in."

"You should have been expecting her. Didn't you notice her sitting in the lobby?"

"There were several people in the lobby."

"Yes, she was the one you hadn't checked in. You have to pay attention Miranda."

The next day, Candice ran to the lobby when she heard loud voices. Miranda was having an argument with Mr. Chatterjee. She turned to Candice and blurted out, "I can't understand him. He's talking gibberish."

"Gibberish!" thundered Mr. Chatterjee. "I only asked about what the test is for!"

"I don't know what his test is for," Miranda said. "Tell him to ask the doctor."

"I will tell him no such thing," said Candice. "Mr. Chatterjee, please come with me," she said just as Dr. Rao arrived in the lobby to see what the shouting was about.

"Miranda, you're fired," Candice said. "Get your things and get out."

QUESTIONS FOR THOUGHT AND REFLECTION

1. What did Candice fail to evaluate when she hired Miranda?
2. What clues did Candice overlook as she gave Miranda her orientation?
3. Should Miranda be working in health care?
4. Can Candice recover from her mistake?

⭐ EXPERIENTIAL EXERCISES

1. Watch an episode of CBS' *Undercover Boss*, in which a chief executive officer of a major corporation assumes a position among employees on the frontline and interacts with the corporation's customers. Typically, this experience produces amazing insights for the corporate executives, because they develop empathy for their employees and the customers they serve.
2. Spend some time in a hospital lobby. Can you discern people's roles by observing their dress, body language, and interaction style?
3. Face a friend and mimic each other as you change expressions. Then, try to mirror each other with more subtlety, as if you were engaging with a new acquaintance.
4. Pick a program on TV or a movie with an appealing character. Watch it and observe the empathy you develop with this character. What habits and behaviors can you learn from this character?

⊘ CROSS CURRENTS WITH OTHER SOFT SKILLS

ACHIEVING HONESTY AND INTEGRITY: This core of your character enables you to be empathic. (pp. 18-25)

ADOPTING A POSITIVE MENTAL ATTITUDE: A positive mental attitude is easier to adopt and maintain if you understand the mechanics of empathy. (pp. 2-11)

STRIVING FOR TOLERANCE: Tolerance is easier with empathy. (pp. 29-35)

CONTRIBUTING AS A MEMBER OF A TEAM: Know how showing empathy can help transform your team and organization in to a deeply caring group. (pp. 336-342)

READING AND SPEAKING BODY LANGUAGE: So much of what makes up empathy is unspoken. (pp. 277-284)

CHAPTER 7

Dealing with Others

- Consider conflict as a neutral aspect of the workplace, capable of producing innovations or difficulties.
- Understand the role of ego in conflict and in dealing with difficult people.
- Develop a general strategy for dealing with difficult people of all types.
- Explain the current status of racism, prejudice, and bigotry in our society.
- State the importance of multicultural competence to health care.
- Create a thoughtful, consistent, and positive way to answer the phone.
- Try to separate emotions from problems.

Managing and Resolving Conflict

The art of being wise is the art of knowing what to overlook.

—William James

LEARNING OBJECTIVE 1: MANAGING AND RESOLVING CONFLICT

- Name the five conflict management styles.
- Explain the four generations of workers as a source of conflict.
- Name other sources of conflict in the workplace.
- Explain how reframing can eliminate conflict.
- Gain insight into four conflict resolution skills.

Is This a Fight or a Conflict?

What do you think of when you hear the word "conflict?" Do you think of angry people fighting and arguing? Maybe you even think of warfare, as in a military conflict. Many people avoid conflict because they tend to think of conflict as something personal—people fighting against other people. The truth is, conflict can be functional instead of personal; it arises because the timing and goals of events or procedures sometimes overlap. For example, a patient may be scheduled to have a meal just before a procedure that requires him to have fasted for 12 hours beforehand. That's a scheduling or procedural conflict: it's not personal. No one is angry at or opposed to someone else. Anger and confrontation are not always part of conflict, especially if you approach it correctly.

Later in this chapter, interpersonal conflict with co-workers or patients are covered. But first, let's examine conflict organically, as a normal feature of daily life in the workplace, without any judgments.

WHAT IF?

What if you found that conflict was conducted with politeness and civility in your workplace? Would that surprise you? Is that really possible?

Don't Take This Personally

Even though conflict can be positive, we are conditioned to think it's going to be a negative experience—something involving winners and losers—so it can be difficult to keep our egos at bay. Instead of seeking solutions, we expect to win or lose, to hurt or be hurt. People tend to resort to one of several conflict management styles according to the Thomas-Kilmann Conflict Mode Instrument: avoiding, compromising, collaborating, accommodating, and competing (Figure 7-1). Later in this chapter, we look at smart ways to approach a conflict objectively and constructively. Before we can develop smarter strategies, however, we have to learn to recognize old habits—good or bad.

Which of the following is your most common knee-jerk reaction to conflict?

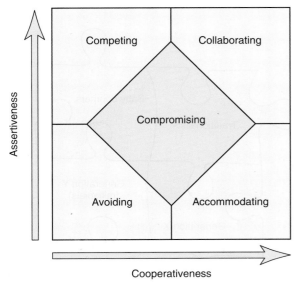

FIGURE 7-1 Adaptation of the Thomas-Kilmann Conflict Mode Instrument.

Avoiding

Normally an ineffective conflict management approach, avoiding can nevertheless be appropriate when the outcome of the conflict doesn't matter to you. You may feel it's trivial, so you simply withdraw. However, when you feel there is something at stake, avoidance becomes a poor strategy. The other party may be unaware of your concern, which can leave you feeling powerless.

Compromising

Compromising can be an effective approach if the outcome is satisfactory to all parties. As a starting point, compromise can foster creativity and teamwork, which can be positive approaches to a solution. Conversely, compromising will be unsatisfying if one or more of the parties are unhappy with the compromise. In these cases, the parties have settled merely to avoid further conflict.

JOURNALING 7-1

Think about a compromise you have made recently, and describe it in your journal. How did it come about? Are you satisfied with it? Should you have handled the conflict differently?

Collaborating

Collaboration is the optimal approach in most cases. It involves seeking the input of all parties involved in the conflict, which makes everyone feel validated. It incorporates the positive aspects of compromising because it encourages developing a broad range of potential solutions, through teamwork and creativity. Although irrational parties may never agree to a reasonable solution, this approach uses problem-solving to implement solutions even over the objection of irrational parties, in the interests of a higher goal such as patient safety.

If you tend to be a problem-solver, try not to get pigeon-holed. You'll wear yourself out if you become the "go-to" person for conflicts, and you could even be perceived as controlling or interfering. Encourage others to take the lead.

Accommodating

Accommodation takes compromise one step further by addressing the concerns of the other party rather than your own. Although this approach pays off if the other party possesses the optimal solution, be careful not to be too accommodating. If you always accommodate the needs of others before considering your own, people may see you as indecisive or easily manipulated. This perception can prevent you from advancing or achieving your goals.

Competing

Competing is not a productive conflict management approach because its aim is control rather than progress. Sometimes competitive people have no idea what they want, just that they want to win. Although being assertive can help you reach your goals, blind assertiveness that lacks cooperation is detrimental. Don't forget that providing health care is a team effort and that your colleagues have valuable wisdom to share.

Identifying Sources of Conflict at Work

So how should we approach conflict when we encounter it?

The first step is to understand how the conflict arose in the first place. Recognizing these sources of conflict will put things in perspective right away.

People, disagreements, situations, policies, and workload stressors can lead to conflict at work. Some days are worse than others and some sources of conflict are worth constructive engagement; others are not. You don't have to engage in conflict every time a situation with the potential for conflict arises. In most cases, it's up to you. Choose wisely.

Four Generations at Work

As seen in Chapter 4, four distinct generations now share the workplace for the first time in history, bringing different sets of values, norms, and expectations to the job. In health care, where teamwork is so important, members of different generations might clash from time to time. In fact, a generational tidal wave is hitting the workplace with a force not seen since Baby Boomers arrived at their desks in the early 1970s. Plus, the Millennials, born after 1980, challenge the workplace like never before.

Although they are becoming less numerous due to retirement, members of the "Great Generation" who came of age during World War II tend to occupy positions of importance and authority. These "traditional"

workers value hard work and may be less flexible than their younger colleagues. Still, they are a great source of wisdom, which provides a valuable perspective when solving problems. Younger generations should treat these senior colleagues with respect, if not deference. In fact, part of their value in the workplace is in the maturity they demand of younger workers.

Baby Boomers were born between 1946 and 1964 and often work 60 hours a week to succeed and advance in their professions. They are loyal to their employers, often building a career at the same company until retirement.

Generation X workers were born between 1965 and 1980 and may feel left out of the 21st century workplace as many Baby Boomers earn available promotions. This generation also seeks flexibility in their workplace in order to gain a better balance between work and personal life.

Generation Y workers, or Millennials, share many of the same attitudes as their Baby Boomer parents, with whom they typically have close relationships. They are comfortable navigating technology and prefer working in groups. Figure 7-2 shows generations working together to achieve a common goal.

These generations are also discussed in Chapter 9.

JOURNALING 7-2

What generation are you a member of? Record some strategies for interacting positively with members of the other three generations you will encounter in the workplace.

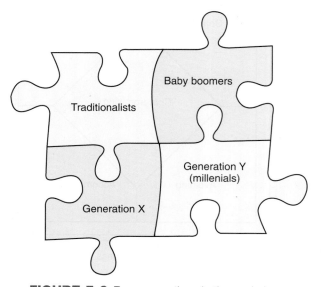

FIGURE 7-2 Four generations in the workplace.

Stressful Economic Conditions

Today's stressful economic realities are intruding into the workplace. Even though the health industry offers incredible growth opportunities for health professionals, this progress is stop-and-start. Although an aging population of Baby Boomers will demand excellent health care, and medical research is proceeding at an incredible pace, the financing of health care remains uncertain. As a result, some health professionals are competing with one another to avoid layoffs.

Health care facilities are also undergoing unprecedented consolidation through mergers and acquisitions as health care transitions from nonprofit to for-profit entities. Suddenly, there is a new emphasis on cost-cutting, productivity gains, and efficiencies through automation, such as electronic health records. All this change, often unwanted by workers, can lead to conflicts.

Difficult Personalities

Difficult co-workers and patients add stress and conflict to any workplace, and health care is no exception. Develop skills and strategies to combat these sources of conflict.

> *Nothing gives one person so much advantage over another as to remain always cool and unruffled under all circumstances.*
>
> —Thomas Jefferson

In a customer-oriented environment like health care, conflict arises among co-workers when someone fails to act because he or she believes a task is not their responsibility—a response seldom acceptable when it comes to patient care (Figure 7-3). Patients and their families are the reason your employer exists, and their care is the focus of your work. Patients and their loved ones are often in personal crisis or acute stress, and their behavior can lead to conflict with the health professionals they encounter. Working collaboratively, you and your colleagues are in the business of managing and resolving these conflicts. In health care, customer satisfaction is everyone's job, although people can be difficult at times.

Additional factors that contribute to or intensify conflict are listed in Box 7-1.

Strategies for Managing Conflict

Once you have identified the source or cause of your conflict, you can choose from a number of management strategies before it becomes a bigger issue. Once you set your emotions aside, the key is to focus on strategies under your control—reframing and action.

Let's examine some more specific strategies now.

Reframe to Eliminate Conflicts

The first step of conflict resolution is to focus on things that are within your control. This choice will divert

FIGURE 7-3 Two coworkers disagree about work duties (Copyright © istock.com).

BOX 7-1

Sources of Conflict at Work

- Assumptions and expectations both cause conflict when they are not commonly understood.
- Core values, such as honesty, are not being met. Many conflicts appear to be over surface issues, but these often mask deep issues.
- Different personal lenses and interpretations of the world based on insensitivity to other's religion, political beliefs, or moral convictions can lead to conflict.
- Emotions: Once emotions are engaged, logic and common sense can get lost.
- Gossip and cliques: Whether you're in high school or at work, gossip and "in" crowds are destructive.
- Miscommunication and vague or thoughtless language can lead to unnecessary conflict. Try to pause and choose the right words the first time. It is extremely difficult to correct a misimpression that you caused with careless language.

your attention from the negatives and give you something positive to focus on.

* *Change your perspective.* In cognitive psychology, this is called "reframing." What if you no longer cared how a dispute turns out? What if you viewed circumstances from a different perspective? You don't have to be a prisoner of your own preferences or biases.
* *Review your personal goals.* Goals are aspirations that are truly important. How does the outcome of the conflict fit into your larger goals? This perspective might change the importance you attach to a particular conflict, position, or solution.
* *Change your response.* Visualize what happens if you choose a different response. Listen and then restate your colleague's or patient's concern. Ask yourself if you are responsible in a significant way for what has happened. Are your expectations for a resolution unrealistic, out of line, or just not that important? What can you learn from this calm analysis? What solutions might arise from your thoughtful considerations?
* *Check your impulse control.* Ask yourself why some people you know don't seem to get caught up in certain kinds of conflicts. Ask them for their perspective and advice.
* *Finally, act like a third party mediator* in your own mind. Step outside of yourself for a moment. Ask questions. Why is this issue so important? If you were a disinterested bystander, what could you see that might help resolve a conflict?

Conflict Resolution Skills

If addressing the issue still feels important once you have tried reframing the conflict, it probably is. In this case, it's time to take action, often collaboratively. Negotiators all use well-established skills to help end conflict. By now, these may seem like common sense to you, but it is worth examining them from a health care perspective.

Finding Common Ground

Conflict is centered on disagreements. Therefore, take a moment to review what people in the dispute *do* agree on. This helps create a context in which the disagreement seems a little smaller in scope and importance. For instance, a dispute might arise in the

FIGURE 7-4 A nursing assistant changes bed linen, setting a positive example of patient care (Copyright © istock.com).

waiting room as to who arrived first. Assure everyone that they will see the doctor shortly. The dispute has not been resolved, but the common ground makes it seem less important.

Setting a Positive Example

You can exercise leadership simply by holding your own behavior to a higher level. Suppose two other nursing assistants are standing outside of a patient's room, arguing over whose turn it is to clean the room. "I'll help," you say, going into the room. The conflict is likely to dissipate because of your positive example (Figure 7-4).

Facilitating the Exchange of Ideas

You can elevate a negative, ego-controlled conflict into a positive and productive conflict by refocusing the discussion on the issues rather than the people. Andy wants to sterilize the instruments at the beginning of the day, but Susan wants to do it at the end of the day when she has more time. "Has anybody asked Dr. Day what she prefers? How long does the sterilization take? Does it matter how recently the instruments were sterilized?" By asking questions about the process and best practices, you have introduced new considerations that may help remove egos from the discussion.

Consulting Evidence and Documentation

The same resolution process can be facilitated by referencing documentation. By referring to an objective source, ego-based positions can be abandoned more readily. If the conflict has to do with infection control practices, you might suggest that everyone examine the latest Universal Precautions issued by the Centers for Disease Control and Prevention to determine whether the issue is covered.

Collaborating to Analyze

Finally, try an open-minded approach by listening to the other person's viewpoint objectively. Then consider all the factors to either adjust your own viewpoint or support your point of view.

For instance, let's say you have a co-worker who objects to the holiday work schedule. Christmas falls on a Saturday this year, so the following Monday will be an observed holiday. You have Christmas off, but will have to come in on Monday. Your co-worker is scheduled to work Christmas, but wants to be off too. You point out that since Christmas is on a Saturday, he'll get Sunday *and* Monday off without it counting toward his holidays. In some ways, then, he is getting the better end of the deal.

What You Can Learn from a Conflict and Its Resolution

Can you learn anything from a situation that will help you avoid being drawn into these kinds of conflicts in the future? Almost always, each situation offers insights for the future. The more thoughtful you become about managing, resolving, and reviewing conflicts, the less likely it is that your next conflict will be quite as negative.

CASE STUDY 7-1
Slow Down

Dominick DelVecchio decided to see a counselor at the hospital's Employee Assistance Program before making a final decision about his career. He had been a first responder and paramedic for the Spring Valley Medical Center for almost 15 years, and he would really rather not resign, but he had been pushed to the limit.

He could admit it. Lately, he had been a little hard to get along with. Over the past year, he had gotten into numerous arguments with his co-workers. Lately, the tragedies that were just supposed to be part of the job were getting to him, especially accidents involving children.

Ten days ago, he had been in a really foul mood, and he didn't even know why. A call came in as soon as he arrived. It was an early labor in a remote area. He jumped behind the wheel and started driving way too fast for the dark conditions and winding roads.

"Slow down!" yelled Dave, as they slid on some gravel along the edge of a curve.

On the way back to the hospital, he was even worse. Sally kept pounding on the window, signaling to slow down.

Soon enough, they screeched into the ambulance dock, and the baby was born 15 minutes later, perfectly fine. The father told everyone that he saw the birth but it was nothing compared to the ambulance ride.

Two days later, Dominick received an email from Alfred Singh, the head of the Emergency Department, informing him that he was not to drive pending further notice.

Dominick explained all of this to the EAP counselor.

"What did Dr. Singh say when you talked to him about it?"

"I didn't talk to him about it. I'm not talking to some guy who delivers that kind of a notice in an email!"

"That doesn't seem right," the counselor agreed.

"No, it's not right."

"You seem very angry about it."

"Yes, I've been angry a lot lately," he said, almost surprised at his confession.

"Then let's talk about that," she said.

Dominick filled her in on the past year.

"I suggest you de-stress and reframe," she said.

"I'm open to anything," said Dominick. "I'm not myself."

She taught him to take some deep breaths. She urged him to hold his reactions to stressors and to think about his response. She suggested that he apologize to some people who were on the receiving end of his rage. Finally, she urged him to talk to Dr. Singh.

Dominick made an appointment to see Dr. Singh in his office.

"Dominick," said Dr. Singh. "I owe you an apology."

"You do?"

"Yes, one of the guys, I forget who, told me he thought you were driving recklessly, and I should have talked to you. I've been so stressed out recently, I don't know. I just fired off that email. I shouldn't have done that." After they finished talking, Dominick decided he was not going to be so unhappy. He was going to apologize to Dave, and some of the others. He also decided to keep seeing the EAP counselor.

QUESTIONS FOR THOUGHT AND REFLECTION

1. Did Dominick feel that he played a role in the conflict he was experiencing?
2. What part did emotions play in his conflicts?
3. Should Dominick have consulted the EAP counselor?
4. Why did Dr. Singh's apology make Dominick feel better?
5. Do you think Dominick will be happier on the job now? If so, who should get the credit for that?

Down a Dark Road

Southwestern Physical Therapy had just acquired five new continuous passive motion (CPM) machines for total knee replacements. Rick Cervantes, the owner of the practice, was psyched.

"By working with Orthopedics Southwest, we can rent these puppies out for $350 a week—that's twice the rate that the local medical supply outfits charge. We'll roll it into all the other billing, and nobody will be able to tell."

"I don't know," said Gary Loo, one of the therapists. "Since Frank Ramsey left, we don't have anyone trained on these things."

"These are patient controlled," scoffed Rick. "Look. They can operate them by themselves."

"It says here you can lock the patient out," said Gary, looking at the manual. "You can set sequence codes that keep the patient from fiddling with the settings. What about the Interferential Therapy units? Are you going to use them to subdue the pain?"

"Great idea, Gary. Really. We can add the IT units to the package and charge $450 a week. I can get portable IT units online for a hundred bucks apiece."

Gary shook his head.

"Now what?"

"I only brought up the IT units because, if you suppress the pain, the patients won't know that the settings are wrong. That could really damage a knee replacement."

"And what is the probability of that happening, Gary?"

"I really don't know, Rick. But it could happen."

"Low," said Rick. "That's the probability."

Gary just lowered his head.

"OK Gary. Do you have any other concerns here? We're just trying to make a little money, if that's OK with you."

"Well, what if Orthopedics Southwest notices we're gouging the patients on these devices. That's not going to sit too well."

"Are you kidding me, Gary? Do you think Art Kreutzer cares what we charge? It's the insurance that pays, Gary. Do you think Art Kreutzer keeps his fees low? Don't you think he charges $500 to sterilize his instruments afterward? Do you think he sends in a bill that says 'Sterilization, $500?' We're not going to itemize this stuff, Gary."

He fell silent and looked around the room. "OK, Gary, we'll train the patients on the CPM, if that will make you happy. They'll come here directly from the hospital anyway. We show them how this thing works and send them home."

"Maybe we should train the spouse or whatever. The patient will be out of it."

"OK, Gary, we'll train the spouse. We'll train the spouse, the daughter, the next-door neighbor, the family dog. Whatever makes you happy."

"I still think we should learn how to get the sequence codes and lock out the patient," said Gary.

"That'll take weeks, Gary. Meanwhile, these units are sitting right here, gathering interest charges, and Art Kreutzer is doing knee replacements all day long today. We're not going to wait around. You got your way on training the patients and their tennis partners, Gary. Just be happy about that."

Within a week, a CPM from Southwest Physical Therapy tore up a knee replacement, and the patient couldn't feel it because of the Interferential Therapy unit. Art Kreutzer summoned Rick Cervantes to a meeting at Orthopedics

Southwest. "Why weren't the sequence keys used to lock out the patient operation?" Kreutzer demanded to know.

Rick explained that they trained the patients on the CPMs.

"That's it," said Dr. Kreutzer. "There are plenty of PT providers. We're not using Southwest anymore."

"Are you kidding me, Art? You are our biggest customer. We get almost 70% of our referrals from you guys."

"I'm sorry, Mr. Cervantes. I've made up my mind."

After Rick left, Dr. Kreutzer told his colleagues. "You know, he was charging $450 a week for the package. Let's put the PT out to bid, and keep the cost no higher than $250 a week."

QUESTIONS FOR THOUGHT AND REFLECTION

1. Should Gary have been more assertive?
2. Was Gary satisfied with the compromise that they would train the patients on the CPM machines?
3. Rick sounded confident, but did he know enough about his customers, therapists, and patients to make these decisions himself? What could he have done to make this new stream of income work effectively?
4. What conflict resolution style did Rick use?
5. Why was Rick unable to retain the business from Orthopedics Southwest?

⭐ EXPERIENTIAL EXERCISES

1. Locate someone who seems to be able to avoid conflicts. Ask them about their strategies.
2. Watch a political debate or a news program featuring people with conflicting views. How much of the exchange is about issues and how much about egos. Were any of these conflicts resolved?
3. If you know a law enforcement officer, ask him or her about techniques they use to contain and resolve potential conflicts with the public.
4. Notice conflicts as they crop up in your life. Deliberately choose how you will respond.

🔄 CROSS CURRENTS WITH OTHER SOFT SKILLS

MANAGING STRESS: Managing conflict shares a lot with managing stress. (pp. 203-210)

LISTENING ACTIVELY: Conflict cannot be effectively managed without listening. (pp. 263-269)

CONTRIBUTING AS A MEMBER OF THE TEAM: Whether it is contributing to positive conflict or defusing negative conflict, managing conflict is part of your responsibility to your co-workers. (pp. 336-342)

SHOWING EMPATHY, SENSITIVITY, AND CARING: These skills will enable you to manage conflict caused by sick, anxious patients and their families. (pp. 218-222)

Dealing with Difficult People

No one cooperates with people who seem to be against them.

—Rick Kirschner

LEARNING OBJECTIVE 2: DEALING WITH DIFFICULT PEOPLE

- State why extremes of behavior can become problematic.
- Name four approaches to dealing with difficult people.
- Recognize the range of difficult behaviors.
- Connect patterns of dysfunctional behavior with their best remedies.
- Identify general tactics for dealing with difficult people.

At work, you will have to interact with dysfunctional people. In the past, you may have been able to avoid difficult people, but being a health professional requires collaboration with all team members and patients. You don't get to pick the people you work with, and you certainly don't get to pick your patients. You don't have to like everyone at work. You do, however, have to find a way to work with everyone.

For the most part, your co-workers will be excellent to work with and your patient interactions will be rewarding. However, in every job, you will sometimes encounter people who are difficult to work with. Even those who mean well can take a positive trait too far: good workers may become perfectionists; responsible people may become controlling; sociable people may want more than their share of attention. Sometimes nice people will still simply rub us the wrong way.

The trouble with people who have no vices is that they have some pretty annoying virtues.

—Elizabeth Taylor

Approaches to Difficult People

Earlier, we examined some normal, temporary stressors in everyone's life that can contribute to conflict now and then. Sooner or later, we will all encounter someone whose behavior itself is genuinely problematic or dysfunctional. What do you do then?

Let's examine several ways to deal with difficult people. All of them are effective at one time or another, and some are more effective than others as general approaches. Your response will depend on the type of behavior you are confronted with.

> **→ JOURNALING 7-3**
>
> Record where you think you are on the passive-to-aggressive continuum. Decide what your goals are at work. What kind of a mix is it: getting the work done, getting the work done correctly, socializing, or seeking recognition?

Control Your Own Response

As with any conflict, concentrate on issues directly under your control. When dealing with difficult people, you control your own behavior, attitude, and approach. Do not reflect the same behavior coming at you, as tempting as that may be. This is the worst thing you can do. By responding in kind, you validate the behavior and encourage the person to continue their inappropriate behavior. Moreover, responding with anger impairs your judgment. You will regret your own behavior later. It is best to withhold your reaction until you can rationally choose your response.

Ignore the Behavior

In many cases, your best bet will be to ignore the inappropriate behavior and simply plow ahead with the work at hand. This is the best approach, for instance, with whiners and complainers. You are not likely to stop these people from complaining. Ignore the complaining and refocus on the work at hand.

Walk Away

In extreme cases, walking away is your best bet. If your co-worker is angry, threatening, insulting, or irrational, remove yourself from the situation. They are out of control and the problem is not being effectively addressed.

Change Your Attitude

Once you examine your own role in a difficult relationship, you may find that your bias is contributing to the problem. This calls for a change in your attitude. Other times, you will find that you can improve the situation by simply being more empathetic or understanding. Certainly, empathy is usually the best approach to a difficult patient. Listening actively, validating the patient's concerns, acting calmly, and placing yourself in their shoes will ease the frustration the patient is displaying.

Change Your Approach

Changing your approach is like pressing the rewind button. First, identify the behavior that is difficult and see it in its more general pattern. Try to understand why that behavior is meeting the person's needs, and gain some insight into what those needs are. Then, choose an approach or a strategy that is most likely to be effective, given the dynamics of the behavior you are being confronted with. Many such behavior patterns and their possible remedies follow.

Problem Behaviors in Co-Workers and Patients

You will encounter many different behaviors at work. Each type of person, whether a co-worker or a patient, presents special issues for you to deal with, and each issue calls for its own approach.

The Bully

Bullies are usually intelligent and talented, and they often consider themselves much more so than anyone else they have to deal with. Conversely, they may be very insecure. They can be quite charming in the presence of their superiors but they intimidate their co-workers and subordinates by invading personal space.

Usually, bullying does not have much to do with an actual work issue, although a work-related issue may spark the behavior. Bullying has more to do with a need to dominate. Bullies work by homing in on your weaknesses or sensitive spots. If you submit to their behavior, the behavior will continue.

If you are in the presence of a bully when his or her bad behavior starts, you must calmly defend yourself. You can listen to gain information, but you must look the bully in the eye and speak in a calm voice without focusing on the bad behavior. Provide facts if the bully doesn't have them and ask questions to clarify issues. Give the bully feedback on the behavior by saying things like, "You seem very angry about this. I wish I understood your concerns better." If the behavior is way out of hand, make that observation: "Your anger seems much worse than the actual problem here. Is something else bothering you?" Often, acknowledging the bully's behavior will shock them into controlling their anger.

Being the victim of a bully in a meeting or a public place is a different problem. The bully's behavior is even more inexcusable because a greater element of humiliation is involved. Ask to speak to the person in private in order to resolve the issue. If you are being bullied via electronic communication, take the time to calm down before responding. For instance, don't reply to a threatening email right away. Before you reply, gather all of the necessary facts to develop a solution to the problem. Wait until you can craft a diplomatic response. Of course, forward the message to a supervisor if the message is abusive or threatening.

In the end, bullies can be pushy because they want to achieve results, even though they are approaching this desire with an unproductive pattern of behavior. If the bully is right, defuse his or her behavior by saying, "You're right. Here are the steps we're going to take to achieve these results." If the bully is wrong, you can gain respect by presenting your ideas calmly and firmly without being confrontational.

Verbal Abusers

Bullies often cross the line from dominating behavior to abusive behavior. You do not have to tolerate abuse. In a calm but firm voice, insist that the bully end the abuse. "Stepping up" preserves your confidence and self-esteem, and signals to the bully that you are not a target.

Do not respond in an angry, argumentative manner. People who approach life from a hostile perspective love to argue, and if you fall into that trap, you lose. If necessary, leave. Approach the person later when he is in a more rational, receptive frame of mind. Don't be afraid to point out that it is never acceptable to be rude at work. Ask if something else is going on that could have accounted for such rude behavior. If you receive an apology, accept it. However, you want to make it clear that rude, hostile behavior is not acceptable. Pretty soon, you will no longer be such a target.

The Provocateur

Provocateurs operate in the background, sniping at others, making them look foolish in public, lowering others' credibility. They may appear to be innocent contributors, simply bringing up issues or information. "It looks like everyone but Mary signed up for the training," "Gary, do you think all these x-rays are necessary?" After raising an uncomfortable issue, the provocateur sits back and watches the action. Sometimes the provocateur operates by gossiping, spreading rumors, and circulating inaccurate information.

If you are the victim of this behavior, confront the person. Do not let provocateurs retreat into the background once they have fired their shot. Ask them what their purpose was in bringing up this issue. Ask them what they would have done instead.

The Know-It-All

The know-it-all is a person who claims to know everything. They have a need to feel right and a compulsion to offer their advice on virtually any subject, because they are so knowledgeable and well informed. This person can be more of an annoyance than a danger. Ignoring him, however, even though it may seem the obvious strategy, often provokes an even more assertive effort on the part of the know-it-all to convince you of his vast knowledge. That is because the know-it-all craves attention and appreciation. They usually suffer from low self-esteem and need to be praised.

Now that you know this person's hidden motivation, you are in a position to respond effectively. If the know-it-all is truly knowledgeable, the person can be irritating, but also helpful. If you are interested, ask specific questions, not open-ended ones that will prolong the display of knowledge. If you are not interested, don't probe. Change the subject or direct attention elsewhere. If you value the friendship or working relationship with this person, you simply may need to be patient.

On the other hand, if the know-it-all is really a know-nothing, their hunger to be recognized for their supposed knowledge could be dangerous. They could give incorrect information or advice to a patient, for instance. In these cases, you need to calmly challenge their knowledge. Where did they get that information? You don't have to be obnoxious about this process, just inquiring and persistent. Once you demonstrate that you can't easily accept the know-it-all's hearsay, they will think twice about giving you information that is based on little more than "well known facts."

 WHAT IF?

What if a co-worker you cared about became angry because she wasn't receiving the attention she was seeking? How could you make her feel better without encouraging chronic attention-seeking behavior?

The Liar

People will lie to protect themselves, avoid embarrassment, and take credit for others' ideas and words. Your best defense and response to a person who lies is in the facts. Try to avoid a confrontation, which can lead to arguments, defensiveness, personal attacks, and more lies. Rather, calmly stick to the facts. If you are confronted in public by a liar, ask hard-hitting questions. "Did you record the vital signs, or did you think I was going to do that? Why would you think that?" Offer logic or proof. "Nothing I said should have led you to that conclusion."

If a colleague has proven to be unreliable, document their commitments. Send an email stating your understanding of the commitment and ask if any clarification is needed. In an email, you can state the facts and document your own ideas, contributions, and statements. In a verbal encounter, try to have a witness on hand. Liars will not last long, and neither will their lies, but your careful clarifications and documentation will prove effective as you respond to lies.

The Manipulative or Unreliable Person

Passive aggressive manipulators have an agenda, but they keep it a secret. Instead of being direct, they are scheming and deceitful. They may try to position you into taking on their work or responsibilities, or they may omit information to get you to do what they want. Don't try to psychoanalyze them or change them, which can only lead to frustration and even more conflict. However, as with liars, monitor them relentlessly. When they tell you something that will have a negative effect on you and your workload, demand proof. Don't make assumptions. Ask questions to reveal motives.

Unreliable people are famous for their excuses. They have excuses for every problem and shortcoming, but they rarely include their own behavior among the causes. They find it much more comfortable to use external explanations for everything: the weather, the traffic, the lack of equipment, someone else's tardiness, the lost chart, the unreasonable patient. As the section on *accountability* in Chapter 11 explains, excuses are for ineffective people who are poor problem solvers. Box 7-2 offers some insights for combating excuses.

Don't back down from people who have excuses for everything. Is their excuse the real cause of the shortcoming? Could something else have been done? What actions did the person take to deal with the situation? If you make it clear that you are not the kind of person who accepts excuses, the other person may think twice before abandoning a problem.

With patients, more often than with co-workers, challenging excuses related to health issues is seldom helpful. Neither you nor the patient can change the parents, the genes, the cause of the accident, or the source of the disease that is often offered as an excuse for the current state of the patient's health. As a health professional, though, you can counsel the patient to take responsibility for his or her future actions. The patient can take medicine, get exercise, eat better, or socialize more. Ignore excuses rather than challenge them, and focus on the personal responsibility that can be assumed from this point forward.

The Complainer or Whiner

Complainers seldom seem happy. Every problem, issue, or change elicits a complaint. Ignore the complaints. Do not engage. Change the subject to work. Stay focused on the message.

Tips for Dealing with Excuses from a Lazy or Manipulative Co-worker

- Don't let co-workers get under your skin or distract you from your own job.
- Don't let a lazy co-worker negatively impact your attitude by making you hostile; hostility is as bad as laziness, and it's much more visible.
- Don't worry that it's not fair; life isn't fair. Focusing on fairness makes you feel bad without changing the situation. Be the best you can be.
- Don't let lazy people set the norm. Don't follow their example.
- Don't do their work for them.
- Don't gossip, complain, or whine about your co-workers.
- Don't tattle or report their laziness to your supervisor or theirs. If their laziness is negatively impacting your ability to get your work done, present it as a business problem to your supervisor and ask for advice.
- On the other hand, don't let your co-worker's laziness hinder your progress. Refuse to take blame when somebody else is slowing down the work.
- Recognize that your "lazy" co-worker may just be disorganized, unaware of deadlines, or preoccupied with a personal problem.
- Communicate and reinforce deadlines.

One way to call a whiner's bluff is to suggest that he put his complaint in writing and give it to his supervisor. You can also ask him what solutions he envisions. Whiners love to complain, but they don't plan on generating any ideas to address the problem. These suggestions will reinforce your lack of receptivity to their complaints, and they may spare you future whining.

The Silent Type

The introverted, incommunicative person can be tough to deal with because there is so little communication. Is she shy, or does she lack confidence? Is she manipulative and withholding? Is she bullheaded, insisting on doing everything her own way or a way

FIGURE 7-5 A patient expressing anger. (From Proctor DB, Adams AP: *Kinn's the medical assistant: an applied learning approach*, ed 12, St Louis, 2014, Elsevier.)

she feels comfortable with? Does she feel she will not be heard or appreciated if she speaks up? Perhaps her valuable skill makes her feel like she doesn't need to interact with any co-workers.

Try to find a common interest with this person. Ask her about her background, interests, or expertise. Most of the relationship-building will be up to you. Often, your efforts will be rewarded with the friendship of a person who possesses many hidden strengths and talents, as well as an appreciation for your efforts in drawing her out. At the very least, you will gain insight into her behavior.

The Social Butterfly

When networking becomes constant socialization, the otherwise charming social butterfly can become a pest, interfering with your own work. The solution? Every time he arrives in your work area for a chat, ask him to do some of your work. He will soon skip you on his rounds.

The Difficult Patient

A difficult patient, client, or patient's family member warrants a special approach. As someone who is sick or injured, in pain or under stress, a difficult patient is a person who most health care professionals can understand, forgive, and deal with. The same holds true for loved ones who are worried about the patient. Worry and anxiety can make them agitated and seem more impatient than they really are. We recognize that they are not in their normal state of being, and we are there to help this person, as depicted in Figure 7-5.

It is very likely that you have been a difficult patient at some point in your life. All of us have been dissatisfied or angry customers, justifiably upset over the poor performance of a product or bad service. In the case of an anxious patient or loved one, follow the same strategies you use in dealing with anyone who is anxious—but with an extra dose of compassion and patience. Start by listening—ignore the displaced anger to get to the heart of what's needed.

You might say, "I can see why you're concerned. Let's see what we can do about this." Often, acknowledging their feelings and offering to help can help you move forward. Of course, if the caller, patient, client, or family member becomes verbally abusive, don't allow the conversation to continue. Politely end the conversation by saying something like, "I can see you're still very upset. Let's give you time to work through your feelings."

Justified or not, upset patients are simply customers with grievances. Box 7-3 suggests ways to deal with difficult patients.

I do desire we may become better strangers.

—William Shakespeare

In the end, there are innumerable types of difficult people. If you take the time to see the pattern and understand the motivation, however, you can devise an effective strategy for dealing with all kinds of difficult people.

BOX 7-3

Tips for Dealing with Difficult Patients

- Remain friendly; indicate that you want to help if you can.
- Focus your attention entirely on the patient. Offer to sit together and discuss the issue if necessary.
- Remember that your behavior reflects on your employer.
- Be sympathetic but honest. If you cannot move the patient ahead of others, explain so.
- Promise only what you know you can deliver.
- Be empathetic and on the patient's side to search for a solution.
- Learn the patient's expectations. Ask, "What would you like to see happen?"

- Ask clarifying questions to show interest in understanding the patient's problem or complaint.
- If the patient is being irrational, you may not have uncovered the real problem.
- Thank the patient when the patient shows signs of reasonableness or understanding.
- If you make a mistake, admit it, apologize, and move on.
- Seek information or training that will equip you to handle particular problems better in the future.

CASE STUDY 7-2
Fresh Start

Things were going downhill fast at Banker Street Dental. Last year, there was the IRS audit. Dr. Ivan Billingsley had to pay a huge amount in back taxes. Dr. Billingsley became an angry man with a forced smile on his face. As a result, he lost some of his longtime patients and experienced rapid turnover among his assistants.

Rae Martin knew none of this when she accepted the position as Dr. Billingsley's new dental assistant. To her, Dr. Billingsley seemed like a pleasant, if overly formal, person in the interview. On Monday morning, Rae introduced herself to the receptionist, who also handled appointments and insurance. "I'm Mildred," she said. "We won't see the doctor for a half hour yet."

The first day was not what she expected. Dr. Billingsley's idea of training Rae was to berate her. "Stand over here, young lady. I like my assistants to stand here, where I can reach them but don't have to look at them." Then he would smile at the patient, as if what he had just said was a joke. The dentist reprimanded her when the tray wasn't quite right, when the suction didn't please him, when there were not enough cotton pads. "Didn't they teach you this in school?"

That night, Rae reflected on her new job and told herself that she deserved to be trained correctly. She needed the job, and she needed to find a way to make it work.

The next day started the same way as the first. "Arrange my instruments like I showed you yesterday," he barked at her. "It's not that hard is it?"

"Dr. Billingsley, you never showed me how to arrange the instruments," she said.

"The matter is resolved," he sneered. "Just get the set-up ready."

"Actually, this matter is not resolved," she said firmly. "The unresolved matter is your behavior, Dr. Billingsley."

"What?"

"Yes. From now on, you do not have my permission to speak to me like that."

"What? Like what?"

"You may not raise your voice to me. You may not berate me. You may not embarrass me in front of the patients or the other staff members."

"Look here, girlie—"

"That's just what I'm talking about. You may not call me 'girlie' or address me in a demeaning tone of voice."

"Young lady, you may not address me with this insolent manner of yours."

"I have nothing but the greatest respect for your skills, Dr. Billingsley. I can see that you're a good dentist. But I won't be treated like this."

He didn't know what to say. Actually, he had never fired a dental assistant. They all walked out on him. "I would like a moment of peace, Rae," he said, calling her by her name for the first time. He went into the bathroom and closed the door.

It was 15 minutes before Dr. Billingsley came out of the bathroom.

"Rae," he said. "I would like to apologize. I hope you will forgive me. Can we start over?"

QUESTIONS FOR THOUGHT AND REFLECTION

1. What kind of a difficult person is Dr. Billingsley? Why do you think he thought he could act like he did?
2. What did Rae do to deserve being berated and yelled at?
3. What plan do you think Rae arrived at the evening after her first day at work?
4. Why was Rae's plan effective?
5. Do you think Dr. Billingsley will change?

Down a Dark Road

Anne was a new mental health worker in a locked ward at the state hospital. The security department issued Anne a bulky ring of keys, but she didn't really have a place to carry them, so she just clutched them as she made her way through the day.

Anne was having a hard time being accepted by the staff, but that was nothing new for her. She was introverted and had a difficult time forming new relationships. On the other hand, she had always been empathic, sympathizing with the plight of patients.

One day Anne was clutching her keys as usual while she was supervising lunch in the kitchen. When everyone had their meal, she circulated among the tables, making small talk, asking about the food, and finally stationed herself at the milk machine.

One of the patients, Mick, who also had cerebral palsy, needed some help with his tray, so Anne set her keys on the counter by the milk machine and went over to help Mick. Anne's co-worker, Ben, scooped up Anne's keys and slid them into his pocket. A moment later, Anne went back to retrieve her keys, and Ben made sure he caught the look on her face when she realized they were missing.

"Ben," she hurried over to him, to keep out of the patients' earshot, "have you seen my keys?"

"Your keys? Oh my God, you lost your keys? I have to report this." Ben left the room knowing Anne couldn't follow because the patients were still eating and had their utensils, which had to be collected before they could leave the kitchen. Later that day, it didn't surprise Anne when she was told that "a patient turned your keys into the nursing station."

QUESTIONS FOR THOUGHT AND REFLECTION

1. What factors do you think led Anne to become a victim of bullying?
2. Was the incident really about the keys?
3. What constructive actions do you think Anne could take to deal with her difficult co-workers?
4. What would you do if you were Anne?

1. One of the biggest know-it-alls in television history is the letter carrier on Cheers, Cliff Clavin. Cliff is sure he knows everything. Watch an episode of Cheers to see the effect a know-it-all has on the people around him.
2. Apologize to someone. Reflect on how that makes you feel.
3. Practice ignoring complaints. What happens?
4. Approach a provocateur with calm, direct questions about his or her behavior.

🌀 **CROSS CURRENTS WITH OTHER SOFT SKILLS**

LISTENING ACTIVELY: With difficult people, one of the best things you can do to manage them is listen to their content, and understand their motivations. (pp. 263-269)

EXUDING OPTIMISM, ENTHUSIASM, AND POSITIVITY: This is the opposite of being difficult, and signals that you are not open to the tactics of difficult people. (pp. 380-384)

Valuing Multicultural Competence

The order is rapidly fadin' and the first one now will later be last for the times they are a-changin'.

—Bob Dylan

LEARNING OBJECTIVE 3: VALUING MULTICULTURAL COMPETENCE

- Define multicultural competence.
- Describe current trends in demographics.
- Compare and contrast pluralism with assimilation.
- Indentify the multicultural competence needs of health care professions.
- List several ways you can enhance your own multicultural competency.

Racism and intolerance are still very much alive in American society. Expressing prejudices is unacceptable, but many people still practice intolerance covertly through seemingly polite exclusion, hidden motives, and ignoring or fearing others not like ourselves. These are difficult issues to address. However, complying with and embracing multiculturalism are two different things.

In this section, you will learn to gain appreciation for the diversity you encounter as a health care professional. You will also learn how to navigate and thrive as a member of your diverse community.

What Is Multicultural Competence?

Cultures are groups with a common outlook. They may be racial or ethnic; male or female; of a certain sexual orientation, religious belief, or age. Diversity means that all cultures are welcome and valued. Multicultural competence is the ability of individuals and organizations to appreciate, value, interact with, and benefit from the presence of many different cultures and their individual members.

◀ **JOURNALING 7-5**

Describe your heritage. What do you know about it? How can an understanding of your own cultural identity help you gain perspective and acceptance from people of different cultures?

Diversity in the United States

It is illegal and improper to discriminate against anyone. People with talent and education can achieve great things and rise tremendously in society, whatever their race, ethnicity, nationality, gender, sexual orientation, age, or religious beliefs.

Many Americans identify closely with their cultural backgrounds and many younger people represent a wider variety of ethnic groups who will contribute to the expanding diversity of America as the century progresses.

Hispanic Americans are now the largest minority ethnic group in the United States, many occupying positions of power and influence. Asian Americans come from 20 different countries. Gay and lesbian people are 15 million strong and contribute $700 billion to our economy, according to David R. Morse, author of *Multicultural Diversity*. The 21st century is an exciting time for diversity, and for the changing face of America.

Benefits of Diversity

Diversity is an opportunity, not a problem. In a shrinking world, where transportation is fast and communication is instantaneous, exposure to diverse cultures helps make us better world citizens.

Pluralism

In a pluralistic society or workplace, minority cultures interact with the dominant culture in ways that preserve the uniqueness of each culture while enabling the functioning and operations of the main culture. Only behavior matters in work settings, not beliefs, dress, or rituals. Of course, in health care settings, the nature of the work demands conformity in some areas. For example, the demands for infection control or sterility call for the wearing of scrubs or lab coats in most settings, English must be spoken, and Western medicine and the scientific method is the norm. However, head coverings dictated by religious beliefs are permitted, and speaking languages in addition to English can be valuable. Finally, alternative medicine is more widely accepted.

The United States used to be called a "melting pot," where immigrants came and, within two generations, had totally assimilated into the mainstream of American society and culture. Now, America is better described as a "salad bowl," where immigrants join in the mix of American society and culture but retain their own unique cultural identity.

Perspective and Experience

When our co-workers represent many different cultures, we have much more experience to draw from. We will make better decisions and be more inclusive in our thinking. Exposure to people from a variety of cultures helps build empathy, and makes health professionals more effective.

Threats to Diversity

Stereotyping

Stereotyping is associating the attributes of a group to an individual. Stereotyping is a mental shortcut that enables people to classify others. Unfortunately, stereotypes are based on impressions, opinions, misconceptions, myths, prejudices, and fears rather than research. Although research can identify dominant traits in any group, it does not mean that any given individual will have any or all of those traits. In the end, whether the generalizations you believe in are based on myths or research, they are not helpful in forming relationships with individuals.

Bias and Prejudice

Whether it is recognized or not, bias is unfortunately a major force undermining multicultural acceptance and tolerance. Human beings are not born biased. Bias is an attitude that is learned. Therefore, biases can be unlearned. Once you are aware of your biases, you can overcome them by subjecting them to facts. You may dislike an individual because of what the individual does, but it is unfair and wrong to dislike a cultural group.

Assimilation

Assimilation is an acculturation process that demands that minority cultures adapt to the dominant culture in order to succeed. It is the opposite of pluralism. In the past, immigrants to the United States valued assimilation highly. Immigrant groups tended to congregate and live together just to survive. In many cases, nobody spoke English and learning was difficult. The cultural groups were already composed of adults who had been raised in a foreign culture. It was important to them that their children speak English, play baseball, wear American styles, and eat American food. Assimilation was the goal.

Assimilation into the dominant culture of America is still important to many new arrivals, but now there is a desire to retain some aspects of the old culture as well. When assimilation is so complete that it separates a person from their former cultural identity, many feel that they have lost an important part of who they are. Now, a retained cultural identity is seen as an asset instead of a liability.

The Face of the Progressive Multicultural Health Care Organization

Culture is important to everyone. Culture defines whether you are a member of a group or excluded from a group. It prescribes behavior, defines values, and takes a stand on the function of families, order, and obligations. Health care facilities must show respect for cultural differences. To achieve this, staff members must take on the responsibility of learning all they can about the cultures of the people they typically serve.

For a health care organization to truly create a welcoming, culturally diverse environment, everyone must agree that cultural acceptance is core to the mission of the organization (Figure 7-6). The lobby, waiting room, and staff should reflect cultural diversity as much as possible. If possible, decor and art should reflect the diversity of the clientele. Box 7-4 suggests other actions you can take to welcome different cultures.

What You Can Do to Increase Your Multicultural Competence

American mainstream culture is transforming so rapidly that multicultural competence is essential to being an American, and a necessary attribute of health care professionals.

You can increase your multicultural competence by learning about minority cultural groups. Abandon old stereotypes and get to know individuals from groups other than your own. Make no assumptions. Read books, ask questions, and attend diversity and tolerance workshops to raise your cultural intelligence. In the spirit of getting to know members of minority groups as individuals, you must recognize that it also matters whether the person is a man or a woman, young or old, recently immigrated or an American for many generations.

Use language with caution. If English is not your colleague's or patient's native language, misunderstandings can occur. Always take measures to ensure comprehension. Avoid the use of slang, colloquialisms, metaphors, and even humor, which can complicate communication.

What if you encountered a patient who spoke very little English? What efforts could you make to maximize effective communication?

Mindfulness is a key in becoming more aware and accepting of cultural differences. A mindful person does not deny having biases and uncomfortable feelings in the presence of someone from an unfamiliar culture. Instead, mindful people make themselves aware of their feelings and approach unfamiliar territory with an attitude that allows learning. The more mindful you are of others, the more insight you will have into yourself.

BOX 7-4

Actions You Can Take to Improve Your Multicultural Competency

- Learn to correctly pronounce the names of co-workers and patients from other cultures.
- Introduce yourself, and explain your role.
- Explain what patients can expect, because they are likely to be uncertain about what to do.
- Recognize that direct and prolonged eye contact may be offensive in some cultures.
- Be sensitive to personal space and touching, which varies by culture.
- Teach important American cultural concepts, like punctuality, directness, informality, and equality of gender, age, and social class.
- Pay more respect than usual to older people, who are highly valued in many cultures.
- Define medical terms, which may be a mystery to patients whose first language is not English.
- Learn to say "Hello" and "Thank you" in the languages of the people you serve.
- Be careful of gestures; they can mean different things in different cultures.
- Smiles are universal.

FIGURE 7-6 A young phlebotomy student draws blood (Copyright © istock.com).

Getting To Know You

Emilio was the practice manager for the satellite clinic established three years ago in an underserved community along the waterfront. He had worked hard to relate to the community, which was always in transition with waves of immigrants from different nations. He met with civic and business groups, explaining the mission of the clinic and describing their services. He had gone to bat to get the money to hire interpreters to meet the needs of Spanish-speaking, Korean-speaking, and Arabic-speaking communities.

Still, after 3 years, the clinic was underused. He felt that he was doing something wrong, but he couldn't think of what.

He was absorbed in his thoughts as he walked to his car one evening. He saw a homeless man sitting at a bus stop with bloody scrapes all over his face. The man was watching Emilio. "Are you OK?" Emilio asked him.

"Yeah."

"You need to see a doctor, mister."

"Yeah, that's why I'm at the bus stop."

"There's a clinic right here. Come on in."

"Nah, I don't go there."

"Why not? You're already here."

"You're the first guy I ever saw there that looks like me."

"OK," said Emilio. "At least let me give you a ride."

The next morning, Emilio looked up his friend, Father Anselmo, and asked him to help recruit a focus group from the community. "I'm having a lunch catered for it on Friday," he said. "I want about eight people, including some Korean-, Mexican-, and Iraqi-Americans. You come too, Father."

Use of the clinic doubled over the next 6 months. The faces of the people at the reception desk mirrored the faces of the community members. The bland lobby now sizzled with bright tapestries. Two vans were parked outside, marked as transportation to and from the suburban hospital. Emilio spoke at PTAs, nursing homes, and church groups.

Emilio also even started "Getting to Know You" sessions for the staff. He invited members of the community to teach the staff about their ethnic backgrounds. An Iraqi woman explained how Moslimas dress. A Mexican man explained health beliefs related to hot and cold food. A Korean woman talked about respect for the elderly, politeness, and personal space. At the end, she surprised Emilio with a big hug. "See," she said. "I am learning to be an American. Thank you for learning about me."

QUESTIONS FOR THOUGHT AND REFLECTION

1. Were interpreters enough to make the community feel comfortable with the new clinic?
2. What was it about the encounter with the homeless man that changed Emilio's thinking?
3. Why did Emilio give the homeless man a ride to the competing clinic?
4. Why weren't Emilio's talks to business and community groups enough to attract people in the community to his clinic?

Down a Dark Road

The chain drug store was open until 9:00 on Sunday night, but the pharmacy closed at 6:00. Just at 6:00, William Parker ran into the store waving a prescription and asked the cashier if the pharmacy was still open.

"Let me check," said the cashier. She said on the intercom, "Pharmacy customer."

Back in the pharmacy, they were just closing, and the pharmacist and the pharm tech, Karen, were just about to begin their counts. "Well, go up there, Karen, and see what it is."

Karen walked double-time to the front of the store and saw Mr. Parker pacing around the front. Karen made eye contact with the cashier, and she glanced at Mr. Parker, confirming that he was the customer.

"Can I help you, sir?" said Karen to Mr. Parker.

"Oh yeah, is the pharmacy still open?"

"I'm sorry, sir. We just closed."

"Oh, can't you just fill this prescription? It's eardrops for my daughter. She has a terrible earache."

Karen looked at the prescription, then handed it back to him. "I'm sorry, sir. The pharmacy is closed."

"Please, lady. I'm begging you. We had to wait so long in the emergency room. My daughter hurts so much."

Karen hesitated. But she replied. "I'm sorry, sir. I wish I could help you. The pharmacy is closed though, and we won't be open again until 9:00 tomorrow morning."

Mr. Parker just looked at her. He could see it was no use arguing.

When Karen returned to the pharmacy, the pharmacist asked her, "What is it?"

"False alarm," said Karen. "You ready for the count?"

QUESTIONS FOR THOUGHT AND REFLECTION

1. Was Karen using "sir" as a title of respect?
2. Could the prescription have been filled?
3. Why did Mr. Parker decide not to argue with Karen?
4. Was Karen telling the truth?
5. Will Mr. Parker patronize this store again?

EXPERIENTIAL EXERCISES

1. Think back on a time in your life when you didn't fit in or experienced prejudice. Recall how you felt, and see if you have raised your empathy for others who may live a different life.
2. How many cultural groups do you belong to? Think broadly and write a list. Include beliefs, activities, affiliations, habits, preferences—everything you can think of.
3. Examine a globe to refresh your memory of world geography.
4. What is your place of employment doing to welcome a diverse patient population?

CROSS CURRENTS WITH OTHER SOFT SKILLS

STRIVING FOR TOLERANCE: Tolerance is the prerequisite for multicultural tolerance. (pp. 29-35)

TAKING ACCOUNTABILITY: Only you can increase your multicultural competence. (pp. 333-336)

COMMUNICATION SKILLS

CHAPTER 8

Speaking and Writing Professionally

THEMES TO CONSIDER

- Learn how to speak in a professional manner.
- Communicate effectively through writing by using and following grammar and spelling guidelines.
- Adopt a writing style that is suitable to your audience.
- Use your writing skills to contribute to your profession.

Speaking Professionally in Your Workplace

To speak and to speak well are two things.
A fool may talk, but a wise man speaks.

—Ben Jonson

LEARNING OBJECTIVE 1: SPEAKING PROFESSIONALLY IN YOUR WORKPLACE

- Recognize the value of speaking professionally at work.
- Determine the difference between professional and casual speaking.
- Use language appropriate for business and health care environments.
- Learn new words and use them in everyday speech in the proper context.
- Censor the content of your conversations at work.
- Speak with purpose.

Right or wrong, we are often judged by the way we speak. When you use proper grammar, tone, and vocabulary for work-related conversations, the chance that you will be heard, respected, and understood is much greater. However, one of the best ways to become successful in your field is to use the language of your profession appropriately and speak professionally.

Mend your speech a little lest you mar your fortunes.

—William Shakespeare

When the language you use is incorrect, you may appear to lack knowledge or credibility, which can make your audience feel uncomfortable. You don't want to elicit these feelings from employers, co-workers, or patients. Fortunately, you can practice to improve the quality of your speech at work.

? WHAT IF?

What if a co-worker was describing the busy morning schedule to the office manager and you overheard her say, "Then I had four stupid calls in a row!"

What do you think of how your co-worker expressed herself?

What do you think the office manager is thinking about your co-worker?

How would you explain to your co-worker that her words may have offended the office manager? What might she have said instead?

Speaking at Work

Consider all the different types of speaking you engage in at work, and estimate how much time you spend talking, listening, and interacting. You communicate all day long. You interact with your supervisor and co-workers to learn, exchange information, and advance your causes and concerns. In meetings, you will be called upon to offer your ideas and input regarding the issues of the day. You may be called upon to make presentations, short and long. You may present a patient's case or explain your ideas and proposals. Most importantly, you interact with patients by welcoming them, collecting their information, assessing their needs, preparing them for treatments, explaining procedures, and scheduling their appointments (Figure 8-1). Finally, you speak socially to inform, communicate, share, and even entertain. Speaking well at work is key to your effectiveness, success, and career.

FIGURE 8-1 An optician helps a patient choose a pair of glasses (Copyright © istock.com).

Aspects of Professional Speech

Casual Speaking Is Not Professional Speaking

Think about conversations that you have with family and friends throughout the day. These conversations are likely to be casual and contain familiar language that you use when speaking to people who already know you. Do you use certain popular words, such as "whatever?" Using slang is inappropriate in the workplace, so you might have to reword some of your favorite phrases. Of course, profanity is never acceptable at work.

⟲ JOURNALING 8-1

Describe the way you speak. Are you too formal or familiar? Differentiate between speaking with friends and with co-workers. Make a list of common phrases you say when you are not at work, state their meaning, and write out substitutions using more professional language.

When health care team members speak to one another, many levels of communication occur. Some experts believe that what you say is less important than your tone of voice, your word choice, and your body language. In addition, your audience, location, and comfort level will affect the quality of your communication. You can see these differences for yourself if you pause to notice that your break room conversations are casual, in contrast with discussions in front of patients. Speaking professionally requires you to stop and think before you speak. You will have to rephrase what you might be thinking to express only those thoughts that are acceptable in professional situations. The first rule of all communication is to always identify your audience, so you may speak appropriately in all situations.

The Sound of Your Voice

The tone of your voice affects how people will perceive you, although there is a limit to what you can do to change the sound of your voice. If you have a high-pitched squeaky voice or a low-pitched gravelly voice, try to develop a pleasing tone somewhere between the two extremes. The manner of your speech is important as well. Speaking too fast or too slow, too loud or too soft, can be off-putting to your audience. Maintain eye contact with your audience, and remember that smiles are universal.

It's not what you say, it's what people hear.

—Frank Luntz

When interacting with patients, you want to instill confidence by sounding authoritative, both in what you say and how you say it. Your voice should be strong, delivered with a confident smile. Pronounce words correctly, starting with the patient's name. If you don't know how to pronounce the patient's name correctly, ask. Patients are pleased that you care enough to ask. Using words such as "uh" to fill silence is a defense mechanism you might use to hold the floor while you gather your thoughts. You can still command attention by speaking slowly and pausing frequently. Become aware of these fillers and work to purge them from your speech.

Your Attitude Toward Your Listener

One of the best ways to set yourself apart from the crowd is to be gracious. Saying "please," "thank you," and "you're welcome" is an easy way to ensure that people will remember you in a positive light. Many patients will be unfamiliar with your facility, and your welcoming demeanor will make them feel at ease.

Part of catering to your listeners involves taking cues from their behavior. If they speak softly, lower your volume as well. If they are embarrassed, move to a private place. If they are emotional, be calm, make eye contact, nod affirmatively, and listen. Avoid interruptions, which may suggest that you are not listening.

Speaking the Language of Your Profession

While you are learning about your chosen field, practice your medical terminology as much as possible. Educators will tell you that these words are the new language you need to use in the workplace, but you may not fully realize the importance of pronunciation and usage until you are in clinical situations. Learn all the words you can, and the proper way to say them. Play vocabulary games with a group or read health care journals to immerse yourself in the language.

Using medical terminology correctly marks you as a professional and instills confidence in the

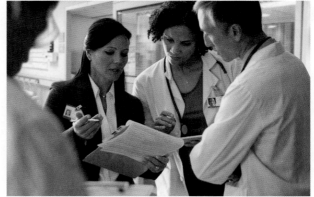

FIGURE 8-2 Hospital staff members discuss patient charts (Copyright © istock.com).

patients you are speaking to, as well as their family members (Figure 8-2).

Read to Speak, Read to Succeed

Reading helps you build the tools you need to become a better speaker.

Employers and co-workers value employees who are well read. Read a newspaper every day or watch the evening news to raise your awareness of current events and advances in medicine. You will always have something interesting to talk about, and you will be aware of what others are talking about. Being informed is the best way to contribute to conversations at work.

Read to Build Your Vocabulary

Reading is the single best way to improve your vocabulary. When you know more words, you have more ability to gain insight. You can differentiate more finely between similar characteristics. For instance, if you know the difference between a pale and an ashen complexion, you know whether to be concerned or not.

Moreover, a more diverse, colorful vocabulary commands attention and makes you more interesting. Instead of concentrating on big words that others will not know, use smaller words that are heard less often but convey the same meaning.

Expanding your vocabulary means reading more challenging material, which can be difficult. If you're not comprehending the message, examine the context. The words used around an unfamiliar word or concept will usually give you clues to the meaning of the new word. Bookmark a dictionary website on your computer and stick it on your toolbar so you will always have immediate access to it. You may also want to keep a print dictionary nearby while you are reading to reduce frustration when you encounter new words.

Keep a list of unfamiliar words handy. In your spare time, review them, pronounce them, and use them in a sentence. Research shows if you use the word seven times, it will become part of your vocabulary. Additional tips for building your vocabulary are listed in Box 8-1.

Edit Your Own Talk

Too Much Information!

Conversations with supervisors, co-workers, and patients may include many topics both personal and professional. It is acceptable to share small details of your life with those you see every day. In fact, you might be thought of as rigid if you did not share some aspect of your life. Don't share too much. A detailed conversation about last night's escapades is never appropriate at work. Likewise, discussions about your health, salary, or relationships should be reserved for friends and family.

The New Cool

At an early point in your formal education, you may have learned or felt that using an advanced vocabulary word to describe something was considered "uncool." As we grow older, we need to command the English language to achieve success. Employees who use a wider vocabulary are usually more successful than those who have limited vocabulary. In other words, saying a little eloquently is better than saying a lot with words that are used improperly. Make it a goal to build a well-balanced, professional vocabulary.

> *Communication takes place in the mind of the listener, not the speaker.*
>
> —Peter Drucker

A Note to Non-Native Speakers of English

If English is not your first language, you have both an advantage and a disadvantage. Speaking another

language fluently is often desirable in health care, but if you have a pronounced accent, people may have a difficult time understanding you. Speak slowly and clearly.

Note that speaking in a language other than English in the workplace may alienate co-workers and patients. Right or wrong, the perception is that you must be saying something negative when you exclude others from conversation. Plus, you cannot tell who can understand you based on appearances. If your office is bilingual, it is considered a courtesy to switch to English if you are joined by those who speak only English. Still, co-workers will appreciate it when you help them communicate with a patient whom they are unable to understand.

CASE STUDY 8-1
The Best People in the World

Dr. Avila was nervous about introducing his new office manager to the medical assistants and the support staff. As the managing partner of a large practice of over 75 physicians, Dr. Avila was acutely aware of the importance of this position and the success of the person chosen. He had passed on several senior staff members who had long been trusted employees of the practice, because they just weren't quite what he felt the practice needed. He wanted a real professional, an excellent communicator, and a warm individual to fill the position.

He was about to introduce his choice, Robert Candalaria, to the group of almost 200 staff members. Although Dr. Avila was uncomfortable in front of large audiences, he mumbled his way through an unremarkable introduction. He felt relieved to walk off the stage to the sound of applause, shaking Robert's hand as they passed at the corner of the stage.

Robert stepped quickly to the podium. "You know, the best thing that any of us can do is give our very best to care for the people we actually come into personal contact with. Those are the people we are in the best position to help, the ones who come to this practice for help. They are our customers. We are here to serve them." He had walked up the aisle and stopped next to a middle-aged man whom Dr. Avila said was one of the people who had applied for the job that went to Robert. "I'm Robert," he said, extending his hand. "LeRoy," said the man, surprised and annoyed.

"LeRoy Walker?" asked Robert. The man nodded. "LeRoy, haven't you been managing things on an interim basis since my predecessor left?" LeRoy nodded again, a little less annoyed. "Thank you, LeRoy, for your service," said Robert. "I already know you've made my job easier."

Robert paused briefly before making his way back to the podium.

"I'm a Certified Medical Assistant, CMA, AAMA," he said. "How many of you are certified in your profession?" Most of the hands went up. "That's great," he said, "I think we owe it to our customers to give them the best our profession offers, don't you?"

"As you know, this practice already sponsors many CMA continuing education programs. In addition, if you are an AAMA member, the practice will pay your recertification fee. If you're not an AAMA member, we'll pay the portion we would pay if you were. We will reimburse you for any preapproved continuing education. If you're not certified, we will work with you to get you certified, including offering tutorials for the CMA exam. I want our patients to know that they are being cared for by some of the best professionals available."

By now, Dr. Avila was feeling a lot better.

QUESTIONS FOR THOUGHT AND REFLECTION

1. What was Robert's challenge in making this speech?
2. Do you think Robert had given thought to the needs of his audience in planning his speech? Why or why not?
3. Do you think Robert was being manipulative when he approached LeRoy?
4. Would you like to work for Robert?

Down a Dark Road

Kristen and Erika, both medical assistants, and mutual friends outside of work, were huddled at the front desk on Monday morning at about 7:30. No patients were expected for 30 minutes and they were ready for the day, so they began catching up on the social events of their weekends.

"Where'ya go last night?" asked Erika.

Kristen whispered, then Erika squealed, "Seriously?"

Erika leaned in for more details, and soon the women were engrossed in their conversation. They did not hear Mrs. Long, the 8:00 patient, enter the reception area, and had just about finished their conversation when Mrs. Long cleared her throat.

"Are you girls finished? Great. Now where is your supervisor?"

Kristen and Erika tried to calm down Mrs. Long, but in the end they were forced to knock on the doctor's office door and ask Ellie, the office manager, to come and speak with Mrs. Long. Ellie heard the patient's story, and apologized for their rude behavior. Kristen and Erika also apologized. The doctor, no stranger to their behavior, had a big decision to make.

QUESTIONS FOR THOUGHT AND REFLECTION

1. What exactly is the problem? State the many levels of communication operating in this example.
2. How should the office manager and doctor handle this problem?
3. Should you discuss the details of your social life in the workplace?

⊛ EXPERIENTIAL EXERCISES

1. Spend a half-hour in the lobby of a hospital or medical office. Observe the language used between co-workers. Note words or conversations you feel are professional and ones that are not. Can you spot patients and staff as being different by the way they speak?
2. Review your medical terminology textbook. Write down all the terms you forget. Ensure that you know what they mean and how to pronounce and spell them correctly. Do the same with medications you use frequently.
3. Read a health care related article. Write down at least five words you're not familiar with. Write a sentence with clear meaning for each word, and practice using it.
4. Play a word or vocabulary game with a group of friends. Playing games is a valuable way to increase your vocabulary, and the more diverse the people you play with, the more exposure to new words you will have.
5. Do you wish you had a dime for every time you said "um" when you are speaking? These habits will not go away without your intervention. Buy an inexpensive click-counter that you can keep discretely in your pocket. Count every time you hear yourself using filler words. At the end of the day, fine yourself a dime for every instance. When you've kicked the habit, buy something nice for yourself.

◎ CROSS CURRENTS WITH OTHER SOFT SKILLS

LISTENING ACTIVELY: To speak effectively, you should be listening more than speaking. (pp. 263-269)
READING AND SPEAKING BODY LANGUAGE: Sometimes the key to communicating is the things we don't say. (pp. 277-284)
SHOWING EMPATHY, SENSITIVITY, AND CARING: You can demonstrate empathy and caring to others professionally. Professionalism can be warm and comforting. (pp. 218-222)

COMMITTING TO YOUR PROFESSION: Good, knowledgeable speakers will always be in demand in your profession. (pp. 342-348)
EXUDING OPTIMISM, ENTHUSIASM, AND POSITIVITY: Smiles can be heard in all languages, and it is amazing what a positive attitude will do for your communication skills. (pp. 380-384)

Writing, Grammar, and Spelling

Writing is easy: all you do is sit staring at the blank sheet of paper [or your computer screen] until the drops of blood form on your forehead.

—Gene Fowler

LEARNING OBJECTIVE 2: WRITING, GRAMMAR, AND SPELLING

- Think about your audience before you write anything.
- Learn to communicate concisely in your writing, respecting your reader's time.
- Use correct grammar and spell every word correctly.
- Learn how to identify and create your individual style.
- Understand how to adjust your tone so you convey the attitude you intend.
- Arm yourself with email best practices.
- Gain familiarity with writing for social media and cyberspace.

Did you know that writing is not really about writing? Writing is all about your reader. You are not writing to write. You are writing to communicate. If you make one change now in how you write, it should be to always have your reader in mind, no matter how easy or difficult writing is for you. Constantly ask yourself, "What would the reader make of this? What does the reader want to know? Will this be clear to the reader?" Reflect on what you want from someone's writing when you are the reader. Writing should be clear, interesting, informative, and concise.

Words and sentences are subjects of revision; paragraphs and whole compositions are subjects of prevision.

—Barrett Wendell

Basic Aspects of Good Writing

Whether you are writing nursing notes, problem-oriented notes, general documentation, thank-you notes, or reports, you are leaving behind a permanent record that will always reflect on you. If the grammar and spelling are correct, the tone appropriate, and the words concise and well chosen, you will be seen as a person of intelligence and professionalism.

Grammar

Grammar provides the rules for any language, but there are a huge number of exceptions in English. This book cannot teach you grammar, but you can improve your skills by taking classes or reading one of the books recommended in the Bibliography. In the meantime, write simple sentences that have a clear subject and an active verb. Short, simple, direct sentences minimize errors and delight your readers.

? WHAT IF?

What if you received a note from a co-worker that was so garbled you could not even figure out what the person was trying to say? What kind of an emotional response would you have to that? What impression would you have of the writer?

Spelling

Spelling is almost always black and white, either correct or incorrect. In health care, you are writing to an audience that knows correct word spelling. Therefore, when you misspell a word, it distracts from the message you are trying to communicate. Plus, misspelling medical terms can result in incorrect dosages or treatments.

Recognize that spelling is something you can master with simple analysis and repetition. When you first encounter a new word, take a few seconds to examine it carefully. What are its syllables? Is there anything weird about the word, like surprising combinations of letters, letters that don't match how they are pronounced, double letters, or letters that are not doubled when you would expect them to be?

Let's apply this process to the word *parallel*. The first half, para, is easy. It is just like all the other instances of para you know: parasympathetic, paranormal. The last four letters might trip you up if you don't learn them now. There is no particular rule that justifies the double "L" so just remember it: *llel*. In fact, when you think of these four letters standing alone, they look so weird that they just might stick in your memory.

Tone

Think of your writing tone as your manners. How do you come across to your reader? Polite? Respectful? Sarcastic? Hostile? Your tone reflects your attitude. The nuances of tone can be subtle. Word choice affects it. For example, do you see problems, or disasters? The way you frame ideas and experiences can affect the outcomes. Box 8-2 explains how to manage tone.

Word Choice

Words are charged with meaning and with mood. Think about the difference between the synonyms *angry* and *enraged*. Most people can deal with anger,

BOX 8-2

Elements that Contribute to Tone

- Short sentences suggest simple, often powerful ideas.
- Long sentences suggest complicated, nuanced ideas.
- Is the vocabulary appropriate for the audience?
- Active voice seems personal: "I thank you."
- Passive voice seems impersonal: "You are to be thanked."
- To increase formality, eliminate contractions.
- To decrease formality, use slang and lingo.
- Avoid overuse of the exclamation point, and never use emoticons as substitutes for tone.

but they steer clear of rage. Word choice can make your reader think you are condescending or pretentious, as in these examples:

"I told you to stop this."

"As previously discussed, you have been instructed to desist."

English is such a rich language because it is comprised of many words that express similar things. This can be a blessing and a curse. With so many words available, we have to choose wisely to convey the meaning, tone, and emphasis we desire to communicate.

Brevity

Some people think that lengthy discourses, complicated sentences, and fancy words equal good writing. Nothing could be farther from the truth. It takes time and thought to chisel your message down to its final length.

I didn't have time to write a short letter, so I wrote a long one instead.

—Mark Twain

Every one of your readers is as busy as you are, so get to the point. State the information you are trying to convey in as few words as possible. This requires some effort and thoughtfulness on the writer's part. For some writers, it's easier to get all the information down on paper quickly and then review it to tighten the piece. For others, it can be more helpful to begin by thinking instead of writing. If you're one of these writers, Box 8-3 contains questions to consider before you write anything.

Your Writing Style

Your writing style is as unique as your fingerprint. Even though you need to use proper grammar and spelling, the prose you write will still reflect your personality. Your writing style is made up of the sentences you construct and the words you choose. Your style is also reflected in the quality of your thoughts and insights, and the effectiveness and clarity you use to communicate.

◀ JOURNALING 8-2

Describe what is unique about your particular writing style.

BOX 8-3

Questions to Ask Yourself Before You Begin Writing

- Who is my reader? Who will read this?
- What does my reader need to know about this subject?
- How can I put the essential information in the first sentence?
- What tone or attitude should I adopt?
- How can I create that tone?
- What is my intention: to inform, persuade, amuse, applaud?
- Am I making a request or call to action?
- How can I keep this as short as possible?
- How can I end on a strong note?

The Sound of Your Voice

Have you ever had "writer's block," where you know what you want to say, but you can't seem to get it down in words? Here's a quick tip: Ask yourself how you would say it if you were just talking to a friend. Then write that down. Your spoken voice is a good guide to your written style. Eventually, you will want your written style to have its own voice, but your spoken voice is a great place to start when you hit a rut.

Look for Models You Can Emulate

Much of what you write, at least at first, will be documentation of patient care. These are legal documents that serve as reference for the entire patient care team, now and in the future. The tone should be respectful, factual, and free of opinions. Beyond these basics, you should familiarize yourself with the style of documentation you see as you review patient charts. For instance, do the writers use full and complete sentences? In other words, is it typical to write:

"The patient received a bed bath. Her vital signs were taken, and her BP was 110/64."

Or, is a more abbreviated style acceptable:

"Bed bath given. BP 110/64"

Whatever elements of style you see, incorporate them into your own, so you contribute to the consistency in these important documents. Often, physicians and others will scan the notes to get information and a sense of how the patient has been doing since the last visit. They will expect to see the "house style" and any deviation will slow them down.

Electronic Writing

Writing a letter on paper might seem old-fashioned, but there are few better ways to deepen a relationship. One area that still demands written notes is patient documentation. However, most writing is done electronically.

eMail

Every email is an opportunity for you to present yourself in a positive light. However, email requires special attention and involves additional constraints.

First, when you write email, ensure that your message is concise and free of emoticons, garish colors, and backgrounds. Your recipients may receive at least 50 emails each day, so be concise. Begin your emails with the most important details and follow up with any necessary information. Make any requests early in the email so they will not be overlooked. If possible, state your message in the subject line. "Keep a close eye on Mr. Souza today" conveys the most urgent part of the message instantly, but the reader can open the message for additional information.

Second, use email for its intended purpose of instant communication and not as a substitute for face-to-face communication. Remember to keep your audience in mind and write accordingly.

Acronyms like "lol" have no place in professional emails. Even common business acronyms are out of place if your audience does not know them. Use work-related acronyms only if they hold meaning for everyone who may read your email.

Do not write anything in an email that you would not say to someone in person. And do not write anything you may regret later. Do not write emails when you are emotional. Take advantage of the time that electronic communication allows. Remember, emails last forever. They can be used as legal documents and as evidence in court. Box 8-4 suggests additional email practices to avoid.

Blogs, Twitter, and Cyberspace

If you are a good writer and have something important to say, you may want to expand your writing to the web. In no way, however, can you appear to represent your employer unless your employer explicitly authorizes you to do so. Nevertheless, social media are here to stay, and it is likely that health care facilities will increasingly use Facebook, blogs, Twitter,

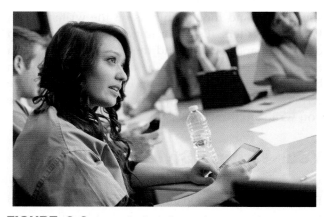

FIGURE 8-3 A medical staff member uses her personal mobile device during a staff meeting (Copyright © istock.com).

or LinkedIn to market themselves and interact with their customers.

Of course, you can make personal use of social media, but you still have to take care not to do or say anything that would embarrass your employer or raise concerns with your supervisor. The advent of social media calls for incredible maturity, restraint, and intelligence (Figure 8-3).

Twitter is a particularly good place to start. Your Twitter messages are limited to 140 characters, which is great training for concise communication. Moreover, figures in your field use outlets such as Twitter to share articles, blogs, and websites.

The key to writing online is having something of value to say. Your readers won't tolerate boredom. On the other hand, if you consistently offer information and views that others value, you will attract an audience and be in a position of influence.

The First Draft

Over the course of your career, you will be asked to write a long piece, such as a report or an important letter. How would you start? Each writer must experiment and find the style that works best for them. Try one of the following methods to see which approach fits you best.

The Color Code Approach

Some writers must write fast to catch their thoughts as they come. Then, once captured, the writer follows these steps:

* Highlight the various thoughts in different colors, according to their focus, to form connections.
* Group like colors together.
* Number thoughts within each color section.
* Determine the order in which to present each section.
* Organize each thought to achieve a unified flow.
* Create an opening and ending.
* Edit the final read-through.

Mapping and Webbing

Does forming a sentence onscreen or on paper just feel totally paralyzing? If so, mapping might work best for you. Forget the computer screen or lined paper at first and instead make a "thoughts web" or "mind map" to act as your first draft before you write. To try your hand at mapping or webbing, start with a blank sheet of paper:

* In the center of a sheet of paper, write down a single word or phrase that is central to what you want to say. Then circle it.
* Next, as other thoughts about your message come into your head, jot these down at random around your central word, making a spider web of words. Include phrases that occur to you or words you want to use as well. Take your time.

The more thoughts you can capture in these circles, the better.
* Now draw lines between all of them that connect.
* Look for meaningful links. Do you see connections and patterns that you want to talk about?
* Later, you can link these connections to make larger webs until you have cohesive paragraphs. This usually frees you to connect and construct a solid first draft.
* Once you are satisfied that you have covered everything, make a short outline.

Mind-mapping is a valuable technique because it uses the spatial, creative, imaginative part of your brain and enables you to make more connections in this stage. Figure 8-4 is an example of a mind map; you can explore this topic in more depth online.

The Diving Board Approach

Many people simply plunge into writing, whether it is a report or a thank you note. They may think about their audience and start "talking" to them on paper; they may like starting with an interesting first sentence that will grab the attention of the reader. Others know right away how they want their document to end and write from there. Later, after this "diving in" approach, they find it easier to go back, fill in the blanks, rearrange things, choose words thoughtfully, and edit.

Advanced Elements of Style

Although patient care notes and other documentation, emails, and tweets all need to be brief and concise, there is, in contrast, a shift to an emphasis on style and expressiveness when it comes to writing longer pieces like articles.

Powerful Verbs and Punchy Words

Verbs are essential to any language. They are the action words that drive your thoughts forward. Writers who make an effort to choose interesting verbs will have an engaging writing style. Instead of writing, "He sat up straight," you might consider "He sprang to attention."

Modification

Modifiers add details. Not surprisingly, modifiers modify meaning. It wasn't just a shirt, it was a yellow

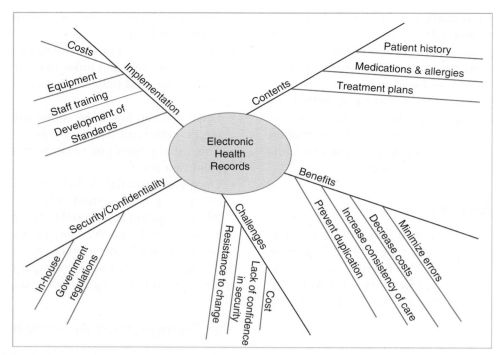

FIGURE 8-4 Mind map. (From Haroun L, *Career Development for Health Professionals: Success in School and On the Job*, ed 4, St Louis, 2016, Saunders.)

shirt. The patient didn't just shuffle, she shuffled precariously. These are examples of adjectives and adverbs, respectively, adjectives modifying nouns, adverbs modifying verbs. If you don't overuse adjectives and adverbs, they can add personality to your writing.

Phrases or clauses can also modify to add meaning, color, and precision. You can modify phrases and clauses in three places of a sentence: before the subject, between the subject and the verb, and after the verb. Here are some examples:

* "Before surgery, the patient signed the consent form."
* "The patient, with little hesitation, signed the consent form."
* "The patient signed the consent form, after consulting his wife."

These modification strategies add color, meaning, detail, and rhythm to your writing. You can improve your style by placing modification phrases throughout your sentences to achieve variety and interest. The great thing about modification is that there is no limit to the kind of variety possible and the ways it can contribute to your style. When you ask yourself how you might modify a word or a sentence, you are actually asking yourself for additional observations, important details, and vivid language to help achieve the purpose of your writing assignment.

Transitional Words

Transitional words are signposts that help the reader follow your logic. For example, to remind your reader that you are making the second of three points, start your second point with "Second." To announce a conclusion, write "Therefore." To move on to your next point, write "Next." To show that you are wrapping up a list of steps, write "Finally." To introduce an exception or a contrasting view, write "However." Transitions keep the reader on track to grasp your message and keep them engaged.

A Note to Non-Native Speakers and Writers of English

If English is not your native language, it can be difficult to learn. It's a tough language. One thing that may differentiate you from native speakers is that you may write better than you speak. There will be no accent in your writing if you use correct grammar, spelling, and tone. You may find that written English is a strength for you that does not come as easily to native speakers.

This is the sort of bloody nonsense up with which I will not put.

—Winston Churchill

CASE STUDY 8-2
Donna Wong, PhD, RN

Dr. Donna Wong wrote the best-selling nursing textbook of all time, *Nursing Care of Infants and Children.* Like you, she started out as a health care professional and only later came to see writing as a way to contribute to her profession.

When Donna met someone for the first time, she would often say, "Were you expecting a little Chinese lady?" In fact, born in 1948, Donna looked a lot like her Italian-American mother. She was raised in New Jersey, and became a nurse after attending Rutgers. In 1971, she married Dr. Ting Wong, a Chinese immigrant who became an officer in the Air Force.

As a young nurse working with children, Donna was dismayed to encounter children with serious illnesses who were not being treated effectively for their pain. In fact, in those days, it was not widely recognized that infants even experienced pain since their nervous systems were not fully developed. Moreover, young children could not effectively communicate the level of pain they were experiencing, and they were usually under-medicated. While this was one issue that concerned the young nurse, there were many others, and she often thought how poorly student nurses had been served by the pediatric nursing textbooks of the day. Soon, she earned a master's degree in nursing from the University of California at Los Angeles and began thinking seriously about what could be done to better educate student nurses in the field of pediatric nursing. Through a series of fortunate coincidences, she teamed up with Lucille Whaley and wrote the now-famous textbook *Whaley & Wong: Nursing Care of Infants and Children,* first published in 1979. Now in its ninth edition, this book is still a treasured reference.

Donna went on to earn a PhD in child development from Oklahoma State University. She was a professor at the University of Oklahoma Medical Center, at Oral Roberts University, and the University of Oklahoma School of Nursing. For many years, Donna was a nurse consultant at the Children's Hospital of the St. Francis Medical Center in Tulsa.

Donna had an amazing ability to synthesize new knowledge reported in the literature and translate it to nursing practice in her books. These assimilations went into her files, one for each chapter in the forthcoming edition. Donna published extensively in the journals herself and peer-reviewed articles for the journals. She formed an organization called Pediatric Nursing Consultants, teaching some of the most talented pediatric nursing researchers about writing and publishing. She became a popular speaker at conferences and conventions. She started an ongoing conference on pediatric pain.

Donna is also known for the Wong-Baker FACES Pain Rating Scale (Figure 8-5), which is now used worldwide to assess children's pain. Recognizing that children were inconsistent in how they reported their pain, resulting in inconsistent treatment for pain, Donna and her colleague Connie Baker extensively researched graphic representations of faces expressing comfort and pain.

Donna encouraged friends and colleagues to research issues that needed answers. Donna talked to kids about what it felt like to have a cast removed, get blood drawn, or experience chemotherapy. Moreover, her book reflects the very latest in the pathophysiology of disease, explaining the mechanisms of disease, and what that means for treatment and nursing care.

Donna came from humble beginnings, but her passion for nursing and her extraordinary ability to write clearly and accurately, helped her succeed and receive recognition,

0	1	2	3	4	5
No Hurt	Hurts Little Bit	Hurts Little More	Hurts Even More	Hurts Whole Lot	Hurts Worst

FIGURE 8-5 Wong-Baker FACES Pain Rating Scale. (From Hockenberry MJ, Wilson D, *Wong's Nursing Care of Infants and Children*, ed 10, St Louis, 2015, Elsevier.)

including the first Audrey Hepburn Award for Contributions to the Health and Welfare of Children.

On May 4, 2008, Donna Wong died of leukemia, a disease she had fought bravely for 3 years. She packed an incredible amount of life into her 60 years, and improved the treatment and lives of millions of children.

QUESTIONS FOR THOUGHT AND REFLECTION

1. What role did writing play in Donna Wong's life?
2. What impact did her writing have on others?
3. What inspires you about the life of Donna Wong?

Down a Dark Road

The hospital's general counsel, Arthur Adams, was reviewing a patient's chart, which had been subpoenaed by the patient's attorney in connection with a lawsuit that the patient had filed. The patient, Mrs. Roberta DeMasi, alleged that she received substandard care at Buchanan Hospital, which led to the amputation of her left foot. Mr. Adams was dumbfounded by what he saw. In particular, there were four nurse's notes by an "M. O'Brien, PCT"—Patient Care Technician. The first one, dated April 2, read:

"The patient has a sticky wound on the bottom of her foot with this black stuff oozing out. Charlie, one of the dietary aides, helped me take off the bandage for changing. What a terrible smell. I squirted some crème on it and covered it up as fast as possible. M. O'Brien, PCT"

The next one was worse.

"April 4. Roberta was in a cranky mood tonight. Constantly complained about pain in her foot. RN gave her PRN pain medication. Patient still complained. M. O'Brien, PCT"

The next note was the biggest liability:

"April 7. Patient's foot worse than ever. I had RN take a look, and she called DOC. MD arrived and said it was the worst he's ever seen. He said she had "green." He had to debride the wound. Patient squealed like a pig. MD put on cream, re-wrapped bandage. Patient's temperature elevated. M. O'Brien, PCT"

"Elevated?" thought Mr. Adams. Elevated to what? The last note didn't help.

"April 8. Somebody said they might have to amputate. MD changes bandage now. Roberta in a nasty mood. Medical students observed wound. Patient complained she didn't give consent for this. M. O'Brien, PCT"

Mr. Adams met with the president of the hospital, his legal team, and the vice president of human resources.

"We have no choice but to settle this case. Once the plaintiff's attorney sees his patient's chart, he'll know we have nothing," Mr. Adams said. It was a somber meeting.

Mr. Adams told the human resources vice president: "Find this M. O'Brien and have him or her terminated, and locate the supervisor, and put the supervisor on probation. The only thing we can do now is eliminate future liabilities."

QUESTIONS FOR THOUGHT AND REFLECTION

1. Name the mistakes M. O'Brien made in the documentation.
2. In your opinion, what was more damaging, the patient's medical care or the way she was characterized in the chart? Which was the most offensive, in your opinion?
3. Do you think that M. O'Brien ever imagined that his or her words would ever be read by the hospital's president and general counsel?
4. Was the decision to terminate M. O'Brien based on anything besides the notes written in the patient's chart?

1. Determine if your employer or externship site has any written policies on documentation. Ask the charge nurse for an example of what she considers good documentation.
2. Explore mind mapping online.
3. Read a short story by Ernest Hemingway or James Joyce. Observe their use of language, their word choice, their attention to details, and how the details contribute to the tone and meaning of the story.
4. Read a journal related to your field. What kind of observations can you make about the writing style you encountered there?
5. Ask a friend to critique an email you wrote. Did it seem to address its intended audience? Was it clear and concise? How was the tone? Was it interesting? Any suggestions for improvement? Return the favor.

CROSS CURRENTS WITH OTHER SOFT SKILLS

THINKING CRITICALLY: Thinking is a prerequisite for writing. (pp. 320-325)

COMMITTING TO YOUR PROFESSION: Writing and researching are key components to advancing knowledge in your profession. (pp. 342-348)

Professional Phone Technique

Tomorrow you might get a phone call about something wonderful and you might get a phone call about something terrible.

—Regina Spektor

LEARNING OBJECTIVE 3: PROFESSIONAL PHONE TECHNIQUE

- Know how you are going to answer the phone every time.
- Convey emotions through tone, pitch, and volume.
- Know what kinds of calls to expect, and how to handle them.
- Defuse emotional callers.
- Commit to learning the technology associated with the telephone.

When you answer the phone, it is a mistake to think that your voice is doing all the work. Your posture, breath, smile, tone, and attitude are conveyed through your voice.

Preparing to Answer the Phone

Who are you when you answer the phone? You get to choose. It is almost as if you choose a persona, like an actor in a play. Make sure your phone persona is the best "you" it can be, and then use that version of you every single time. Your professionalism is challenged every time you answer the phone at work. Every caller will judge you and form an opinion of your employer based on their interaction with you. Plan your phone presence. At health care facilities, callers may be anxious or ill. So be sensitive to their needs.

Planning Well Ahead

You should have a well-rehearsed greeting when you answer the phone. Of course, you will want to follow any policies and practices in place at your place of employment, but you will probably want to identify the facility, followed by your name: "Hello, Riverside Labs. This is Lori." You want to speak slowly and clearly, so the caller knows immediately that he has reached the right place.

Prepare your telephone voice ahead of time. You will want to speak moderately loudly, in case the caller has a hearing deficit or a poor connection. Plan to enunciate and speak directly into the phone. You can train your voice to sound clear and professional by humming for a minute at the lowest register of your voice. That is also an effective way to clear your voice after you have consumed dairy products or other foods that can produce mucous around your vocal folds.

Keep a notepad near the phone and plan to take notes, like the health professional in Figure 8-6. Write the caller's name, affiliation, and the time on the notepad. That way, you can clarify the caller's name right away if you need to, and you will have it to refer to later in the call without forgetting it. Write down any important information.

Just Before You Answer

Just before you answer the phone, sit up straight to open the full capacity of your lungs. You want to have your whole breath available to you. Smiling, with your posture and body language in ready position,

FIGURE 8-6 Health professional on phone, taking notes. (From Proctor DB, Adams AP: *Kinn's the medical assistant: an applied learning approach*, ed 12, St Louis, 2014, Elsevier.)

state your rehearsed greeting directly into the receiver. The greeting and introduction should be identical every time. You will have practiced it to get as much inflection, warmth, and enthusiasm into your voice as possible.

Your main job as the recipient of a phone call at your health care facility is to listen. You should verify the caller and listen for the purpose of the call. Do not interrupt. Take a breath before you speak to ensure that it is your turn. Obviously, your caller will be seeking information, but very often your answer will be in the form of a question, because you want to clarify the caller's need and get as much information as you can. Quite often, you are going to take a message, transfer the call, or arrange for a callback from one of your colleagues. It is your job to anticipate the questions your colleague will have and record that information.

Kinds of Calls

You should answer the phone as quickly as possible, before the third ring. You never know which calls will be an emergency.

WHAT IF?

What if the call is an emergency? What actions are you prepared to take?

Routine Calls

Most calls, of course, will be routine. Box 8-5 offers a list of typical calls. The telephone is for exchanging information, and the need for information in health care is fast-paced. You are likely to spend a significant amount of time on the phone every day. Be prepared to make this time as economical as possible.

For many health care professionals, a flurry of information is exchanged over the phone every day. Many times, callers will miss you, or you will be unable to reach your parties, and follow-up calls are needed, adding to the confusion. You will need a system if there isn't one already. Regardless of whether you have to create your own system or whether you use the existing system, it will only be successful if you use it every single time. It must be a habit. You cannot suspend the phone record or phone log system just because it gets busy. It is precisely at these times that the system is most needed.

Difficult Calls

Follow-up calls are not difficult, unless they are not made. When you need to or promise to follow up, something is at stake. Information must be obtained or clarified to ensure the smooth operation of the enterprise. Somebody is waiting to hear back from you, and their impression of your employer depends on whether you meet this obligation.

Confidential calls also require special attention. When what you say should not be overheard, try to move away from others or lower your voice (Figure 8-7). If the situation is seriously confidential, arrange to return the call in a private setting. Care should be taken that any notes are conveyed verbally or transcribed to the appropriate record, and the notes destroyed.

Complaints are part of any enterprise. Mistakes will be made. Misunderstandings will occur. And when they do, you will receive a complaint. Health care professionals deal effectively with problems all day long. Develop solutions by examining the problem itself rather than its delivery.

Angry callers are a special class of patients. Try to defuse the emotion surrounding the problem. Speak in a calm voice, and indicate a willingness to assist. Usually, you are not the reason the person is angry; you have simply answered the phone. However, you are your employer's representative, and so it is your job to deal with the angry caller. Say something reasonable, such as "I can understand your frustration. Let's see what we can do about this." Listen actively and ask good questions so you have a good grasp of the caller's problem.

If the anger persists, you should deal directly with it. "I'm having a hard time trying to help you. Would it be better for you if we discussed this issue when we can focus on finding a solution?" Arrange a callback, either from yourself or from someone who can address the problem effectively. If you transfer the call, do your colleague a service by trying to defuse the anger to keep it from transferring.

Of course, if the angry caller is abusive, uses coarse or offensive language, or is completely consumed with rage, you are not required to continue the conversation. Use the following explanation to communicate with the caller: "Unfortunately, I am not able to assist you when you're speaking to me this way. Please call back when you're ready to focus on a solution. Goodbye." Your duty is to follow procedures and protocols, while doing your best to meet the caller's needs. Firmly repeat the policy, and offer to do what you can do. "Sir, I cannot put you through to the doctor. However, I would be happy to take a message for her."

> ### JOURNALING 8-3
>
> Think about telemarketing calls you have received at home or at work. Write down the kinds of techniques the more aggressive callers use. How have you responded? Think about how you might respond even more effectively. Write down the words you would use.

Doctor shopping, unfortunately, is one of the problems associated with drug addiction. Drug addicts will stop at nothing to obtain drugs, and may call complaining of pain to see if someone there would be open to writing them a prescription. On the other hand, the person may simply be a prospective patient seeking information about a physician, dentist, or other provider. A prospective patient will be willing to give you their name and other contact information and will ask general questions about the provider's expertise. If addicts meet resistance, they will usually move on to an easier mark.

Emergencies demand special skills. You should always be prepared to respond effectively to an emergency call. As soon as you realize you are dealing with an emergency, ask "Please state the nature of your emergency." Emergency callers are often quite emotional, so you should use some of the techniques you use with any other emotional caller. Concentrate on getting the facts. If possible, get the person's name and location, or the exact location of the emergency.

FIGURE 8-7 A nurse calls a patient with confidential information (Copyright © istock.com).

The caller's number should be recorded on your telephone equipment, but try to obtain it anyway. Ask the person to tell you what you can do to effectively respond to the situation. Identify the severity of the situation, and identify others who may be in the best position to help, whether it is the police, an ambulance service, the poison control center, or the attention of a physician or other emergency professional.

Making Calls and Leaving Messages

When placing calls, clearly identify yourself, your role, your employer, and the person (such as a dentist) on whose behalf you are calling. Make an effort to engage with the person you're calling and smile while you are talking; often people can "hear" that you are smiling and this encourages their cooperation. Be precise about the information you are seeking or the request you are making. Write down any information you receive. Arrange any follow-up which may be needed. Thank the person for their help or kindness.

The people you call in your capacity as a health care professional are as busy as you are. Frequently, you will have to leave a message to achieve the purpose of your call. Box 8-6 offers suggestions for making your message effective.

Phone Technology

In this age of global telecommunication and technological advances, all of us are challenged to master existing technologies and learn new ones. Functions you will have to learn include transfers, holds, call waiting, conferencing, voicemail, answering services, caller ID, call forwarding, pagers, faxes, international calling, and operating headsets. Reliable

communication is essential to the safe and efficient delivery of health care. Therefore, technological skills are required of you. You must take this training very seriously and practice it. Identify more than one mentor or resource you can consult until you are comfortable with the technology used at your facility.

Finally, keep frequently called numbers on hand so you can access them easily and quickly, whether your calls are routine or emergencies.

The telephone is an amazing invention,
but who would ever want to use one?

—Rutherford B. Hayes

CASE STUDY 8-3

"Get him on the phone NOW!"

Charlissa had just arrived for her night shift in the Emergency Department when the phone rang. She took a deep breath, put a smile on her face, and said "Community General Hospital. This is Charlissa speaking. How may I help you?"

"I'll tell you how you can help me, Charlissa," said the caller, an agitated male. "You can put me on the phone with Dr. Horace Skinner RIGHT NOW."

Charlissa took a deep breath before she replied. "Sir, could you give me your name?"

"Tell him it's Jerry Pacheco, and put him on RIGHT NOW!"

She wrote his name down on her pad. "Mr. Pacheco, Dr. Skinner is unavailable just now. Could I help you or take a message for him?"

"Is he there?"

"I believe so, however—"

"Then put him on!"

"Sir, I would like to help you."

"Put Skinner on this phone, RIGHT NOW."

"Mr. Pacheco, I'm sure I can help you. Please give me some information about your situation."

She heard a deep sigh on the phone. Then the male voice, softer, controlled, between gritted teeth, continued. "I am out of town. My wife was taken to your emergency room. Dr. Skinner spoke to me and told me she was stable. He said he would call me back. I HAVE NOT HEARD FROM HIM!" he finished, returning to his original state of agitation.

"I can certainly understand why you're concerned, sir. Could you tell me your wife's name?"

"Lisa," he said.

"Sir, can you hold? I'll see what I can find out."

"Of course. Put me on HOLD."

Charlissa pressed the mute button. She checked her procedures and Ms. Pacheco's privacy statement. "Does anybody know where Dr. Skinner is?"

"In surgery," somebody said.

"Does anyone have a condition report on a Lisa Pacheco?"

"In surgery with Dr. Skinner."

Charlissa pressed the mute button again. She was able to relay an update to Mr. Pacheco. "Mr. Pacheco. Your wife is in surgery with Dr. Skinner."

"Oh God, oh God."

"Mr. Pacheco, I know you are very anxious. I am going to find out what is going on in surgery and call you back. Will that be all right?"

"Oh, God, yes. Call me back. Please call me back, Charlissa."

She took down his cell phone number, which matched the number on her display. "Give me ten minutes, Mr. Pacheco."

Five minutes later, she dialed his number. "Mr. Pacheco, your wife is fine, and she's just coming out of surgery. Dr. Skinner will call you as soon as he is out of the surgical unit. That's why he didn't call you before. I gave him your cell number."

At first, she thought she might have been disconnected. "Mr. Pacheco?" Then she heard he was there.

"Thank you, Charlissa," he said, barely audible. "Thank you."

QUESTIONS FOR THOUGHT AND REFLECTION

1. How did Charlissa prepare for this call?
2. What did Charlissa do when she realized the caller was agitated?
3. Did Charlissa show mastery of her equipment?
4. At what point did Mr. Pacheco stop acting angrily?
5. What more could Charlissa have done?
6. How do you think the rest of Charlissa's shift went?

Down a Dark Road

Brittany was chatting with the other medical assistants when the phone rang. She picked it up before she really finished talking. "Tell him to buzz off," she laughed. "Hello."

"Hello?" said a male voice.

"Hello? This is Brittany."

"Is this Dr. Lorris' office?"

"Yup. What can I do for you?"

"Well, actually, I have terrible pain in my hip joint. I know I have to have a hip replacement eventually, but right now, I'm in a lot of pain. Do you think Dr. Lorris could help me?"

"I don't know. He's a GP, you know, not a bone and joint doctor."

"That's OK," said the voice. "I just need help with the pain, until I can get the hip taken care of. I'm in a lot of discomfort. Do you think your doctor can help me?"

"Sure, I guess so. Do you want an appointment?"

"No, I'll just stop by."

"Ok. He's not that busy today."

"Does it matter which pharmacy I use?"

"Not that I know of. It depends on your insurance."

"I'll be right over."

QUESTIONS FOR THOUGHT AND REFLECTION

1. What was the caller's name?
2. Did Brittany do anything right?
3. Was there anything suspicious about the caller? Can you identify any concerns you would have had?

1. Watch a local newscaster. Notice the animation in her voice, and how that is achieved with facial expressions.
2. In a mirror, talk to yourself as if you were answering a phone. Exaggerate your vocal inflections and your facial expressions.
3. Record yourself taking a phone call. Play back the recording. What observations can you make about your voice and the messages carried along with it? How could you improve your phone voice?
4. Familiarize yourself with office policy regarding phone calls, including answering protocols, screening procedures, emergencies, and complaints.
5. If you know a 911 operator or a person who answers calls in an emergency department, ask them what techniques and tips they use to get structured information from an anxious caller.

CROSS CURRENTS WITH OTHER SOFT SKILLS

LISTENING ACTIVELY: Your main function on the phone is to listen. (pp. 263-269)

ADOPTING A POSITIVE MENTAL ATTITUDE: Your attitude is the foundation of your voice and your message. (pp. 2-11)

MODELING BUSINESS ETIQUETTE: The principles of courtesy and professionalism should guide your phone presence. (pp. 170-178)

SPEAKING PROFESSIONALLY IN YOUR WORKPLACE: Speaking on the phone is an important part of your workplace speech. You want to convey warmth, caring, and helpfulness. (pp. 244-249)

Bibliography

Flower L, Hayes JR. The cognitive process theory of writing. *College Composition and Communication* 32(4):365-387, 1981.

Strunk W and White EB. *Elements of style,* 4th ed, New York, 1999, Longman.

CHAPTER 9

Interacting Successfully

THEMES TO CONSIDER

- Take responsibility for the success of interactions between you and your clients and between you and your co-workers.
- Uncover more information by being an active listener.
- Listen to drive conversations forward.
- Recognize communication challenges related to people with disabilities or language barriers, and know what to do to solve them.
- Use communication strategies to respond to diversity in the workplace.
- Become aware of the power of body language.
- Empower your communication strategies with body language.
- Use body language to strengthen rapport with others.

Communication is a two-way street. When communication is working really well, the message sent is the same as the one received. Communicating effectively involves choosing your words carefully, saying them clearly, and supporting them with appropriate body language. The other half of good communicating involves paying attention in order to accurately interpret the other speaker's words and body language.

The importance of having great interpersonal communication skills is often underestimated. Many people think that if they keep their heads down and do their work, everyone should be satisfied with their performance. In reality, nothing will contribute more to your chances of being hired, your job satisfaction, and the respect you receive, than your ability to communicate effectively. Employers know this. They know, too, that they can teach job skills but they can't teach interpersonal skills. Interpersonal skills are especially essential in the health professions because health problems can make it difficult for people to communicate effectively. Health professionals must listen carefully, read body language, and develop intuition in order to detect problems.

It may take time and experience to develop interpersonal skills, but embracing any on-the-job communication challenges as learning experiences will accelerate your development.

Listening Actively

The most precious gift we can offer anyone is our attention.

—Thich Nhat Hanh

- Understand the essential role of listening in conversations.
- Listen as a strategy to keep conversations moving forward.
- Listen actively to uncover important information.
- Defuse conflict with listening strategies.
- Learn to ask great questions.

Yogi Berra said, "You can see a lot just by observing." He could have said, "You can hear a lot just by listening." Listening is an art that enables you to hear a lot more than what is being said. Only a portion of what people say is actually heard, and different listeners hear different amounts, depending on their listening skills.

Instead of worrying about what to say next, good listeners ask questions based on what they are hearing. Good listeners are curious. They want to learn more, understand, and gain insights they can use in the future. As a health professional, you should listen for context, anticipate, project warmth, and be helpful even while you are listening. Good listening skills are the foundation for all the positive and effective interactions you have as a clinician and as a co-worker.

JOURNALING 9-1

Complete this sentence: "Today I learned …" Plan to practice your listening skills during a conversation with a friend. Record what you learned about your friend as a result of your new skills.

Starting a Conversation

In order to listen, you have to be in a conversation, and you will often initiate the conversation. After all, to a patient visiting a health care setting, you will be the host.

Introduce Yourself

Did you know that there is more than one way to introduce yourself? There is definitely more than one side to you, which is apparent during your daily interactions. For example, you should have a specific short introduction ready to use every time you greet a new patient, focusing right away on your name and your

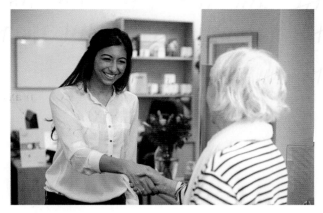

FIGURE 9-1 A receptionist introduces herself to a patient (Copyright © istock.com).

role (Figure 9-1). Plan what to say in advance, so it comes automatically. On the other hand, introducing yourself to co-workers requires a more detailed approach. For example, when you meet people at a new job, you might use a longer introduction because your new co-workers want to get to know you.

? WHAT IF?

What if you encounter a co-worker at your new place of employment and he doesn't introduce himself? How would you handle that situation?

Here are a few tips that can help new colleagues get to know you:
- Do you have an unusual name? Be prepared to spell it and pronounce it clearly. Share a few details about its origin. Remember to be patient and keep a sense of humor if someone has trouble pronouncing or remembering a name that is new to them.
- Say where you went to school, or share some of your work-related accomplishments.
- Humor can break the ice. A mildly self-deprecating joke can make your new co-workers feel at ease around you. Of course, be sure to stick to appropriate humor.

What kind of sharing fits your personal style? Consider using three or four sentences to introduce yourself to a new colleague. Be ready to share this information naturally, with a smile on your face and a handshake. From there on, listen, answer questions, and ask questions.

Other Conversation Starters

Giving a sincere compliment to someone you have just met is a great way to begin a conversation and be an active listener, because you have already demonstrated that you are a good observer. You have also started the conversation by focusing on the other person, which gives you an opportunity to listen actively and learn more about her.

Many conversations begin with a question. You might ask for information such as directions, advice, or guidance. Then, listen.

The Listening Process

Why is it so easy to get lost in your own thoughts when you are supposed to be listening to someone? Distraction has a lot to do with the difference between the speed of speech and the speed of thought. You usually think at a rate of about 500 words per minute, while most of us speak at about 130 words per minute. People who speak at 150 words per minute are fast talkers. It is impossible for humans to speak at 200 words per minute and still be intelligible. Because we think at 500 words per minute, we must concentrate in order to actively listen to someone speaking at a much slower pace than our thoughts.

Teach yourself powerful concentration skills by practicing the art of mindful listening—a three-phase conversation that goes deeper than the surface layer of conversation to understand a person's feelings, identify common ground, and make a plan to go forward.

The three phases of a productive conversation are listening, summarizing, and asking questions (Figure 9-2). As a conversation deepens, you will often repeat these three phases. We'll look closer at all three phases now.

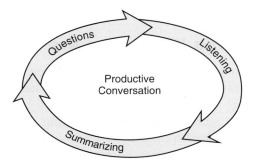

FIGURE 9-2 The listening process will repeat itself several times in a conversation.

Listen

The listener propels the conversation by making gestures and interjecting to encourage the speaker to continue. Typical expressions for encouraging a speaker are listed in Box 9-1. Give speakers all the time they need to express themselves. You want them to say as much as possible, to unearth as much information as possible. As you listen, observe body language and assess the speaker's emotions.

JOURNALING 9-2

Think about three significant conversations you have had today. Summarize them in your journal, just as you would summarize them to ensure that you understood what was being said.

Summarize

Once the speaker has expressed himself, clarify what you have heard with statements such as "If I understand you correctly," followed by key phrases or ideas you have heard. This validates the speaker because it demonstrates that you have been listening.

Another benefit of repeating the speaker's ideas is that it helps you avoid misinterpreting the speaker by making assumptions that may or may not be true. You are not just reacting to the person and thinking about your response.

Question

When you are sure that you understand the speaker, ask open-ended questions beginning with who,

BOX 9-1

Gestures and Interjections to Keep a Conversation Going

- Nod
- "Uh-huh."
- "Yes."
- "Go on."
- "Tell me more."
- "Then what?"
- "I see."
- "Mm-hmm."
- "I hear you."
- "Oh."

FIGURE 9-3 Two health professionals listening to a patient.

what, where, when, how, and why. However, ask one question at a time. Every time you ask an open-ended question, one that can't be answered with a simple "yes" or "no," you repeat the listening process.

The Pause

The pause—a natural break in conversation—is a signal to change speakers and listeners. Never interrupt; wait for that pause. People who interrupt have already stopped listening. They have already decided what they want to say in response, even before the other person has completed her thought and paused. Even an encouraging interjection, like "Uh-huh," should wait for a pause. If you speak after a pause, it shows that you were listening actively, especially if you make a logical comment, make an observation, or ask a relevant question. Then, once *you* pause, you have invited your partner to respond, and you can again encourage them to continue. Figure 9-3 shows two health professionals listening successfully to a patient.

Two monologues don't make a dialogue.

—Jeff Daly

Listening to Someone Who's Upset

Listening is the best approach to resolving conflict or responding to strong emotions. When a patient or co-worker is angry or emotional, your job is not to solve their problem or even get the facts (which will surface in due course), but to first simply support the

person who is experiencing such discomfort. Their feelings are real and part of their current experience. At this point, they are not looking for advice, pat answers, or an easy dismissal of their feelings or problems. They want to be accepted and understood. Encourage them to vent first, then ask thoughtful questions when they're done.

Once you have finished listening and eliciting all the information you can, summarize what you have heard. Summarizing clarifies issues, validates the speaker, and calms emotions by remaining neutral. Start by saying, "If I understand you correctly …" followed by your accurate summary.

 WHAT IF?

What if you don't understand what someone is saying? What strategies could you use to get the conversation back on track?

Your real objective is not to solve the person's problem or stop any irrational emotions, but to help the person do that for themselves. Here's the difference: Solving someone else's problem for them can foster a dependent relationship in which the other person approaches you to resolve every problem they encounter. By simply listening and questioning, you empower them to solve their own problems. Besides, if you're tempted to give the person advice and your advice doesn't work, you will own the person's problem.

Listening patiently helps the person talk themselves into a calm state—like the state you are modeling as you listen—and develop their own solutions. You cannot reason with an emotional person, but you can help an emotional person calm down and become reasonable. Once you master this skill, encourage your co-workers to observe your communication style as you interact with patients.

Listening When You Are Busy

Sometimes we feel we don't have time to listen. Health care settings can be chaotic. Who has time for listening?

A 1984 study examined the listening behavior of doctors in a health clinic by measuring and recording the time patients were permitted to speak at the beginning of their appointment. Although the doctors were aware of the study, they only let the patients talk for an average of 18 seconds before interrupting them. The doctors responded to the findings by denying that they interrupted their patients that quickly. They also explained that they were busy and that patients would talk endlessly about their problems if they weren't interrupted. The researchers repeated the study, but instructed the doctors to let the patients speak without interruption, no matter how long the patients took. The average patient only talked for 30 seconds, and the longest amount of time only lasted 90 seconds (Beckman and Frankel, 1984).

So are you really too busy to listen? Will you interrupt your patients to speed things along? Are you willing to forego the information you would have gathered, if you had listened just a little longer?

CASE STUDY 9-1
A Deep Discovery

Alicia was dreading her 3:00 appointment with Mr. Cruz. Her employer, Dr. Lin, charged a $75 fee when a patient missed a dental appointment without 24 hours' notice. Mr. Cruz had missed an appointment several months ago, and exploded at Alicia when she told him about the fee. She couldn't get him to calm down long enough to explain that the fee was waived the first time it happened.

Unfortunately, Mr. Cruz also missed his next appointment. Alicia thought they had seen the last of Mr. Cruz, but then his wife called and rescheduled.

Mr. Cruz seemed to be in a good mood when he arrived. He even waved at Alicia. Alicia thought he might not even be aware he had missed his last appointment, even though she called him the day before to remind him.

Mr. Cruz was still smiling as he approached her counter. "Good afternoon, Mr. Cruz. How are you?"

"Better than you might think for somebody who has to see the dentist."

"That's great," said Alicia. "Now, when was your last appointment?"

"I was here in September or October, I think. I'm not quite sure."

"Hmmm," said Alicia, looking at his chart. "It says here that you had an appointment in December, but you didn't come." She looked up at him with a neutral expression.

"I don't see why I have to pay this $75 penalty," he said as he recalled his missed appointment. "Things come up, you know. Nobody's perfect. My schedule is very unpredictable."

Alicia suspected that Mr. Cruz's unexpected friendliness was probably a ruse, but she forced herself to hear him out.

"I'm an insurance adjuster," he was saying. "When there is a claim—an accident, a flood, a fire—I have to be on the scene right away, while the circumstances and evidence are still fresh. I have a responsibility to my company," he said. "I try to keep these appointments, but my job is a higher priority."

Alicia noticed that he was talking faster now, and more color rose in this face, but she just nodded and said, "Uh-huh."

"I always have my cell phone," he said. "I guess I could have called, but would that have helped? I mean, if I called, and it wasn't the day before, you would still charge me, right? Even though I called?"

At this point, he paused, and Alicia knew she had to choose her reply carefully. She saw that he was trying to contain his emotions, but she knew that he had a short fuse.

"I think you are right," she said. "Calling always helps."

"But you still would charge me the penalty if it wasn't the day before, right?"

Alicia smiled at him. "Mr. Cruz, what we really want to do is treat as many patients as we can. We don't want to charge penalties. I would be happy if we never had to charge a penalty."

Mr. Cruz took a deep, deep breath. "I understand."

The waiting room was empty, so Alicia joined Mr. Cruz in the lobby. She asked Mr. Cruz to sit in a chair so they could face each other. "Mr. Cruz, do you know why we have this policy?"

"Yes, but I don't see why you have to charge money for nothing. That is a steep price to pay."

Mr. Cruz seemed a bit calmer now and the edge had gone out of his voice.

"Mr. Cruz," she said, lowering her voice a bit and pointing to the sign taped to the window that stated the policy, "We don't charge if you call the day before. We would not charge you a penalty if you called ahead of time because we might be able to schedule another patient in your place. Unfortunately, Mr. Cruz, you didn't call."

"I understand."

"Thank you for understanding," said Alicia. "I think the doctor is ready to see you know. We can make payment arrangements when you are through."

QUESTIONS FOR THOUGHT AND REFLECTION

1. What tactics did Alicia use to avoid getting into an argument with Mr. Cruz over the penalty fee?
2. What role did body language play in this exchange?
3. Why did Alicia enforce the penalty fee?
4. What information did Mr. Cruz disclose as a result of Alicia's listening ability?
5. What statement did Alicia repeat to convince Mr. Cruz that it was only fair for him to pay the penalty?

Down a Dark Road

Prima finally got a job as a sonography technician at the obstetric practice of Drs. O'Malley, Kendrick, and Anselmo. She had done very well in her program, but she knew she had a lot to learn on the job. She had already learned how to use a more advanced sonography imaging machine than the ones she had seen at school and at her internships. She had encountered some anomalies—that was what Dr. Anselmo called them—in some of the sonograms she had taken. She wasn't sure Dr. Anselmo was using that term correctly. Some of the patients had to have amniocentesis, and it struck her that there were many more complications than she had originally anticipated. Prima pursued sonography because she liked babies, and she thought it would be a very positive profession, with a lot of happy moms as well as opportunities to learn and advance. She had not seen a miscarriage yet, but she dreaded the day when that would come. She told her boyfriend that the job was a lot more complicated than she thought.

At the end of her third week, Prima did a sonogram for a woman who was logged in as Dr. Alison DeMoure.

"Are you a medical doctor?" she asked when Dr. DeMoure arrived.

"No, I teach engineering at the University. You can call me Alison." She pointed in the direction of the man who was with her. "That's Mitch, my husband." She was soft-spoken, and she seemed to lower her voice even more as she shared that this was their first child.

"Wow, that's great," said Prima. "Let's see, your birth date is April 2, 1971—is that right?"

"Yes."

"Wow, and this is your first baby? You're getting a late start."

Alison exchanged a glance with Mitch, who stepped forward. "The baby will be fine," he said to both of them.

"Sure she will," said Prima with sudden enthusiasm. "What are you guys hoping for, a boy or a girl?"

"A healthy baby," said Alison.

"We don't care about the gender," said Mitch. "We want to be surprised." He nodded at Alison, as if to reassure her.

"Well, you're far enough along that we can probably tell," said Prima.

"We don't want to know, one way or the other," said Alison.

"Sure, you want to have a healthy baby. Let's get started."

Pretty soon, they all heard a healthy heartbeat. "He's got a great heartbeat," said Prima. "Oh my God, look at him!" Prima felt happy that the baby seemed healthy. "Do you want to take a print of this, so you can put the little guy on your refrigerator?"

Alison and Mitch seemed relieved that the baby seemed healthy, but Alison said she didn't want the image.

A half-hour later, Dr. O'Malley came out and asked to speak to Prima in his office. "Did you tell the DeMoures that they are having a boy?"

"No, I mean, they were so happy about the heartbeat. I hope the little guy is going to be OK."

"The little guy?"

"The baby. You know."

"Didn't they tell you they didn't want to know what the sex was?"

"I don't think I heard that."

"No, you didn't listen."

"Well, the important thing is that the baby is OK, right?"

"Yes, the baby is fine, but you didn't listen to them and respect their wishes. That's not the way we do things around here. Make sure it doesn't happen again," said Dr. O'Malley, and he rose from his desk, indicating their meeting was over.

1. What do you think Prima's main concern was when she realized the age of the patient?
2. What, if anything, did Prima do to reassure the DeMoures?
3. How could Prima have handled the issue about the baby's gender?
4. Prima kept saying that it was good that the baby seemed healthy; why do you think she kept repeating that?
5. What do you think the DeMoures talked about in the car on the way home?

⭐ EXPERIENTIAL EXERCISES

1. Listen to your friends or clients talk without interrupting them. How long do they talk before they pause?
2. Write two introductions for yourself, one introducing yourself to a patient and one introducing yourself to a new co-worker. Memorize them and say them out loud until they sound natural.
3. Use your "co-worker" introduction on a partner. Observe where the conversation goes from there.
4. Compliment a friend or family member. Observe where the conversation goes from there.
5. Watch the evening or Sunday morning news. Pay close attention to the questions the reporters ask. Are they open-ended questions? Are they good questions? Do the questions elicit interesting or revealing information?
6. Watch a late night talk show. Evaluate the questions asked in a similar fashion.

🔄 CROSS CURRENTS WITH OTHER SOFT SKILLS

MODELING BUSINESS ETIQUETTE: What is the connection between listening and etiquette? (pp. 170-178)

TALKING TO YOUR BOSS, MANAGER OR SUPERVISOR: This is when listening can really pay off for your career. (pp. 325-333)

GAINING ENERGY, PERSISTENCE, AND PERSEVERANCE: Learn how listening fuels your energy. (pp. 190-197)

MANAGING ANGER AND STRONG EMOTIONS: Why is listening a good strategy here? (pp. 375-380)

Communicating with Special Groups of Clients

Something there is that doesn't love a wall.

—Robert Frost

LEARNING OBJECTIVE 2: COMMUNICATING WITH SPECIAL GROUPS OF CLIENTS

- Rapidly assess special communication challenges.
- Have strategies at hand to communicate effectively with hearing-impaired clients.
- Know how to gain the attention of people with hearing and visual impairments.
- Empathize with the needs of disabled people, so you can anticipate these needs.
- Know how to guide and seat a visually impaired person.
- Know when to treat an older person like anyone else, and when they require special communication techniques.
- Help people with speech impairments to express their needs and thoughts.
- Use an interpreter correctly.

We take our sensory organs and communication abilities for granted until we encounter someone who has lost these senses. What a gift we have in being able to hear, see, and speak! Keep in mind, however, that people with disabilities take pride in their many abilities; many have creative ways to accommodate for a particular challenge and may not want help if they don't need it. Always take your cues from the person, and ask before helping.

Communicating with People Who Are Hearing-Impaired

People who are hearing-impaired have made many adjustments that make it easier for them to function. Nevertheless, they frequently encounter ignorance and rudeness that can create feelings of helplessness. Be empathetic to these challenges.

Recognizing People with Hearing Impairments

The first challenge is to recognize that a person is hearing-impaired. For instance, some people still have trouble hearing even with hearing aids, while hearing aids can actually correct hearing for others. These days, hearing aids are so small and discreet that many people do not even notice them.

You also cannot tell by speech quality alone that a person is hearing-impaired. For example, if a person loses hearing after age 12 years or so, his or her speech is likely to be unimpaired. If a person loses hearing after age 5, he or she will have some noticeable speech impairment, but will likely be easy to understand. People who are born deaf or lose their hearing early in life will have significant speech impairment, and you may have great difficulty in understanding them.

A hearing-impaired person who visits a health care facility usually simply tells you that he or she cannot hear normally. If you do encounter someone with speech impairment, it is important for you to understand that the impairment is the result of hearing loss and not intellectual disability.

Strategies for Communicating with Hearing-Impaired People

Once you realize that you are communicating with a hearing-impaired person, adopt a strategy to communicate effectively (Figure 9-4). It is natural for you to raise the volume of your voice, and this may be helpful for some hearing-impaired people. It is best, however, to simply ask such clients how they prefer to communicate.

> *The problem with communication is the illusion that it has taken place.*
>
> —George Bernard Shaw

Some hearing-impaired people rely on their lip-reading abilities. This form of communication is

FIGURE 9-4 A nursing assistant speaks to a hearing impaired nursing home resident (Copyright © istock.com).

helpful, but medical terminology can be confusing. It is therefore important that you confirm comprehension. If you ask, "Are you having a hard time understanding me?" and your patient continues to smile and nod, you should be concerned about the quality of communication taking place.

JOURNALING 9-3

Think about a time when you experienced bias, prejudice, or discrimination. Write about the experience and emotions related to it. How do you feel about it now, after all this time? Record your thoughts about how and how often a hearing-impaired person may have these experiences, and how they may feel about it.

Writing is one way to avoid confusion. Writing can be slow and awkward at times, but your client may be used to the pace. You can supplement written communication with signage or objects that will clarify the message you are trying to send. If your place of employment often serves people with hearing impairments, suggest installing a series of helpful signs created specifically to enhance communication with the hearing impaired.

Body language and gestures, discussed later in this chapter, are great tools for communicating with hearing-impaired patients. Even with people who are not impaired, body language can convey as much as 70% of the communication. Use body language to aid your communication with hearing-impaired clients, especially in adding the nuances that words and voices usually carry, such as warmth, urgency, or seriousness. Exaggerate gestures to help your words carry more meaning.

> *Deafness has left me acutely aware of both the duplicity that language is capable of and the many expressions the body cannot hide.*
>
> —Terry Galloway

Finally, remain alert to your client's use of body language. Additional suggestions to facilitate communication with people who have hearing disorders are listed in Box 9-2.

Using Interpreters

Many people with lifelong or profound hearing impairments know American Sign Language, or

Ameslan. Many health facilities employ professional interpreters, including those fluent in Ameslan. These expert interpreters not only translate between languages but also *interpret* language for clients, explaining medical terminology, answering simple questions, and clarifying any confusion between the patient and the health professional. Interpreters aid communication with hearing-impaired patients, as well as patients who speak little or no English.

If no professional interpreter is available, determine whether there is someone in your office who may know some sign language. Just as you would seek a Spanish-speaking colleague to assist a Spanish-speaking patient, you should treat Ameslan as the native language of hearing-impaired people, and seek an interpreter if possible.

When Friends and Family Offer to Serve as Interpreters

Many hearing-impaired individuals—as well as people with speech impairments and language deficits—bring along friends or family members who serve as interpreters. Although it is thoughtful for a friend or family member to offer support, be careful of relying on them as an interpreter. As a health professional, you must protect the privacy of the patient's confidential medical information. Having a friend or family member act as the interpreter might also result in misinterpretation, especially if they have to explain information rather than just translate it. Moreover, this dynamic presents a conflict of interest because the friend or family member may have his or her own agenda, or may not be objective. Sometimes, sensitive information, perhaps involving contraception or a poor prognosis, is information that a translator in a personal relationship with the patient might not share, and you may not know it.

You need to gain the patient's approval directly from the patient if a friend or family member is to serve as an interpreter. You must do everything you can to support the confidentiality and best interests of your patients, especially those with disabilities. Finally, you should document in the medical record any information you received from the patient that was provided by an interpreter, and express any concerns you may have about the accuracy of the information.

Communicating with People Who Are Visually Impaired

People who are visually impaired usually have excellent hearing. There is no need to raise your voice to be understood. There are many degrees of visual impairment. Many individuals are able to discern movement, shapes, and contrasting colors. Take as much advantage as you can of whatever abilities the person may have, while also being prepared to interact with a person who is totally blind.

Identify yourself and your role. Address the visually impaired individuals by name, so they know you are speaking to them. People who are visually impaired don't have access to facial expressions and body language that aid comprehension. As a health care professional, you have to recognize this and be able to put yourself in your client's shoes. Ask yourself what you need to do to be considerate. For instance, explain any sudden loud noises. Don't be afraid to use touch because it indicates that you are listening and paying attention.

Assisting Visually Impaired Individuals in Moving Around

When escorting the visually impaired person, to an examination room for instance, allow him to take your arm (Figure 9-5). Give verbal directions as you move together. Describe any obstacles. When you arrive,

FIGURE 9-5 A nursing assistant directs a blind patient (Copyright © istock.com).

explain the layout of the room if necessary. When you offer a seat, place the visually impaired person's hand on the back of the chair, which enables him to navigate the seating. When you leave, tell the person you are leaving the room, and introduce him to people who will be with him.

Don't be afraid to use words or phrases like "Look out" or "I see what you mean." Speak directly to the visually impaired person, not through an intermediary. Treat the visually impaired person like any other patient.

Some people with severe visual impairments will have professionally trained guide dogs. The dog is "on the job;" leave the dog alone. Do not make eye contact with the dog or interact in any way with the dog unless you have the owner's permission.

Communicating with People Who Have Speech Impairments

Causes and Types of Speech Impairments

There are many reasons why people are speech-impaired. They may have been born deaf or lost their hearing before they developed the ability to speak. They may have uncorrected or untreated speech impediments. They may have disfiguring injuries affecting their tongue, mouth, teeth, or jaw. They may be recovering from a stroke, or aphasia, when they have trouble recalling or forming words. They may

be suffering from a neurodegenerative disease such as cerebral palsy or Parkinson's disease. Or, they may stutter. Remember that speech impairment and hearing impairment do not go hand in hand, and resist the temptation to speak louder than normal. Some people are offended by this unnecessary gesture.

Strategies for Communicating with People Who Have Speech Impairments

Do not pretend to understand something the individual says. Ask the individual to repeat what he or she said, and then repeat it to confirm your understanding. Be patient and take as much time as necessary. Concentrate on what the individual is saying, moving closer or to a quieter location if necessary. Resist the temptation to speak for the individual or attempt to finish the patient's sentences. People with speech impairments have to exert tremendous effort to speak and be understood. It would be frustrating and even insulting to have someone fill in their thoughts, as though they are not already making a monumental effort to do so for themselves.

Instead, ask questions that require only short answers or a nod. Consider writing as an alternative means of communication if you are having difficulty understanding the individual, but first ask the individual if this is acceptable.

❓ WHAT IF?

What if, despite your best efforts, you simply cannot understand what a patient with a speech impairment is saying?

Communicating with People Who Speak Little or No English

Our diverse nation is full of innovation. As trade, education, and transportation have become more global in the 21st century, people from all over the world have come to live, work, study, or visit in the United States. The complex mosaic of these cultural and linguistic patterns in American society places new demands on health care professionals, who must effectively communicate complex medical information to people who speak little or no English.

Strategies for Communicating with People Who Speak Little or No English

As you can imagine, it is extremely difficult to communicate with someone when you do not share the same language (Figure 9-6). Accurate communication is essential in a health care setting, where many words and concepts are unfamiliar to the patient. The best solution is the utilization of a professional interpreter. If a friend or family member accompanying the patient serves as a translator, you must consider the concerns discussed earlier in this chapter.

Refer to the suggestions in Box 9-3 when communicating with people who speak little or no English.

In Extreme Cases Where Little or No Verbal Communication in English Is Possible

In the absence of an interpreter and in the case of complete inability to communicate in any common language, it is best to try to reschedule the appointment until suitable communication arrangements can be made. Measures might include arranging for a dial-up interpreter service. In an emergency, however, you will have to communicate as well as possible, using body language to reassure the patient.

Communicating with Small Children

Most health care professionals have an affinity for small children (Figure 9-7). However, communicating with them may not always be so easy. Children may be shy, fussy, tired, or uncooperative. Children who are sick are under added stress, and children with autism may find it difficult to connect with anyone,

BOX 9-3

Suggestions for Communicating with People Who Speak Little English

- Draw an object on paper or write things down. Many foreign speakers of English have larger vocabularies of written words than spoken words.
- Use simple language free of metaphors, slang, or colloquialisms.
- Make simple and direct requests, saying "please" and "thank you," which are universally recognized for their politeness.
- Speak a little slower than normal and articulate clearly, although not in an exaggerated fashion.
- Make many more gestures than normal when speaking.
- If another language is prevalent in your area, your clinic might make a small electronic translation device available to the staff.
- Refer to a pocket dictionary.
- As long as you understand your client, don't correct their English.

FIGURE 9-6 A nurse comforts a non-English-speaking patient (Copyright © istock.com).

FIGURE 9-7 A medical professional calms an anxious, young patient before an MRI test (Copyright © istock.com).

especially strangers. Certainly, the treatment of a sick child is an occasion for anxiety, if not for the child at least for the parents or caregiver. Still, you can increase your chances of communication success by adopting a number of strategies.

Strategies for Communicating with Small Children

Maintain the same level with the child and make eye contact with them. Call them by their name. If the child won't respond to your eye contact, say, "Amanda, can I have your eyes?" Be positive and simple. Try to get your idea across in one sentence, using simple words.

To better gain compliance with a request, use the phrase "I want," as in "Alice, *I want* you to show me which ear hurts." This is not as harsh as a direct order, and it plays into a child's desire to want to please you as an individual. You can gently bargain with a child. For example, you can use the "When-then" strategy: "*When* you have your shot, *then* you can have a cup of orange juice." You can also offer a choice to involve the child in the decision-making. "You can have the insulin shot in your arm or in your leg."

If the child is crying or panicking, calmly ask, "Can I help you?" You can also gently restrain the child.

Communicating with Elderly People

Most of the time, you will communicate with the elderly just as you would anyone else. You may be more alert to the possibility of any of the disabilities discussed previously, such as hearing loss. Keep in mind that most elderly people are as able as anyone else. However, there are certain groups of elderly people who have special communication needs.

People with Alzheimer's Disease, Dementia, and Other Organic Brain Diseases

There are many stages of organic brain diseases affecting memory, functioning, and identity. However, the following strategies are useful for communicating with people experiencing all but the most profound stages of these diseases:

* Approach the person from the front, within his line of vision so as not to startle him, and face him as you talk in order to hold his attention.

* Minimize distracting hand movements and keep in mind that your body language may convey more meaning than your actual words.
* Smile often; a frown could be misinterpreted.
* Speak in a normal tone of voice and greet the person as you would anyone else. If anything, speak at a slower pace and in a quieter, more soothing tone.
* Choose a quiet meeting place, one without a lot of stimulation or distractions.
* Respect the individual's personal space. If she paces, walk with her while you talk.
* Refocus a distracted person's attention by pointing either back to yourself or to a calm feature, such as plants or a window view.
* Ask only one question at a time, and use questions to refocus. For example, "You were telling me about the television show."
* Because many people with dementia have better long-term memories than short-term memories, ask them questions about their past.

 WHAT IF?

What if a patient with Alzheimer's disease is arguing with another patient with the same condition? How would you intervene to defuse the situation?

Communicating with Your Clients and Co-Workers From Different Generations

For the first time in history, Americans share their workplaces with four generations of people at a time. Many traditionalists of the World War II generation have not left the workplace. Many are healthy and vigorous and enjoy working. Baby Boomers, born between 1946 and 1964, remain as a huge presence in the workplace even though some are reaching retirement age. Members of Generation X, born between 1965 and 1980, are assuming senior management positions. Millennials, born after 1980, began entering the workforce around the turn of the Millennium.

As health care professionals, each generation must learn to interact with the others. However, you can only control your own interactions, which should be sensitive to the other three generations. To accommodate all generations, assume a neutral and conservative appearance, behavior, and communication style. Next, appreciate that each person is an individual and should not be stereotyped, while understanding the differences in general tendencies for each of these four generations. These can be summarized, roughly, as follows:

* *Traditionalists* are loyal and hardworking. Their world may be rapidly disappearing, but they have knowledge and wisdom to bring to the workplace. They will probably be less tech-savvy than others, but skilled in face-to-face interactions. You should work hard to break down any barriers with older co-workers, so you can benefit from their strengths and allow them to benefit from yours.
* *Baby Boomers* are achievers, willing to work long hours to gain pay and position. Co-workers can learn a lot from their drive and ambition. They try to embrace technology. They respond to praise and recognition. Many younger workers can form relationships with Baby Boomers based on their willingness to help Baby Boomers with technology.
* *Generation X* workers are a smaller group than the Baby Boomers or Millennials, but they occupy leadership positions in many organizations. Learning from the excesses of their parents, Generation X workers strive for a better work-life balance. They seek flexibility in the workplace and offer ideas that make the workplace a better place to spend time. They value innovation, entrepreneurship, and creativity. They don't like to be micromanaged. If they are not happy with their working conditions, they will consider moving on. Members of other generations can learn a lot from Generation X workers, and it is well worth engaging with them to keep their talents in the organization.
* *Millennials* are digital natives and free spirits. Seventy-million strong, Millennials represent the future of the workforce. They are talented, hard-working, impatient, and learning-oriented. They want to get experience and move up as fast as possible. Giving Millennials as much responsibility and diversity as possible is the best way to keep them engaged and productive.

CASE STUDY 9-2
The Advocate for the Deaf

Eva was an experienced dental assistant. She had been working in Dr. Richter's office for about 6 months, having moved to Rochester because of her husband's relocation. She liked the office and the people there, and she was getting to know the patients. Some of them had already been in two or three times.

Eva was a little apprehensive today, though, because her 1:00 appointment, Millicent Marquis, was deaf. Her husband, Tommy, served as her interpreter. Over lunch, Dr. Richter shared some information with her about Millicent.

"She's just coming in for a cleaning, assuming nothing else has come up," the Doctor told Eva. "I don't bother giving her to one of the hygienists. She is comfortable with me, and I like her. But she's a big advocate for people with disabilities, and she'll give you a piece of her mind."

Millie was a large woman in her 70s with wild red hair. She walked with two canes and the assistance of her husband, a wiry man with white hair. "I can't hear without him, and I can't walk without these," she announced, in a voice that was loud and intelligible but somewhat garbled. Dr. Richter greeted her and escorted her to the closest examination room, helping her, with Tommy's assistance, into the dental chair.

Dr. Richter got in front of Millie and made eye contact with her. "We have a new dental assistant, Millie. Her name is Eva Plume," and she pointed to Eva, who moved into Millie's line of sight.

"I guess I'll have to break her in," said Millie. Dr. Richter raised her arm to get Millie's attention. "Go easy on her, Millie. I want to keep her." Then Dr. Richter said she would be back shortly, and Eva would stay with her.

"I guess you can't hear me," Eva said nervously.

"No, but I can read your lips."

Eva blushed while Tommy gave her a flurry of signs with his hands.

"Oh, she'll survive," said Millie.

"What kind of a dental office is this that I have to bring my own interpreter? He's totally unreliable. You should provide your deaf patients with a professional interpreter."

"That would be nice," said Eva.

"Nice? Did you say nice? It's the law, by gum. I have a right to know what's going on."

"Don't take her too seriously," Tommy said to Eva, signing to Millie at the same time. "She definitely knows what's going on, and I'm definitely unreliable."

That made Millie laugh, but then she got serious. "Can you understand me, Eva?"

"Yes."

"Good, because we need a few rules."

Eva nodded.

"If you or that Dr. Richter hurt me, I'm going to raise my right hand, and you are going to stop immediately, got it?"

Eva nodded.

"If I just want a break from the action, I'll raise my left hand."

Eva nodded again.

"Thank you for nodding, Eva. That's something I can understand."

Just then Dr. Richter came back in. She had been wearing a mask, but she took it off.

"Eva knows the rules," Millie told Dr. Richter, and Dr. Richter smiled and winked at Eva.

Throughout the cleaning, Dr. Richter explained everything she was doing, and Tommy translated it to Millie. Dr. Richter stopped once in a while to ask Millie if she needed a break.

Afterward, everyone helped Millie out of the dental chair, and the whole gang moved into the lobby. The other assistants and hygienists came out to greet Millie.

"Now that I've broken you in," she said to Eva, "I'll expect you to be here when I come back in 6 months." Eva's college roommate had a deaf sister, and she taught Eva how to sign "Thank you."

QUESTIONS FOR THOUGHT AND REFLECTION

1. Would you share Eva's anxiety if you knew you were going to see a deaf patient?
2. What actions did Dr. Richter take to make it easier for Millie to communicate with her and Eva?
3. Did Dr. Richter use Tommy appropriately as an interpreter?
4. Why does everyone like Millie so much?

Down a Dark Road

Robert was nearing the end of a long day as a medical assistant in Dr. Seldek's office. There was just one appointment left, Ms. Moriarty, and he wanted to get her in and out.

"Moriarty?" Robert asked the elderly woman with a cane.

"Yes, that's me." She replied.

"Are you here by yourself?"

"No, my friend is waiting for me in the car. It's hard for her to walk, and I'm just here to get my, uh, thingamajig checked."

"Sit over there, and the doctor will be with you shortly," Robert said, pointing.

She looked at him through her dark glasses without responding.

"What are you, blind?"

"As a matter of fact, young man, I am."

"Oh boy," said Robert as he moved around the desk to help Ms. Moriarty. He grabbed her arm, which startled her. "Sorry," he muttered. He quickly escorted her to the row of chairs, positioned her in front of the first one, placed one of his feet behind hers, and plopped her down onto the seat. "Oh my," she said.

When Robert returned to his station, his colleague Anika approached him. "What are you doing?"

"She's blind."

"I know that. That's not how you treat a person with a visual impairment."

"Oh yeah? What would you do?"

"I wouldn't shove her into a chair, for one thing." She went around the counter and stood in front of the patient. "Hello, Ms. Moriarty," she said with a smile. "I'm Anika, one of the staff members here. Would it be all right if I sat next to you while you wait for Dr. Seldek?"

Robert rolled his eyes at her and glanced at the clock.

QUESTIONS FOR THOUGHT AND REFLECTION

1. When is sarcasm appropriate in a health care setting?
2. What were cues Robert should have picked up indicating this patient is visually impaired?
3. What mistakes did Robert make in the way he physically interacted with Ms. Moriarty?
4. In your opinion, what factors contributed to Robert's behavior?

What if you observed a co-worker mistreating a disabled person? How would you approach the situation? Would you confront your co-worker? Why or why not?

★ EXPERIENTIAL EXERCISES

Along with a partner, put headphones over your ears or cotton in your ears to simulate a hearing impairment. Talk with your partner for 10 minutes.

1. Have a 10-minute conversation with a partner using only written communication.
2. Share stories with your classmates, colleagues, or friends involving communicating with people that have various communication disabilities or challenges.
3. With a partner, take turns guiding each other when one is wearing a mask. Be sure to use touch and verbal cues.
4. Ask friends, classmates, colleagues, and family members for examples of foreign phrases. For example, in Arabic, "Assalamu alaikum" (pronounced: as-salam-u-alay-koom) means "Peace be with you." Can you collect similar expressions in Spanish, Italian, Russian, Hebrew, Hindu, Mandarin, or a language common in your area? Make a list of these expressions, learn how to pronounce them, and memorize them.

⊘ CROSS CURRENTS WITH OTHER SOFT SKILLS

AIMING TO BE ADAPTABLE AND FLEXIBLE: Sometimes you have to think on your feet when communicating with disabled people. (pp. 25-29)
STRIVING FOR TOLERANCE: Disabled people are entitled to the same high quality of health care as everybody else. (pp. 29-35)
SHOWING EMPATHY, SENSITIVITY, AND CARING: Caring for disabled people gives you an opportunity to practice the values that are at the core of health care. (pp. 218-222)
PRACTICING PATIENCE: This is when your patience really pays off. (pp. 361-364)

Reading and Speaking Body Language

There's language in her eyes, her cheek, her lip.

—William Shakespeare

LEARNING OBJECTIVE 3: READING AND SPEAKING BODY LANGUAGE

- Understand the scope of body language.
- Know how to use your eyes in communication, and how others see your eyes.
- Learn how reliable facial expressions are for revealing emotions.
- Acquaint yourself with some common gestures and what they *may* mean.
- Learn how to mirror to build rapport.
- Understand the paralinguistic qualities of your voice.

Have you ever had a conversation without speaking? You may not think so at first, but think about it. How about the times when someone else was speaking, and you and your friend exchanged smiles? These kinds of silent exchanges occur constantly because body language is so subtle and automatic. Even when you are talking, your conversation is peppered with an array of gestures, expressions, and postures. Body language is one of your most accomplished skills and precious assets, but it must be used with purpose and discretion. When it is used involuntarily, as it often is, you must have insight into this special and pervasive language.

Research consistently shows that body language consists of 60% to 70% of the meaning in interpersonal communication. As a health care professional, you must raise body language to a higher level of consciousness. Box 9-4 examines the many aspects of body language.

I speak two languages, Body and English.

—Mae West

Facial Expressions

Many facial expressions are involuntary, appearing all by themselves whenever you experience a particular emotion. Even if you don't want to convey a specific expression, it may be impossible to keep it from surfacing before you have a chance to convey a more suitable expression. For example, you might encounter a client with a disturbing disfigurement and you may look repulsed before putting on your more professional face. These are called "fleeting" expressions or "microexpressions."

My opponent says I am two-faced. I ask you: if I had two faces, would I wear this one in public?

—Abraham Lincoln

Facial expressions and their meaning are universal. The emotions of fear, anger, contempt, surprise, disgust, sadness, and happiness are recognized in all cultures. That is why even simple smiley faces and emoticons, with their raised eyebrows or open mouths, immediately convey universally recognized emotions.

Expressions can be genuine or fake, and people can usually tell the difference. If you do not feel the emotion you want to convey, you are better off maintaining a neutral expression which will at least not tarnish your credibility. A fake smile can just be a courtesy. A real smile is spontaneous, unforced, and something others respond to. The eyes and the mouth are involved in every facial expression. Look at Figure 9-8 and see if you can tell the difference between the fake smile on the left and the genuine smile on the right.

Eye Contact

Eyes have been called the windows to the soul. Any meaningful relationship or interaction can be enhanced by eye contact. Eye contact contributes to first impressions and creates a friendly, welcoming experience. We naturally distrust people who cannot maintain eye contact. The failure to make eye contact can also communicate arrogance, contempt, and disrespect.

At work, establish eye contact with your patients and co-workers for more than 90% of each interaction. In fact, if you are sending a very strong or urgent message, such as a warning or a reprimand, do not avert your gaze so as to emphasize the importance of what you are saying, breaking eye contact eventually.

BOX 9-4

Aspects of Body Language

- Eye contact
- Gestures
- Appearance
- Posture
- Tone of voice
- Pace of speech
- Volume of speech
- Facial expressions
- Smell
- Touch
- Personal space
- Non-speech vocalizations, like sighs
- Drama
- Twitches
- Distractions

JOURNALING 9-5

Recall a time when you had a meaningful exchange with someone that involved eyes only. Maybe it was a confrontation, a flirtation, a reprimand, or a flash of recognition. Describe the circumstances, and write about your feelings at the time.

Breaking Eye Contact

Break eye contact every so often to avoid intimidating your partner. When you do break eye contact, glance left or right, not up or down, and then bring your gaze

FIGURE 9-8 A genuine smile has much more facial muscle involvement. **A,** A fake smile is usually forced and lacks emotion. **B,** The genuine smile involves the whole mouth and the eyes are a little closed.

back to your partner's eyes. A sufficient break can last even less than a second and eliminate any discomfort. When you look down to break eye contact, you are making a gesture of submission or inferiority. Similarly, if you look up, you are quietly disrespecting your partner, looking "over" her or acting superior. Again, this creates a subtext that does not facilitate a deep connection.

Eye contact deepens each person's interest in the conversation and reflects your level of interest. For example, if you want to augment your interest, look back and forth between the other person's two eyes. This will give your eyes sparkle and animation that signals interest and engagement on your part. On the other hand, if you are not responding favorably to what you are hearing, feel poorly understood, or want to discourage the speaker from going on much longer, try gazing at a spot between your partner's eyes or eyebrows. The other person will not perceive that you have broken eye contact, but will feel a vague discomfort that they are not communicating with you as effectively as they could.

? WHAT IF?

What if the person you are speaking with will not break eye contact? What options do you have?

Blinking is also a form of breaking eye contact, in that it can be distracting and take your partner's mind off the conversation. When you don't blink, or when you blink only occasionally, you convey confidence.

Eyes as Guides

People will follow your eyes. When you are distracted in a conversation and look elsewhere, your partner will often look there, too. That is because people watch your eyes for guidance, particularly when they are in an unfamiliar setting, as a patient is in a clinic or a hospital.

Use this information to your advantage to help guide clients, calling their attention to paperwork, charts, visual aids, and directions. The more the patient follows your eyes, the more they feel in need of guidance.

Eye Contact When Speaking with Two or More People

Have you ever sat in an audience and felt that the speaker was speaking directly to you? If so, the speaker was skilled in a particular technique for connecting with an audience. As they speak, good speakers will make eye contact with specific individuals in the audience, for only three seconds each. The speaker's eye contact sweeps from one audience member to another and occasionally glances away from the audience altogether, as if to give the audience the same break in eye contact you would give in a one-on-one conversation.

Because that speaker made eye contact *specifically with you*, even if it was for only 3 seconds, you retain that connection long after she has moved her gaze to another person. When you are speaking to a group, even if it is only two other people, you can use this technique to keep connected with the people and actively involved in the conversation, even when you are listening instead of speaking.

Skillful speakers can even quell a distraction in the audience using eye contact only. If a person in the audience is talking to a neighbor, the speaker can break the behavior by gazing at the person. The longer the gaze, the more uncomfortable the person causing the distraction becomes. In other words, you can command respect simply by making eye contact with someone and not breaking the gaze until you get the response or behavior you seek. This tactic gives you the control and commands the attention of the audience.

Smile

In terms of body language, nothing matters more than your smile. From Texas to Timbuktu, people smile and respond positively to people who smile at them. Babies respond to smiles, and they soon learn that they can elicit smiles from others. Strangers smile at each other. Smiling is one of the simplest ways to elicit a positive response.

As we observed earlier, people can tell when a smile is insincere. There are many ways to smile, and each has its own effect. Smiles can indicate embarrassment, nervousness, confidence, confusion, and surprise. Cultivate your genuine smile. It will light up your face and bring good-will back to you.

Genuine smiles trigger endorphins, chemicals in your brain that make you feel good (Figure 9-9). If you don't smile often, you are depriving yourself of many pleasurable feelings and positive interactions. If you smile easily, you can magnify the positive effects of a genuine smile by bringing it slowly to your face, which deepens its effect and creates deeper feelings of trust and attractiveness.

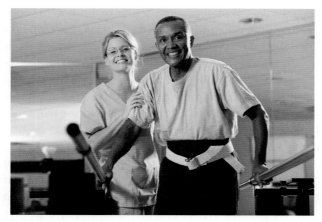

FIGURE 9-9 A smiling physical therapist assistant works with a pleased patient (Copyright © istock.com).

TABLE 9-1
Gestures and Their Meaning

Gesture	Meaning
Steepling (palms slightly apart, fingers spread and touching, making a "steeple" and pointing it at your partner)	Confidence, certainty
Pursed lips	Disengagement
Open hands, palms up	Wanting something
Open hands, palms up	Open, candid
Hands on table, palms down, fingers splayed	I've made up my mind
Chopping gesture with one hand	Emphasis
One small nod	Connected
Head tilt	Interest
Wide stance, big gestures	Power

A smile is the quickest, least expensive way to immediately improve your appearance.

Gestures, Posture, and Body Movements

Gestures, unlike facial expressions, can be culturally specific. For example, a circle formed by the thumb and forefinger can mean "everything is all right" in the United States, but in Italy it means "you are a zero." Be careful with your gestures.

Gestures

Despite distinct cultural influences, gestures can be just as subconscious and revealing as facial expressions. For instance, if someone doesn't trust or believe you, they will usually avert their gaze and often scratch their chin or ear. Boredom is often indicated by a tilted head and eyes that glaze over or lose focus, and both lying and irritation can be revealed by excessive blinking, a hard stare, or touching the face. Table 9-1 lists several common gestures and their meanings.

The language of the body is the key that can unlock the soul.

—Konstantin Stanislavsky

Actors work hard to use the subtleties of gestures to convey meaning and interior states of mind, even without speaking. However, in real life, gestures can be unreliable or hard to read compared to facial expressions, so it is best to take them only as indications and search for confirmation elsewhere. You will want to see three or four gestures, facial expressions, and postures before you conclude that a person is bored, interested, cooperative, persuaded or in any other mental state.

Posture and Body Movements

Dance and ballet are art forms devoted to communicating meaning through body movements, but we all use our bodies to convey meaning. Waving, slouching, slumping, jumping, pointing, and clapping are examples of posture and body movements that have clear meaning to most people. Indeed, we clap to express approval, slouch to indicate tiredness, and wave to greet friends.

The body never lies.

—Martha Graham

As with gestures, some postures and body movements are easily understood, while others are more subtle, unreliable, and subject to misinterpretation. As a health care professional, your goal is to make as full use as possible of all the elements of interpersonal communication to send and receive clear messages. For example, leaning forward can show you are interested and receptive. Walking briskly conveys energy, purpose, and efficiency. Standing tall and making few movements can indicate attentiveness and respect for others. Crossing your legs suggests informality and may lead others to communicate more easily.

Posture, whether seated or standing, can be open or closed. When we cover our neck, chest, or stomach, we seem to be protecting ourselves and projecting a sense of vulnerability; these are said to be closed stances. When people keep their neck on their chest or cross their arms, they convey reserve, unfriendliness, and anxiety. Patients often present a closed stance because they are unfamiliar with the setting or are worried about their health. People experiencing pain often assume a closed body position as well.

On the other hand, an open stance projects confidence and openness. When we bare our throat, take a wide stance, and open our arms to gesture, we convey friendliness, confidence, warmth, openness, trust, and safety. As a health care professional, you will want to deliberately select an open stance as much as possible to convey the kind of welcoming messages that most patients hope to receive.

Two body movements are particularly powerful. When you cross your arms, you may simply be chilly, but most people will think that you are protective, reserved, and closed to communication. Therefore, it is best not to cross your arms at all when you are interacting with someone in a health care facility. Conversely, when you present open hands, you are conveying trust and honesty. You are not hiding anything. You are as open as you can be.

Personal Space

All of us have experienced being in a crowded elevator. Everyone is uncomfortable, and nobody talks. Everyone's personal space has been encroached upon, and everyone looks down or up, to avoid making eye contact with their neighbors. Everyone feels relieved when the door opens and a few passengers step out. It is as if we all have the same magnetic charge, and we repel one another to the maximum degree possible. Personal space, therefore, is a big factor in the body language of interpersonal communication.

Researchers have identified four levels of personal space, and these definitions vary from culture to culture, making it impossible to define just how much distance between any two people is appropriate. People in urban areas who are accustomed to busy sidewalks and subway cars can tolerate less personal space than those in rural areas. More formal cultures like those in England and Germany demand more

FIGURE 9-10 A young massage therapist learns how to administer treatment while respecting a patient's personal space (Copyright © istock.com).

personal space than more informal cultures like those encountered in Italy, Greece, or Turkey.

The most intimate personal space is reserved for loved ones, family members, and close friends. As a general rule regarding personal space, you can get within 2 feet of a friend without causing discomfort. A wider space, the social space, is more appropriate for strangers, where the work of getting to know one another has not yet happened. Finally, the public space allows for the most room and is assigned to speakers, teachers, or facilitators. For most people, following these rules is easy. As a health care professional, your role is to follow these guidelines when interacting with clients and co-workers. As human beings, we seek closeness, but only after much of the other work of building relationships has been achieved (Figure 9-10).

? WHAT IF?

What if you have to invade a patient's personal space? What measures can you take to reduce the discomfort the patient may feel?

Mirroring

When two people really "click," they tend to imitate each other's gestures, body movements, and facial expressions—even their breathing patterns. Sometimes called *blending*, mirroring is not mimicking every movement or expression your partner makes, but taking a clue from their communication style to bring yours into accordance with theirs, to build rapport. To do this, you have to be observant and intuitive. Observe your partner's communication style, particularly when you are meeting someone for the first time and want to connect with the person. This is how you practice empathy, particularly with patients. When you are in sync with their tone, gestures, and expressions, your patients will feel that you understand them better, and you will.

People will not cooperate with others who *seem to be* against them. Their perception may be totally wrong, but if people don't perceive some rapport with another person, they resist. This is an important insight for the way you treat patients. Patients are looking for acceptance and comfort in an unfamiliar setting, and feel anxious and vulnerable. If you can successfully mirror a patient's body language, you will receive the patient's grateful cooperation.

Adjust your pace and volume to match the other person's. Face him or her directly and point your arms, hands, and feet in that direction. Celebrate common interests by smiling. Use your listening skills to learn more about the person, and ask good questions. While you listen, observe. Take in the most holistic view of the person and their body language as possible. Mirroring helps you understand and empathize with other people better.

Volume, Pace, and Dynamics of Speech Patterns

Body language is not about the *words* of speech, yet it does control the dynamics of speech. How loud are you? How fast do you talk? What are your speech patterns? These are all parts of your body language that influence the impact and even meaning of the words you speak.

JOURNALING 9-6

Devote a journal entry to your style of speech. Are you fast or slow, soft or loud? Do you have an accent? If you called a friend on the phone, would they recognize your voice? Why?

For example, your tone can be conveyed to a small extent by the words you choose, but comes across mostly in the sound of your voice itself. You can tell instantly whether a person is disappointed, elated, angry, sarcastic, apologetic, or humorous, based on his or her tone. As a health professional, you can learn to adjust your tone to convey warmth and empathy.

CASE STUDY 9-3
Reaching Out with a Little Body Language

Ingrid Kolsen was smart as a whip. As a Swedish-American she spoke English and Swedish fluently. She went to school at Oberlin College and majored in physics. Eventually, she decided she wanted to become a health professional, so she went back to school to study radiology. She liked the idea of working in a hospital, with all the people, teams, technologies, collaborations, and social opportunities.

She took her studies very seriously and became an expert at positioning and counseling patients. She passed her ARRT certification right away and got a job at the orthopedic department of a large hospital in Minneapolis. After she had been there a few months, she began studying for advanced certification in bone density.

There was one thing she hadn't counted on, though. Over time, she began to feel a little isolated. She was very busy and her days were full of interaction, but the activity was all work-related. She was determined to make more friends at work.

Ingrid started smiling more to strangers and making more eye contact with people in the cafeteria. Her efforts paid off quickly. Someone she met in the lunch line asked if he could sit with her. His name was Rick and he was a dermatology resident. He introduced her to some of his friends, and Ingrid was surprised and pleased that such a small initiative on her part could have been so productive.

One day, Ingrid ate lunch with a radiation oncologist named Teri. Ingrid was really interested in oncology. She had always focused on orthopedics and looked for advancement in that field. Listening to Teri talk about longer and more intensive patient interaction, however, made Ingrid realize that she should keep her options open.

"Teri—I mean Dr. Caralin—is there any way I could get a tour of your center?"

"Sure, Ms. Kolsen," she joked. "I'll show you what we do, you can see our equipment. I'll introduce you to some of the other radiation therapy technicians."

Ingrid had already completed her bone density certification, but now she started to look into certification for radiation therapy. It would take a year, but she thought it would be right for her. She learned that she could eventually become a dosimetrist, and even a medical physicist. What great connections she had made, she thought, smiling to herself as she walked down the corridor.

QUESTIONS FOR THOUGHT AND REFLECTION

1. How did Ingrid use body language to make new friends?
2. What do you think about using body language deliberately to achieve your personal goals?
3. Why do you think Rick and Teri found it easy to approach Ingrid?
4. In your opinion, what is more important to advancing your career, education or contacts?

Down a Dark Road

Andy Samuels was a speech therapy intern at Sterling Medical Center where he hoped to obtain a full-time position when he completed his master's degree. He had done research as part of his thesis, and he had worked with members of the hospital's otolaryngology department to plan the research and analyze the data. He had some interesting results, so with the help of one of the otolaryngologists, he arranged to present his material at an all-hospital grand rounds, held each month and attended by many physicians and other senior health professionals and administrators at the medical center.

He told his friends in speech pathology that he had developed some techniques for helping rehabilitate people who had aphasia as a result of stroke. The medical center was a regional center in stroke care and rehabilitation, and these techniques could be useful to the center's treatments and strategies.

Andy was nervous on the afternoon of the grand rounds, but he felt he was prepared. He had practiced his presentation many times. Just before taking the stage, Dr. Laurence Ponte, head of the otolaryngology service, stopped by to wish him good luck. He was the author of the leading textbook on throat cancer and an expert in treating laryngeal cancer, having pioneered some of the operations that are standard today. Andy was thrilled to meet Dr. Ponte on his big day.

The unexpected meeting made Andy a little more nervous, but it also magnified the importance of the day to him. He was sure of himself, his presentation style, and the value of his research. He strode onto the stage and immediately located Dr. Ponte in the second row. Mindful of his body language, Andy smiled at the audience and stood tall.

He looked up at the screen, clicked to the first slide, and began talking.

Although he consciously made eye contact with audience members throughout the auditorium, Andy constantly found himself glancing back at Dr. Ponte. As the minutes tolled by, he found himself focusing even more on Dr. Ponte, because something strange was going on. Sometimes when he glanced at Dr. Ponte, the doctor would nod and smile and nudge his seatmates approvingly. Other times, Dr. Ponte bore a frown, crossed his arms, and gazed up at the ceiling. The doctor's body language went back and forth and Andy couldn't figure it out. The doctor's approval and disapproval didn't seem to coincide with any particular highlight in his presentation.

The audience, including Dr. Ponte, applauded his presentation. There were a few questions, and Andy noticed that Dr. Ponte left while he was answering them. Andy just didn't know what to make of it, and he went home feeling strangely disconcerted about how everything went.

Meanwhile, Dr. Ponte had gone back to his office for a meeting with the group of residents who had also been at the grand rounds. "Did you see him moving back and forth across that stage?" he asked the residents with a roar. "I introduced myself before his presentation and told him I would be in the audience. I could see that made him nervous, so I decided to have a little fun with him. Every time he took a step to his right, I nodded and smiled and gave him all kinds of positive listening cues. But if he moved to his left, I acted bored, like he was wasting my time. Pretty soon, I had that guy practically dancing across that stage. By the time it was over, he couldn't have moved farther to his right if he wanted to!"

QUESTIONS FOR THOUGHT AND REFLECTION

1. Were you puzzled, like Andy Samuels, about what was going on with Dr. Ponte?
2. Do you think Andy could have been conditioned to move across the stage, just based on Dr. Ponte's body language? Why or why not?
3. What was Dr. Ponte's motivation for doing what he did? How did it affect Andy?
4. What do you think about using body language to manipulate people?

⭐ EXPERIENTIAL EXERCISES

1. List emotional messages that can be conveyed by the eyes alone.
2. When you are speaking with a friend, lean in to see if your friend does too. Do you notice any subsequent changes in the tone of the conversation?
3. How long can you maintain eye contact with a friend before you feel uncomfortable?
4. Find a quiet place in a hospital lobby or other public place and observe the body language of the people you see. How much meaning can you make out? What can you tell about the people just from their appearance and body language? Even if you can't make out the words, can you determine the emotional content of conversations you observe?
5. Practice smiling in a mirror. To see your real, genuine smile, reflect on a positive memory from your past. Compare that smile to your polite or professional smile. Can you tell the difference? Try other smiles—a grin; a smile accompanied by raising one of your eyebrows; a slow smile. Cover your mouth to see how your eyes contribute to a real smile and don't contribute to a fake one. Make sure you know what others see when they see you smile.
6. Record your voice. Notice its pitch, richness, and tone. Can you adjust your voice to get other tonal effects? Record yourself and see.

🔄 CROSS CURRENTS WITH OTHER SOFT SKILLS

SHOWING EMPATHY, SENSITIVITY, AND CARING: It is said that eye contact cuts the distance between you and another person in half. It is virtually impossible to connect with others in a deep sense without eye contact. (pp. 218-222)

DRESSING FOR SUCCESS: Your appearance is part of your body language. (pp. 178-183)

DISPLAYING GOOD GROOMING, PERSONAL HYGIENE, AND CLEANLINESS: Good smells and clean hair are positive body language; bad smells and dirty hair are negative body language. (pp. 183-188)

Bibliography

Beckman HB, Frankel RM. The effect of physician behavior on the collection of data. *Ann Intern Med* 101(5): 692-696,1984.

CAREER BUILDING SKILLS

CHAPTER 10

Planning for Career Success

- Set goals and make their achievement a reality.
- Explain the role of rules in the workplace and the effects they can have.
- Understand your responsibilities under HIPAA.
- Create quality documentation that serves the patient indefinitely.
- Explain the difference between gross and net income and the types of deductions that affect gross income.
- Plan for your retirement and describe the most common pension plans.
- Establish a personal budget.
- Describe ways to build a good credit record and explain how your credit record is used.
- Discuss differences in types of student loans.
- Explain the process for making a loan decision.
- Describe smart strategies for buying a car.
- Detail a solid plan for getting out of debt.

Setting Goals and Planning Actions

Goals are dreams with deadlines.

—Napoleon Hill

LEARNING OBJECTIVE 1: SETTING GOALS AND PLANNING ACTIONS

- Set precise, achievable, written goals.
- Map out action items to progress toward goals.
- Set reasonable deadlines for goals and action items.
- Identify obstacles.
- Intensely visualize the achievement of your goals.
- Schedule time to accomplish action steps toward goals.
- Review goals regularly.

Has anyone ever asked you "What do you want out of life?" Have you ever asked yourself that? Stop and think about how it would make you feel if someone you respect asked you that question.

Now think about this: How does the question, coming from someone important to you, make you feel? Does the question scare you to death? Would you try to change the subject? Or is the question exhilarating? Does it send you off into a breathless conversation?

Whether you are planning your work day or whether you are planning your life, setting goals for your career and then choosing and executing the specific actions that go with them will put you on the fast track to success.

Why Goal-Setting Is Important

Imagine playing a game of basketball without a basket. Your team would be missing its goal. As part of a health care team, your goal is to improve the health of the patient. Whether you are directly providing care or whether you provide support to help someone else provide direct care, you are part of a team aiming toward the same goal. When you don't have a goal, you are aimless because there is no target. Goal-setting in the workplace is important to accomplishing the overall mission of the health care team you work with. If you are doing something unrelated to the mission of the team, you are pulling the team down.

Goals are also important in the context of your life beyond work as well. If you can achieve goals that are related to your health, finances, personal growth, family, social life, and spiritual life, they will also enhance the success of your career goals. When you lack goals, you will not achieve much because you do not have a direction or a destination to pursue.

> *If you don't know where you're going,*
> *any road will get you there.*
>
> —George Harrison

Goals give you purpose; they get work done and they clarify your values and give you a sense of meaning.

Levels of Goals

Goals can be set at many different levels. All of your daily goals should support your long-term aspirations. If you had a long-term goal, for instance, of getting promoted at work, you would want some short-term goals to get you there. These might include

obtaining a specialty certification, contributing to problem-solving at work, understanding your supervisor's challenges, or developing a broader skill set. In this way, your daily short-term goals—such as helping with the day-to-day operations while studying for certification at night—contribute not only to your ultimate professional goal, but your health care team's mission as well.

A complete hierarchy of your goal system, therefore, includes daily, short-term, and long-term goals that are all internally consistent and support one another (Figure 10-1).

How to Set Goals

At work, many of your goals are set for you. Let's say you are a dental assistant and you are assigned to rearrange and organize the dental lab. As you accept this goal, it is important to know why you are doing this. In your mind, establish what rearranging the dental lab does for the dental practice. Does it make things more efficient? Does it create more space for the dentist to do other lab work? Does it ultimately improve patient care? The first step in setting any goal is to look imaginatively at your motivation. What do you want? What needs to be done that will improve your work or your life?

JOURNALING 10-1

Consider a time when you accomplished a goal. What was the goal, and how did you achieve it? Did you write it down or keep it in your head? When you achieved it, how did it make you feel?

FIGURE 10-1 Goal levels.

Visualizing and Feeling the Outcome

Once you have settled on a goal, your chances of achieving it are vastly improved by how vividly you can "see and feel" the result. If you can imagine reaching your goal, you have taken the first step toward fully realizing it. You will know where you want to go and get some ideas about how to get there.

Let's say you are a health information technologist in charge of assisting a surgical practice's move to paperless record keeping. You currently work with more than 4000 patient records, which are taking up a massive amount of cabinet space. First, visualize the entire cabinet space cleared and the cabinets removed. Then, you could feel how freeing it is to have more space and to have the ability to access records at the touch of a finger. Once you feel how great it is to have a paperless office, you will be ready to tackle the next step to accomplish this task. If the outcome feels positive and looks achievable, the steps will follow with greater ease.

JOURNALING 10-2

Think about your career as a health professional. Record what inspired you to pursue this goal. What action steps did you take to pursue your goal? Would you have done anything differently in the way you went about achieving this goal? What has been easier, and what has been more difficult? If you had planned differently or visualized more vividly, could any of the more difficult aspects been made easier?

Writing the Goal and the Action Steps

Once you have a positive and specific goal in mind, it is important that you write it down. Motivational speaker Zig Ziglar said that people should strive to be a "meaningful specific" rather than a "wandering generality." Writing down goals encourages you to state them with great specificity and detail.

Enhance this visualization by writing out what the overall goal looks like once accomplished in the present tense. "I weigh 130 pounds." Imagine how fantastic this will be for you, how great you will look, or how much more energy you will have.

Avoid making negative goals. For example, wanting to lose 20 pounds is a negative goal. Instead, state it positively: "My goal is to weigh 130 pounds." As you execute a plan, you move toward a positive goal instead of away from something that is negative.

When you write down a goal positively and in detail, you take the first step toward accomplishing the goal.

Obstacles

Obstacles are those frightful things you see when you take your eyes off your goal.

—Henry Ford

Once you have set your goal and visualized it in all the detail you can muster, look at the goal achievement process analytically. Realistically, are there obstacles to overcome?

Of course there are. The question is, what are they? This is an exercise in anticipation, knowing what to expect. Be honest with yourself. You must plan to overcome every obstacle, or obstacles will derail your goals.

Successful people aren't people without problems. They are people who deal with their problems successfully.

—Dr. Scott Peck

Next Actions

Achieving goals is a matter of knowing what to do next. Let's go back to your goal of earning a promotion. You have already established some intermediate goals to make your long-term goal more attainable (Figure 10-2). Let's say you want to obtain a specialty certification as well as increase your skills set and understand your supervisor's challenges better. To get started on the advanced certification, buy a review book or research the requirements. There might be additional preparation guidelines and resources on the Web site. Sign up for a review course or talk to a colleague who has already achieved the certification.

Next, schedule these activities. Let's say you want to talk to Mary Alice about her experience in getting the certification because you want to find out how she prepared for the exam. You want to know what a difference it has made in her career. Schedule lunch with Mary Alice on Tuesday. Do the same with all the actions you have selected to help you achieve your goal.

Focus

Realistically, people can work on accomplishing only 10 to 12 goals at a time. Write down 10 goals you are currently working on. Have you vividly imagined

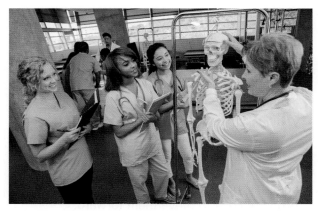

FIGURE 10-2 In an effort to reach the overall goal of becoming a medical professional, students must focus on accomplishing intermediate goals such as learning course material and passing tests. (Copyright © istock.com).

achieving them? Have you written them down in present tense in a positive, specific way? Have you determined what the obstacles are and how you will circumvent them? What about the action steps? Have you identified them and scheduled them into your life?

Review

As a final phase, you must review your goals at regular intervals to sustain them. Planning is not a one-time event; it is an ongoing process.

Every week, maybe on a Sunday night, review your current top 10 goals. Are they still what you want? Are you making progress? Do you see a clear path of achievement through the next actions you have selected? Are the next actions on your calendar for the coming week?

Finally, schedule periodic reviews that are more intensive than usual. People change over time, especially those whose lives are progressing because they are achieving their goals. Over time, some of your goals will lose their appeal as others emerge. Box 10-1 lists tips for achieving a goal.

Your Goal Binder

The key to goal achievement is to make it a persistent, methodical pursuit. The smartest way to stay on track in pursuing your goals is to keep a written record of where you've been, what you've done, and what you want to do next. Studies show that only 3% of Americans have written goals. So, logging your goals and the steps you will take to achieve them will put you far ahead of the game. The goal binder described in Box 10-2 outlines a system for keeping on track.

Only unimaginative people never raise their sights. Successful people are always imagining wonderful new futures. If you are successful, that means you are achieving your goals, like completing your health care education and getting a new job and career. As you grow, your goals will get more daring and exciting. Really, there is no limit to what you can become.

The only thing that has to be finished by next Tuesday is next Monday.

—Jennifer Yane

BOX 10-2

Creating and Using Your Goal Binder

- Brainstorm a list of 100 goals you would like to achieve in your life. Generate the list as fast as you can.
- Divide a three-ring binder into the following sections:
  - Financial goals
  - Personal development and enrichment goals (e.g., education, skill acquisition)
  - Career goals
  - Social and family goals
  - Personal health, wellness, and physical fitness goals
  - Spiritual goals
- Write each of the 100 goals you developed on a separate piece of paper and insert them into the appropriate section of the binder.
- Subdivide each goal into short-term goals you will have to achieve to make the long-term goal a reality.
- Write a "next action" for each short-term or long-term goal.
- Pick 10 goals to achieve first.
- Schedule the "next action" steps for these goals. As soon as you complete one "next action," create and schedule the next one until you finally achieve the goal. Some goals might require hundreds of next actions.
- Review your goal binder regularly.
- Once a week, review the goals you are currently working on to make sure you are taking actions to move them forward.
- As you achieve each goal, replace it with another, so you are always working on 10 goals at a time.
- Every 3 months, review your entire goal binder, being especially open to opportunities that may have arisen for you to speed up a goal that was in the background.
- Schedule an annual goal-setting session, perhaps during a vacation when you are relaxed and have the time. Reevaluate all your goals, deleting those that you no longer want to work on, and add new goals that have become important to you.

CASE STUDY 10-1
Looking for a Lift

Joe started out as a firefighter and eventually became certified as an EMT. When he was 43, he retired from the St. Louis Fire Department and took a full-time job as an EMT with the Green Ambulance Service. He did that for a few years until he was injured and was out for almost 6 months on short-term disability, causing Joe to become unmotivated personally and professionally.

One day, he attended a motivational workshop because his sister bought him a pass for his birthday. To his surprise, Joe found the speaker very motivating. The speaker said that anybody could live a fulfilling, challenging life and that goal-setting and achievement was the way to get it. Joe went home and wrote down his positive and specific goals—everything he could think of that he wanted. He

came up with 85 goals spread across six dimensions of his life. He wrote each goal on a 3 x 5 card and put them in a recipe box.

Joe created a to-do list. It was a modest list that allowed for all the unexpected calls he would get in the ambulance service. One of the goals for the day was to get all his work done, and he made a separate list for that. Another goal involved gaining paramedic certification. He had done some work toward his intermediate EMS certification, but he never sustained his effort.

Joe liked this goal achievement methodology. He latched onto it, and it started to pay dividends. Pursuing goals gave him direction and energy. Even his supervisor noticed his sudden enthusiasm for his work.

Several months later, Joe had his paramedic certification. Why not pursue a leadership role? Joe knew he could be the kind of leader the other EMTs could look up to, so he brainstormed a list of new goals and what he needed to do to achieve them. "There is nothing I can't do," he thought to himself.

QUESTIONS FOR THOUGHT AND REFLECTION

1. What was missing from Joe's life?

2. If Joe was satisfied with his work as an EMT, is there anything wrong with that?

3. What methodology did Joe pursue in reaching his goals?

4. What gave Joe enthusiasm and confidence?

Down a Dark Road

Ivana stopped attending her career college where she enrolled to become a medical assistant. Her counselor called her many times and tried to help her with her problems, but she stopped taking the calls just before the phone company canceled her service.

Ivana had lots of problems. First of all, she was working nights at a nursing home to cover her living expenses and pay for school. It was too much for her, and she slept through her first class more than once. She had also hoped that the job would help improve her English, since Russian was her native language. Unfortunately, there were few opportunities for interactions with the sleeping patients or the busy staff. Finally, she hoped her 1990 Oldsmobile would last a little longer, but it didn't, making it hard for her to get to work and impossible for her to get to school.

Soon, her difficulties with English caused her to lose her job at the nursing home. Some family members complained they could not understand Ivana, and the supervisor let her go. She did not know what to do.

QUESTIONS FOR THOUGHT AND REFLECTION

1. Was it realistic for Ivana to think she could improve her English by working nights at the nursing home? Was it realistic for her to work all night and go to school in the daytime?

2. What should Ivana do now?

 EXPERIENTIAL EXERCISES

1. Watch the movie *Groundhog Day*. Determine how the main character played by Bill Murray manages to improve his daily life through goal-setting.

2. Create a personal Goal Binder.

3. Interview your parents or other respected people about their goal-setting behavior.

4. Pick a goal to work on this week.

CROSS CURRENTS WITH OTHER SOFT SKILLS

MANAGING YOUR TIME AND ORGANIZING YOUR LIFE: Planning goals and actions provides meaning and structure to your time and your life. (pp. 11-18)

THINKING CRITICALLY: Planning is an excellent application of critical thinking. (pp. 320-325)

COMMITTING TO YOUR PROFESSION: This should be reflected as a major element of your goal setting. (pp. 342-348)

Following Rules and Regulations

It's not wise to violate rules until you know how to observe them.

—T. S. Eliot

LEARNING OBJECTIVE 2: FOLLOWING RULES AND REGULATIONS

- Characterize the need for special rules in health care.
- Know the difference between written and unwritten rules.
- Understand why people want rules and want to know what they are.
- Suggest a positive attitude toward rules.
- Understand what it takes to know when an exception to a rule is needed.
- Explain "fit."

Imagine it's your first day of work in a hospital's postsurgical unit. You walk in on time, feeling nervous, but a little excited too. At first, you just stand and watch the staff running around. Occasionally, someone rushes into a patient's room, but others just stand looking around. No one is talking to you, and you're not sure who's in charge. Eventually, you see one guy slip behind the desk at the nurses' station, so you walk up and introduce yourself.

"Hi, I'm Carly," you say. "What can I do to help?"

He shrugs and says, "I have no idea."

You turn and ask someone else, and this time the only response you get is, "How should I know? Figure it out for yourself! That's what I do every single day."

People want to know what the rules are. New employees are especially eager to learn the rules, both written and unwritten, so they fit in and have a sense of knowing what they are doing and how best to do it. Most importantly, rules in health care facilities help patients get the most efficient care and understand how things will work.

A good set of rules should strike a balance between a rigid environment and complete chaos. Workplaces that are too strict lack creativity and individual initiative. Workplaces without rules feel chaotic and anxiety-provoking.

Rules in Health Care

Health care is among the most highly regulated of all industries. Rules govern how health care is delivered, how patients and employees are treated, and how health care is paid for. Much of your education has involved learning the rules associated with your particular health care profession, whether they have been universal precautions, Medicare forms, sterilization techniques, or handling medications.

Best Practices

In fact, best clinical practices in your professions usually involve rules that have been validated by research and effective results. The scientific method is the ultimate rule set in the delivery of clinical health care, generating rules of research, statistical analysis of data, and good practice. These rules are constantly evolving, and that evolution is reported in the journals that support your profession. When it comes to delivering the highest quality health care in your profession, your learning and search for new best practices is never over.

Policies and Procedures

Every health care facility has some form of a policy manual or its virtual equivalent. These detailed rule books cover everything that is important in the smooth, correct, and legal operation of the facility. Large health care organizations likely have an institutional approach to policies and procedures, with established committees and even employees dedicated to creating policies and procedures, publicizing them, and developing the training solutions necessary to implement them.

The implementation of laws and regulations requires policies and training. New employees must be trained in all types of rules, ranging from procedures to safety and ethics issues. New regulations demand site-wide training, and refresher training is always needed. Policies and procedures are constantly being evaluated and improved to strengthen best practices and better ways of achieving goals. These policies provide answers to questions like who gets seen first in the emergency room. How can the identity of new babies be made certain? What obligations are satisfied by the patient discharge process? How can infectious diseases be better controlled? What dental materials should be used? What happens when a patient misses an appointment? For health care professionals, following the rules of policies is a huge and continuous undertaking (Figure 10-3).

Types of Rules

A rule is simply a guideline to follow. They can be written or unwritten and still carry the same force for

FIGURE 10-3 Lab workers follow strict safety and sanitation procedures to ensure accurate results (Copyright © istock. com).

compliance. Some rules are mandatory: "No smoking." Others are not as compelling: "Please use the revolving doors on windy days." Rules also vary in the ways they are communicated.

Written Rules

Written rules take time to work out, often by committees or experts, either inside or outside the facility. Usually, written rules that come from outside have been adopted from organizations that set standards, such as Universal Precautions from the Centers for Disease Control and Prevention or evacuation instructions from the local fire marshall.

Internal written rules are often born of hard lessons learned. How is adequate staffing to be ensured, and how does that affect schedules, holidays, and other expectations? What parking regulations balance convenience with handling the flow of traffic and access to the facility? Is there a need for a written dress code to prevent inappropriate dress? Every employee must be sensitive to the need for new written rules when procedures change, operations are inefficient, or behavior expectations need to be clarified.

Signs

People are likely to follow directions on signs. People want to know what to do, and they are often eager to see a sign that answers, clearly and concisely, basic questions about what to do.

WHAT IF?

What if you went somewhere and felt frustrated that there was no sign to explain what to do? What sign would you want posted?

The most ineffective signs are those that bark an order with no rationale: "Children Not Allowed." Signs are much more likely to gain compliance when they offer details or reasons and make an effort to anticipate concerns: "Children Under 16 Not Allowed Because No Lifeguard on Duty."

Like most written rules, signs appear when it seems necessary to make rules clear to everyone, even those that appeal to common sense, especially when safety is an issue. Signs are so important to safety that international signs have been developed to identify exits, prohibit smoking, and warn of wet floors. Other signs may be unique to a particular facility, governing where lab specimens are to be submitted, how payments are handled, and where to check in. The need for signs, to warn or explain, should be constantly evaluated and improved.

Unwritten Rules

Unwritten rules are interesting because they may carry the force of written rules, but you have to figure out what they are. You do this by observing, asking, and experimenting.

Every workplace has a culture, and the culture is made up of mostly unwritten rules that address such issues as how formal or informal the workplace is, the amount of socialization, the hierarchy and how familiar co-workers are with each other. Are you being micromanaged, or are you expected to take the initiative? New employees have to work hard to gain an understanding of the culture and its unwritten rules.

JOURNALING 10-3

How would you describe the culture at work? List the unwritten rules that govern your culture.

Some of the most powerful unwritten rules are optional (Box 10-3). Go above and beyond, for instance. Volunteer to work on a holiday, or work an extra shift in bad weather when others will have trouble getting in. Establish a useful and unique expertise, such as operating complex medical equipment or learning difficult software. Project enthusiasm. Develop your strengths. Be the best at the most difficult procedures.

BOX 10-3

Useful Unwritten Rules

- Dress well.
- Act every day as you did on the day you interviewed for the job.
- Show respect for patients.
- Don't gossip.
- Don't complain.
- Don't use coarse or profane language.
- Keep your emotions, especially anger, under control.
- Compliment co-workers if you can do so sincerely.

These are the kind of subtle rules which, if followed, will get you recognized, valued, and promoted.

How to Follow the Rules

Following rules has a lot to do with your personality and your attitude. To succeed in your health care profession, you have to be a people person and a team player, an empathetic person who plays by the rules.

Personality

Most people have no trouble showing respect for the rules and following them. Occasionally, a personality adjustment is needed. For example, a person with a rigid personality could follow the rules to a fault, relying on them even in the face of evidence that there are legitimate exceptions. Rigid people can be fearful of any deviation, thinking that they will be safe as long as they follow the rules to the letter. Good judgment demands that rules usually be followed, knowing that there will be occasions for exceptions to the rules. On the other hand, rebellious individuals go out of their way to break the rules, as if they are seeking negative attention. If your personality is extreme in either of these directions, you need to temper your behavior to avoid destructive relationships with others.

Attitude

More people run into trouble with the rules as a result of their attitude, an aspect far more under your control than your personality. Some people not only follow the rules but also think everybody else should follow them, too. It bothers them when others are noncompliant, take a liberal view of exceptions, or seem unfair. This attitude can lead to some slightly antisocial behavior, shunning the perceived rule-breakers, yelling at them, or reporting them to their supervisors. If you have a strongly compliant attitude, restrict it to governing your own behavior and try to let go of any unfairness you perceive in the way others behave.

Others feel that the rules don't apply to them. These individuals create risks for everyone else because they don't appreciate the importance of rules in maintaining smooth operations, safety, and best practices, making it hard to trust them. Unfortunately, these people are the reason that disciplinary procedures have to be developed.

A proper attitude involves a healthy respect for rules as tools to help people get along, work together in teams, perform work safely and efficiently, and deliver the highest quality of care to patients.

Exceptions to the Rules

When you decide to break a rule, you must have an excellent reason that you can readily articulate. It could be something as simple as putting someone ahead of others in a line because of a special time constraint or a more urgent need. It could be something as serious as risking an infection in order to expedite an emergency procedure. Unfortunately, there are few rules governing when to break the rules. As a new employee, you should hesitate to break any rules. As your experience and skills grow over time, you will develop the intuition and clinical judgment needed to identify legitimate exceptions to the rules.

Fit

A contributing factor to an employee's termination can be that they are a bad "fit." Fit doesn't have anything to do with your clinical skills. It has to do with your social skills and your ability to interpret and follow unwritten rules. Many individuals would find it difficult to explain when the fit isn't working. This is a very hard reality for new employees to accept. New employees often think that you should have job security if you work hard, behave, and do your job correctly. The reality is, though, that your co-workers want all of their other co-workers to be the kind of people they enjoy being with all day long. Patients want employees to provide them with a positive, friendly, and appropriate reception. The rules may be unwritten, but they mean everything.

CASE STUDY 10-2
43 Folders

Sue Yang had been a medical assistant at the pediatrics practice for more than a year, and she started to see the same serious issues crop up over and over again. There were missing immunizations. Forms for schools were frequently late, causing a last minute rush that interrupted the flow of work. Appointments were missed or, in some cases, never even scheduled. All of these problems, it seemed to Sue had one thing in common: poor anticipation and follow-up.

Sue discussed her concerns with the managing partner, Dr. Richardson. She agreed with Sue, but she didn't know what to do. "I tell you what, Sue. You're very efficient and observant. I would really appreciate it if you developed some possible solutions."

Sue felt that this assignment could be a good opportunity, but soon realized that it was a difficult assignment. She could come up with ideas for specific problems, but she soon realized that she didn't know how to implement her ideas.

One evening, Sue came across a website called 43 Folders for the 31 days of the month and the 12 months of the year. Sue felt this could be a great solution. Over the weekend, Sue collected and labeled 43 folders. On Monday, she put the folders in her personal file cabinet and started using the system. When a doctor ordered a lab test, she put a note in the folder for the day that the results were due. If a booster shot was needed for a baby, she put a note in the file for the month it should take place. By the end of the week, her files were filling up. She began each day by reviewing that day's file and scheduling its tasks. Then, she scheduled any follow-up appointments and addressed any unfinished tasks. At the end of the day, she moved that day's file to the back, so the next day would be in front when she arrived in the morning.

Sue also added files for the next few years for more long-term reminders. She could see that the August file was filling up with school-related activities, forms, and requirements. Sue made an appointment with Dr. Richardson to share her solution.

Sue explained her version of the 43 folders system. Dr. Richardson loved the idea. "It's a very simple idea, but that's what makes it so brilliant," she said.

Over the next few weeks, Sue continued to pilot the solution she had proposed. She wrote a short manual describing the system and how to use it. She identified all the kinds of documents that would go into the 43 files. She designed a simple form that could be used to record a task or reminder. Finally, Dr. Richardson asked Sue to make a presentation to the staff explaining the system, provide any needed training, and implement it.

By the end of the month, the system was producing results. All the medical assistants were using it, and many parents were complimenting the doctors on the obvious improvements.

One day, Dr. Richardson invited Sue into her office. "Sue, we're going to make you the training supervisor for all the new medical assistants. We've had quite a few recently, and we trust you to ensure that all the rules and procedures are communicated and followed. There's a promotion and a raise involved."

Sue beamed with the knowledge that she had earned her employer's trust. "I will do a good job, Dr. Richardson."

"Sue," laughed Dr. Richardson, you already have!"

QUESTIONS FOR THOUGHT AND REFLECTION

1. Was it Sue's job to solve the poor follow-up problems?
2. Why did Sue try out the idea herself before proposing it to Dr. Richardson?
3. What improvements do you think occurred as a result of the new system?
4. Why did Sue get promoted?

Down a Dark Road

Linda was a bright student who was a natural leader in class, easy to get along with, and helpful to others. Linda was always dressed appropriately in clean, pressed scrubs. On weekends, she loved to escape on her Harley and participate in motorcycle rides for charity. In class, Linda was often the first to contribute with an answer, but her instructor would often rephrase what she had said in a different way. Linda was street-smart, a little tough. It was part of her personality and it was endearing, but she laid it on thick once in a while. For instance, her instructor was always correcting her when she said "tools" instead of instruments to refer to the doctor's set-ups. Near the completion of her program, the corrections had almost become a class joke, but the instructor still tried to teach her the correct use of the language in the workplace.

Linda's first day on the job in Dr. Short's office was hectic and busy, but she felt prepared. She was ready with a smile for everyone. She was exhausted but pleased with herself at the end of the day.

On her third day, Dr. Short pulled her aside. "Linda, your technical skills today were impressive. I love your attitude with the patients, and the staff seems to really feel comfortable with you." Then he frowned. "One problem. My instruments are valuable pieces of equipment. They are not tools. Tools are in my garage."

As Dr. Short strode away, Linda wasn't sure what to think. Was he kidding? If not, was it really a big deal?

A few days later, Linda called out to Dr. Short, who was standing with a patient in the hallway, "What tools do you want for this, Doc? You gonna need a drill?"

Dr. Short's face colored. The patient looked a bit queasy. Linda immediately sat the patient in the chair and began to soothe her. Dr. Short returned with another assistant, and asked Linda to stock the shelves in the supply room.

Linda was devastated. She had been looking forward to assisting this procedure all day. She began stocking shelves, wondering what had happened. It was just a joke. At the end of the day, Linda approached the doctor and apologized, although she was unsure of what she was apologizing for. Dr. Short was kind, but in no uncertain language told her that until she was able to use the proper terminology with him, and with patients present, that he did not feel comfortable with her performing clinical duties.

QUESTIONS FOR THOUGHT AND REFLECTION

1. Why do you think Linda was unable to recognize her errors when speaking about the doctor's equipment?
2. Would you react the way Dr. Short did? What do you think his opinion was of Linda before she repeated her mistake? Why is her mistake so critical?
3. What can Linda do to change her speaking habits at work?
4. What would you do to handle this situation?

⭐ EXPERIENTIAL EXERCISES

1. Find out what written rules you should be aware of at work.
2. Determine how policies and procedures are maintained and updated at your place of employment.
3. Review a recent journal in your profession. Are there new "rules" for best practices being reported?
4. Make a sign needed around your home and put it on the refrigerator. Did you make it as effective as possible?

 CROSS CURRENTS WITH OTHER SOFT SKILLS

ACHIEVING HONESTY AND INTEGRITY: Following rules leads to a positive reputation. (pp. 18-25)
BUILDING TRUST: People who follow rules can be trusted to work more independently. (pp. 212-218)
CONTRIBUTING AS A MEMBER OF THE TEAM: Health care is a team activity, and teamwork requires adherence to the rules. (pp. 336-342)

Maintaining Confidentiality and Discretion

Patients are far more willing to share the intimate details of their private lives when they have confidence that their doctors will not post those details on Facebook.

—Jacob Appel

- Explain the significance of the HIPAA Act of 1996.
- State the rights that HIPAA bestows on patients.
- State your obligations as a health professional under HIPAA.
- Know what is permissible under HIPAA, so your work-related communication is not hampered.
- Understand the importance of confidentiality.

Confidentiality in medicine and health care has never been more important than it is today. Gossip is never professional, but gossip that involves confidential medical information is pure poison because it can come back to you in ways you never intended.

Confidentiality of private medical information has always been a matter of ethics and professionalism. However, with the passage of the Health Information Portability and Accountability Act (HIPAA) in 1996, private medical information is now also protected by federal law.

The Health Information Portability and Accountability Act of 1996

The HIPAA law, like all laws, can seem complicated and extremely detailed at first. However, regulations and other efforts have been made to simplify understanding so that everyone who works in the health care field can understand its requirements. Every health professional must understand the law and implement it in their daily practice. For one thing, every health facility is required to designate a privacy officer who provides training and print materials to support implementation of the law. You should know who your privacy officer is and use that person as a resource in your efforts to comply with HIPAA.

FIGURE 10-4 Health professional explaining a HIPAA form to a patient.

BOX 10-4

Patient Rights Under HIPAA

- Right to receive a copy of your facility's privacy policy
- Right to determine how they receive confidential information
- Right to restrict parts or uses of medical information except those required by law
- Right to review their own private medical information
- Right to request that errors in their private medical information be corrected
- Right to know how and to whom their private medical information was disclosed

Patient Rights Under HIPAA

You are probably already familiar with the practice of providing patients with the facility's policy on handling protected medical information. As seen in Figure 10-4, many facilities also obtain the patient's signed acknowledgement that they received the policy, to further protect the facility. Under HIPAA, patients, too, have rights with regard to this protected information. For instance, patients may elect to protect their privacy by asking that you communicate confidential information to them in a specific way, sending it to a post office box or calling a specific phone number. They can also restrict the disclosure of their private medical information, say to an estranged husband or a divorce lawyer. They can also request that parts of their medical information not be disclosed, such as mental health treatment or medication use. These patient rights regarding medical information are further summarized in Box 10-4.

When patients exercise any of their rights related to how their medical information is handled, the request should be entered prominently into the patient's chart or electronic medical information file. Always review this information for special requests whenever you access a patient's chart in order to avoid any mistakes.

 JOURNALING 10-4

Think about yourself as a patient. Write a directive that indicates how you would want your private medical information protected.

It is important for you to understand that, while your facility owns the patient's medical record, the patient is now entitled to see it. This right was not always honored before the implementation of HIPAA. There should be no question about the patient's right to see their medical information and, if it is incorrect, to have it corrected.

If medical information ever becomes the subject of a lawsuit or legal dispute, you will usually not be involved if you have protected confidential information and observed patients' rights. However, that is why it is important for you to understand and observe these rights.

Your Responsibilities Under HIPAA

Many of your responsibilities are covered in the privacy policy disclosure your facility distributes to your patients. However, the most important aspects of your responsibilities are listed in Box 10-5.

It is certainly permissible for you to check with your privacy officer if you receive a patient request affecting their protected medical information, and you are not sure what is required or permissible. Just tell the patient that you want to observe their rights and need to clarify the details of those rights for your benefit and the patient's. Common sense requests, like the opportunity to confer with a health professional privately, should always be granted immediately.

Activities Not Prohibited by HIPAA

The purpose of HIPAA is largely to put into law what was always widely practiced as a matter of medical ethics. It has also been effective, however, in stopping

BOX 10-5

Your Obligations as a Health Care Professional Under HIPAA

- Inform all patients of their privacy rights under HIPAA.
- Be able to explain the proper use of medical records.
- Protect medical records from everyone not involved in the care of the patient.
- Keep medical charts and records secure.
- Follow the privacy policies created by your facility.
- Know who your privacy officer is and complete any mandated training.

some of the past abuses of how private medical information was handled. Before 1996, it was not uncommon for insurance companies to use private and confidential medical information to deny health insurance to Americans with preexisting conditions. It was used by unscrupulous employers to deny employment. There were no penalties to punish or prevent health workers from sharing health information or gossiping about patients, especially those they may know from other areas of their lives such as church, school, or neighborhood organizations. Box 10-6 identifies common health care practices that are interpreted to be permissible by HIPAA.

This list is far from exhaustive. However, it illustrates the concept that HIPAA is not to be used to restrict the normal communication necessary to carry out high-quality health care. While reasonable precautions should be observed, the law favors the well-intentioned provision of quality care.

? WHAT IF?

What if you receive a call from a newspaper reporter asking for a condition update on a patient in your facility?

State Laws and Ambiguous Situations

In many cases, states laws are authorized to supersede the provisions of HIPAA law and its regulations. For instance, children's private medical information rights vary from state to state. Parental rights,

Common Medical Practices Not Prohibited by HIPAA

- A doctor or a nurse talks to a patient in a semiprivate hospital room, within earshot of the patient in the other bed.
- A patient is not immediately informed of her HIPAA rights in an emergency.
- First responders don't inform disaster victims of their HIPAA rights when they arrive on the scene of a public health emergency.
- A doctor talks to a pharmacist about a patient's medication within earshot of other patients.
- A medical assistant addresses a patient by name in the presence of other patients.

- Patients sign into an office and see other patients' names.
- One patient has an incidental view of another patient's chart or prescription.
- A patient sees other records come up while the dentist is searching for the patient's record.
- A nursing assistant overhears a nurse talking to a patient on the other side of a screen.
- Nurses speak about patient care issues in a nursing station.

guardians' rights, grandparents' rights, the rights of lesbian and gay partners, and the rights of divorced parents—depending on custody and alimony laws—can vary from state to state. Medical records can be shared with insurers in a secure way to facilitate reimbursement, but the concept is that only the most restrictive information should be shared. You should seek guidance about the state laws in effect where you practice.

Frequently, health professionals call patients and clients with protected medical information. Usually, employers will have policies and guidelines for these situations. You should be aware of these policies and guidelines. However, someone else may answer, or you will get voicemail. It is improper to leave private medical information on voicemail; you have no knowledge or control over who has access to that voicemail. When you reach a spouse or caretaker of a patient, however, it could be a matter of judgment, based on your facility's policy and procedures manual, over whether to share private medical information with this person who is close to the patient but not the patient themselves.

General Confidentiality

Confidential patient information does not exist for any reason other than to facilitate the best possible care of the patient. It is not appropriate to share in idle conversation, gossip, or storytelling. Do not discuss patients or their information in elevators, hallways, lobbies, or any other place inside or outside the health

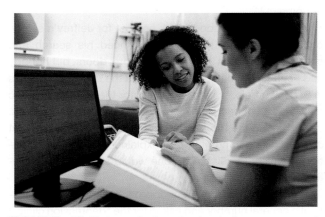

FIGURE 10-5 A medical professional discusses records with a patient (Copyright © istock.com).

facility. You should avoid mentioning a patient's name as well as any other information that could identify the patient. This is especially important when you have patients who may be known to the public or of interest to the media.

Anything you learn about a patient in your capacity as a health professional should be considered confidential (Figure 10-5). If the patient discloses personal information, even in a friendly conversation, you are prohibited from repeating that information to anyone. Information you overhear at work is confidential.

In this age of social media and instant communication, you have a special obligation to protect all confidential information. Information can be dangerous, ruining reputations and "personal brands" in an instant. Your patients depend on your integrity.

St. Nowhere

Al Berks was extremely concerned about his long-time business partner Jeffrey Galloway. They were great friends, but their furniture business had not been doing well, and Al could see that Jeffrey was becoming depressed. He wasn't himself. He spent long days sequestered in his office, but Al had no idea what he was doing in there. Then, Jeffrey started showing up only 2 or 3 days a week. Now he hadn't been seen in a week. Jeffrey was divorced, and his children were grown, and Al had lost track of where they lived, so there was no one he could check with. Al dropped by Jeffrey's house, but there was no answer to his knock, no car in the driveway, and no evidence that anyone was at home.

Al became very concerned, not just for Jeffrey's safety, but for his mental health. Al continued his search and started knocking on Jeffrey's neighbors' doors, but nobody had seen him. Finally, the kid across the street said, "He's in St. Nowhere's," which was slang for the state psychiatric facility. Al went back to his office and start dialing numbers.

Starting at the top, no one would "confirm or deny" that Jeffrey had been admitted. Al explained his business relationship with Jeffrey but no one would share any information with him.

Finally he tried a different approach. He called the hospital's general number and asked for the "depression clinic."

"We don't a have a clinic especially for depression, but we have many depressed patients on many different units."

"Oh," said Al. "Well, I just wanted to talk to someone about possibly getting treated. Could I talk to someone from one of the units?" He was transferred to the Green Unit.

"This is Maria. How can I help you?"

"Oh hi, Maria, this is Al Berks, the furniture guy on TV?"

"You're calling me at work to sell me furniture?"

"No, no, I always say that. That's how people know me. My partner, Jeffrey Galloway, is a patient there, and I need to talk to him."

"I can't confirm or— "

"Oh, I know. I don't want to put you in an awkward position, but please hear me out. Jeffrey doesn't have any family nearby. I know he's been having a hard time. If you see him around, could you have him call me? He knows my number."

Maria was tempted to confirm Mr. Galloway's admission. This guy seemed sincere, and everybody knew about the Berks and Galloway furniture store ads, so they were definitely friends. But she still hesitated. Had Mr. Galloway provided the hospital with the OK to give his personal information to his business partner? What if they're having an argument? How would she really know if they were friends? They could be business partners who had grown to hate each other.

Maria chose her words carefully, not wanting to disclose by omission the protected information Al Berks was seeking. "Mr. Berks, I would help you if I could. The only thing I can do is give you my number. You're welcome to call me back in a day or two if you still haven't heard from your friend."

"OK, Maria. Thank you for taking my call." He took her number and hung up. Al just sat there for a while, gazing over his main gallery, when his cell phone rang.

"Hi Al," said Jeffrey in a sad voice. "I'm sorry you've been worried about me. That was lousy of me. I didn't think anybody would care. I'm in St. Nowhere's."

"Jeffrey, thank God, are you OK?"

"Yes, better, actually. How did you know I was here?"

"The kid across the street. How come he knew?"

"Oh," Jeffrey had to laugh at himself. "I left for the hospital early in the morning. The kid's my paperboy. I practically hit him when I was backing out. I had to apologize to him. I think I told him to hold the paper until I got back from the state hospital. I've been here awhile, three or four days I think, maybe five. The medicine is starting to work. I feel a little better. You talked to Maria?"

"Yes. She was nice, but she wouldn't say you were there."

"She asked me if I wanted to call you. She said it was up to me. I didn't mean to make you worry. Maria asked, so I put you on my list. I signed something so you can visit me and call me. I'll be here for a few more days."

"I'll be over in an hour."

QUESTIONS FOR THOUGHT AND REFLECTION

1. Were you able to understand protected medical information from the perspective of a patient's friend?
2. Did Maria handle Al's call correctly?
3. Did she do the right thing by telling Jeffrey that Al had called, looking for him?

Down a Dark Road

Carlene was filing lab results into charts, when she came across a result for her friend Leslie, who had married Carlene's cousin Bob 2 years ago. They were perfect for each other. Leslie's lab results reflected that Leslie was pregnant. Carlene filed the result away in Leslie's chart. She had to be mindful of Leslie's private medical information. She needed to wait until the doctor had a chance to give Leslie her results. She checked in the appointment book, and sure enough, Leslie had an appointment with Dr. Darby on Friday.

Carlene worked in the back on Friday afternoon. She didn't want to see Leslie, because she was afraid her expression would tip off Leslie as to the results. She didn't want to spoil the surprise. She was proud of herself for keeping such wonderful news to herself. She hadn't said anything at work, and she didn't even tell her mother. Anyway, she would see Bob and Leslie at the bowling league on Monday night.

When Carlene got there, Bob said Leslie couldn't come because she wasn't feeling well. All evening, well into their third game, Carlene kept an eye on Bob. She could not figure this guy out. Here he was, about to be a father, and he acted like this was just another night at the lanes. She figured they wanted to be sure about the baby, though, this being her first, so she didn't bring it up until they were turning their shoes in at the end of the night.

"So how does it feel, Pops?" she finally said to him.
"Pops? How does what feel?"
"The baby, silly."
He just looked at her. He was playing dumb, she figured.
"Look, Bob. I work at the clinic. I saw Leslie's pregnancy test come back positive. You don't have to pretend around me."

Bob darkened. "She's not pregnant," he said. "She just doesn't feel good. You're an idiot. I had a vasectomy five years ago." Then he looked at her again. "What pregnancy test?"

QUESTIONS FOR THOUGHT AND REFLECTION

1. Was Carlene in a tough position with regard to the confidential information she discovered about her cousin's wife?
2. Can you imagine being placed in a compromising position as a result of your exposure to your patients' private medical information?
3. How should Carlene have handled this information?
4. Will Carlene's mother be upset that Carlene didn't share the news of Leslie's pregnancy with her?
5. What will happen to Carlene when Leslie calls Dr. Darby?

⭐ EXPERIENTIAL EXERCISES

1. Review your facility's protected patient information policy. Read the fine print.
2. Find out where special confidentiality requests are entered into patients' charts.
3. Identify your privacy officer.
4. Visit http://www.hhs.gov/ocr/privacy/hipaa/understanding/index.html to learn more about HIPAA. Bookmark the site, and visit it twice this week to broaden your understanding of how to protect patients' protected health information.

🔵 CROSS CURRENTS WITH OTHER SOFT SKILLS

ACHIEVING HONESTY AND INTEGRITY: Protecting confidential information always comes down to your personal integrity. (pp. 18-25)

BUILDING TRUST: Confidentiality only works if, like trust, it is observed 100% of the time. (pp. 212-218)

PROFESSIONAL PHONE TECHNIQUE: Confidentiality is especially challenging when you are on the phone and sometimes are not sure whom you are speaking with. (pp. 257-263)

COMMITTING TO YOUR PROFESSION: Professions are identified, in part, with codes of ethics, which includes confidentiality. (pp. 342-348)

Keeping Records

The shortest pencil is longer than the longest memory.

—Anonymous

- Explain the purpose of keeping records.
- Know the types of records and their formats.
- Adopt documentation best practices.
- Anticipate and describe the future uses of medical records.

The goal of keeping records in a medical facility is to access information easily when it is needed. Other important goals include patient confidentiality, avoiding legal issues, gathering insurance information, processing reimbursement, and addressing financial considerations. A record-keeping system should also account for the needs of those who will use this information, and what kinds of questions they will expect it to answer. All these needs dictate the exact format employees use to ensure readability, compliance with rules and regulations, clarity, and professionalism.

In the past, medical charting and records were maintained by hand. However, electronic record keeping is becoming more common. Electronic records increase accuracy and legibility, and they save precious time. They are easy to use and share with others as needed. If it is easy to electronically record notes and measurements at the time they are observed or taken, the medical record will be more accurate and immediately accessible. However, it is not always possible or practical to record every important piece of information electronically, so you must also be effective and efficient in recording information by hand. Figure 10-6 shows how properly maintained medical records can provide fast access to information when it is needed.

Types of Medical Charting and Record Keeping

One of the main purposes of a good medical record system is to impose logic and order on the patient care process. Practices typically use some kind of problem-oriented charting that states the patient's problem or problems and before explaining the patient care

FIGURE 10-6 Medical charts. (From Proctor DB, Adams AP: *Kinn's the medical assistant: an applied learning approach*, ed 12, St Louis, 2014, Elsevier.)

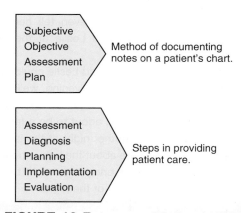

Subjective
Objective
Assessment
Plan — Method of documenting notes on a patient's chart.

Assessment
Diagnosis
Planning
Implementation
Evaluation — Steps in providing patient care.

FIGURE 10-7 Acronyms SOAP and ADPIE.

and planning that is performed in response to the problem. For example, acronyms SOAP and ADPIE are commonly used to explain health care processes (Figure 10-7). Other systems may be used in your facility and it is your responsibility to learn and use that system. Regardless of which system you use, all systems ensure that the correct information is being collected and recorded in an orderly and predictable manner.

In addition to these basic charting approaches, many other kinds of information must be recorded, including progress notes, drug administration records, and flow charts such as input and output or vital signs records. Other systems keep track of appointments, dietary intake, inventory, various dental records, range of motion, respiratory intake and output, speech and hearing changes, images, functional changes, mental status reports, insurance and diagnostic codes, lab results, and use of medical interpreters, among others.

Policies, Procedures, and Conventions

Right away, familiarize yourself with the policies and procedures governing charting and record keeping in your facility. What, when, and how are you expected to record information? Some records such as shift reports are routine in their frequency. Other records are driven by changes in the patient's condition or irregular events, such as diagnostic tests or fire drills.

There will be a policy on making corrections, because medical records are legal documents that cannot be changed or even corrected without following a specific protocol. Sign your entries with your name and title or certification, as dictated by your employer. Your facility may specify proper ink colors or designate different colors for different purposes. Regardless of the policies and procedures, always observe the rules and guidelines for excellent documentation that you have been taught (Box 10-7).

BOX 10-7

Charting Best Practices

- Think about your audience: Who are they, and what do they need to know?
- Anticipate your audience's questions and record accordingly.
- Record only what you did or observed yourself.
- Never make judgmental statements.
- Focus especially on changes in the patient's condition.
- Spell correctly and use only approved or common abbreviations.
- If writing, use legible handwriting.
- Use descriptive words accurately.
- Re-read your notes and make any necessary corrections or clarifications.
- Follow policy in making corrections.
- Chart after providing care only.
- Use the patient's own words when significant; identify them with quotation marks.
- Always sign your entries in the medical record.
- Follow all policies in place to standardize charting.

Style

Your facility will likely have protocols for how information is recorded or charted, beyond the particular system used. For instance, there may be a list of allowable abbreviations. Many acronyms are universally recognized in health care, such as BP, ADL, or HIPAA, and these can be used because they readily communicate their meaning. Certain stylistic conventions may be used, such as elliptical style or sentence fragments, to facilitate rapid access to information. Sometimes, these practices may not be encoded in policies but rather should be inferred from what you see in the records in general.

Accuracy and Consistency of Medical Records

In a field in which change is unavoidable, the one thing that can remain standard and constant over an extended period of time is the patient's record. The patient may be treated in many different places. The patient will interact with and be treated by many different health professionals. Their care may be inpatient care, outpatient care, or home care. They may experience different treatment approaches, tests, and medications. The whirlwind of care surrounding a patient may be confusing, inconsistent, rushed, or chaotic. However, if all these variables are patiently and consistently recorded in the patient's medical record, a coherent picture of diagnosis, treatment, care, and patient responses will exist in a standard, carefully constructed and maintained record for future caregivers.

JOURNALING 10-5

Think about your own medical history. What would you want your permanent, portable medical record to contain? Record the kinds of information and imagine scenarios where the information could prove crucial to your health and well-being.

Habit Formation in the Keeping of Records

Very often, in the methods and practices of medical record keeping, there is a right way and every other way. Start out by knowing the proper and correct procedures for recording medical information.

Date	Time	Nursing Margin	Other Depts Margin
7/8	1700	750 mL tap water enema given with the resident in the L side-lying position.	
		The resident was asked to retain the enema for at least 15 minutes. Bed in low	
		position. Signal light within reach. No resident complaints at this time. Resident	
		informed that I would check on her in 5 minutes or when the signal light was used.	
		Angie Martinez, CNA ———————————————————————	
	1715	Assisted resident to the bedside commode. Privacy curtain pulled. Signal light and	
		toilet tissue within reach. Resident reminded to signal when finished expelling the	
		enema or if she needs assistance. Angie Martinez, CNA —————————	

FIGURE 10-8 Charting sample. (From Kostelnick C, *Mosby's textbook for long-term care nursing assistants*, ed 7, St Louis, 2015, Elsevier.)

For instance, every medical note, event, or recording should have a date and time. Documenting the time when something occurs helps piece together a story that can be used in making a diagnosis or an adjustment to the care program. Timeliness, accuracy, style, and signature are other habits to thoughtfully develop as you establish your reputation for careful, competent record keeping. Figure 10-8 shows a good example of documentation.

Accuracy

Your observations and measurements should be recorded objectively in the medical records. However, your subjective impressions—as long as they are not judgmental—can also be important parts of the medical record, providing clues for accurate diagnosis and treatment. For example, you might note a change in the patient's skin tone, a subtle change in responsiveness, a slight slur of speech. As long as you note the subjectivity of your observation, you are providing data that no one else is in a position to report. Experienced health care professionals are known for their highly developed sense of intuition, which can help save lives.

Use accurate words and appropriate terminology. Try to be your own harshest critic in evaluating whether you have stated your observation accurately. For example, a rash may be red, but how red? Is it warm? Is the skin dry or irritated? You should ask yourself the questions that the reader will ask, and record as much information as precisely as you can. Be wary of words that are relative. It is often not enough to record that something is small or large,

faint or distinct, frequent or occasional. You must always qualify these adjectives to convey the degree that they appear.

Consistency

In the haste and confusion of a moment, it can be tempting to neglect recording patient information when it occurs, thinking you will get to it later. This is a mistake. Long after the moment has calmed, long after you are gone from the scene, the medical record will stand as the only testament of something important. Even if you do record the information later, you might remember it inaccurately, and it will certainly suffer from a lack of immediacy. Moreover, you might never record it at all as you are consumed by the rush of oncoming activities. You must develop the habit of recording information as it occurs. In the long run, recording information may be more useful than the care you are documenting.

 WHAT IF?

What if you forget to document important medical information? What can you do about it? More importantly, what can you do to ensure that it never happens again?

Uses of Medical Records

Purposes of quality medical records include planning, coordinating, and delivering quality medical care. However, as you contribute to all medical record keeping, you should be guided by all the users of the information you compile and keep your various audiences in mind.

Members of the Health Care Team

The primary users of the medical records you create are your colleagues and the members of the health care team treating the patient, now and in the future. Doctors, dentists, lab professionals, imaging technicians and a host of other colleagues need to obtain accurate information quickly and easily from the medical charts. This information is available to them only if you put it there.

Every patient is a puzzle, both from a diagnostic and treatment point of view. Just as soon as a patient comes to a health care professional's attention, the record keeping begins. Every detail, no matter how seemingly unimportant by itself, combines to create a holistic picture of a patient that contributes to analysis, decision-making, and understanding. Whether the patient's condition is accurately diagnosed depends on the knowledge and skill of the clinician, but it is also based on the information that has been recorded. The same is true of the ongoing treatment of the patient, which is constantly adjusted and improved, based on the quality of the ongoing stream of documentation. Finally, at some point in the future, in ways you could never imagine or anticipate, the patient's medical record is likely to prove useful or crucial to understanding a future illness or condition and point the way toward specific, optimal treatment choices. Your documentation is not just for today; it is for forever.

Legal Considerations

Medical records of all types are legal documents. They can be subpoenaed and used as evidence in a trial or civil case. If they are comprehensive, accurate, and objective, they will legally protect you, your employer, and your patients.

Medical records that are inaccurate, incomplete, or judgmental can harm you or your employer and expose you to legal action. More important, poor or sloppy documentation can harm a patient because it contributes to poor decision-making and treatment. Your employer and your patients want you to record the best documentation possible, for everyone's benefit and protection. Nothing strengthens patient care and your employer's legal standing better than great medical record keeping.

WHAT IF?

What if you notice someone else's documentation in a patient's chart that is judgmental, prejudicial, or derogatory? What actions should you take? How can such a record be properly corrected?

Medical Insurance and Reimbursement

Insurers use medical records to reimburse health care providers for the treatment they provide. Without accurate, properly documented information, claims can be denied. When claims are denied, it means either that your employer doesn't get paid for the care they have provided or the costs they have incurred, or else the patient has to pay for care they are insured for, creating a hardship.

Health insurers are businesses that have structured their premiums in a way that allows them to pay fair claims while still making a profit. Insurers act in their own best interests by employing claims people who verify the legitimacy and accuracy of the claims they pay. It is your job to ensure that the documentation you create is clear and complete, recorded in the proper format and place, so that financial issues can be properly managed and promptly paid. The care and quality of your medical record keeping can ensure that financial concerns do not harm your employer or add stress to your patient.

Consultants and Experts

In difficult, puzzling, or complex cases, physicians and others frequently consult with specialists and experts in various areas of health care, asking them for their guidance and recommendations on how to proceed with the treatment of the complicated patient. These experts rely on the patient's chart to gather information and formulate their opinions. This is just one example of the many unanticipated uses of medical records in the future. Charts could be used for teaching purposes, medical history reviews of patients, or research.

In summary, your accurate, complete, and objective documentation is a lasting part of each patient's health care legacy.

CASE STUDY 10-4
Heightened Vigilance

Ken McGuire seemed to be going downhill fast. The staff were commenting on his deteriorating depression, and wondering if they should restrict his activities. "I tell you what," said Gary, one of the workers. "I told Ken I would escort him to the drugstore in the Square. Why don't I do that as an assessment? I've seen him every day this week, and I share the concerns."

"Do you think that's safe?" asked Kathy, the nurse in charge.

"He's safe with me," said Gary.

On their way to the Square, Gary was getting uncomfortable with Ken's condition. Ken walked slowly, as if each step required great effort. He said very little, barely acknowledging Gary's efforts at conversation. At one point, he just stopped, suddenly crying, unable to say why. Although Gary suggested turning back, Ken insisted he was able to go on because he wanted to buy a birthday card for his girlfriend. Gary kept a close eye on Ken the rest of the way. When they reached the bottom of the hill and prepared to cross the street, Ken said, "What if I ran in front of a car? You couldn't stop me."

"Ken, unless you want me to turn you around right now, you are going to have to convince me that you won't do that."

"I won't," said Ken.

"Do you know how I would feel if you did that, Ken?"

"I won't," said Ken. "It was nice of you to take me. You didn't have to. I won't do anything."

In the store, Ken quickly picked out a card, which surprised Gary. Usually, even he would look at several cards before deciding what he liked best. Then Ken filled a basket with candy. "For the others," he told Gary. "They can't get out like me. It's the least I can do while I'm here."

They returned to the unit without incident, but Gary was relieved to be back. He wrote his observations in Ken's chart. While he was writing, he saw another patient, Lou, walk by the nurses' station wearing Ken's fancy Stetson hat. "Whoa," said Gary. "Why are you wearing Ken's Stetson?"

"He gave it to me," said Lou with a grin.

Gary nodded, and added that to his note. He discussed his concerns with Kathy, and she gave Ken a PRN dose of his medication. After an hour or so, Ken said he felt a little better. At shift change, Kathy said, "That's good, and that's bad."

Ella, the night nurse, asked Gary to read his notes again out loud. "We're putting him on 5-minute checks," said Ella afterward.

In the morning, Gary was back for the second half of his back-to-back shift.

"Everybody to Ken's room," shouted a nurse, followed by two shifts of people. One of the night workers was physically restraining Ken. "Found him in the closet tying his shoelaces to one of the hooks," said the worker. The team went into action to place Ken in a safe seclusion room, and the night nurse called the doctor-on-call for the necessary order.

One week later, Ken was safe, but not much better. All his privileges had been revoked, and the psychiatrist in charge, Dr. Pellos, arranged for a clinical review. He began by reading the relevant sections from Ken's chart, including the progress note that Gary had entered on the evening before Ken's suicide attempt. "That was good work, Gary," said Dr. Pellos, looking up from the chart. "You observed and recorded all the pertinent data. Your charting helped alert everyone to Ken's exact state of mind, and resulted in heightened vigilance. That saved Ken's life."

QUESTIONS FOR THOUGHT AND REFLECTION

1. Did Gary describe Ken's behavior objectively?
2. Do you think Gary quoted Ken's exact words about running in front of a car?
3. What was the significance of Gary's observation that Ken gave away his favorite hat?
4. What could have happened at the busy shift change if Ken had not been on 5-minute checks?
5. Explain the connection between the documentation and the teamwork you saw in this case.

Down a Dark Road

Dr. Raj was angry. The medical chart for Ms. Gillespie was full of gaps. He was trying to determine the extent of changes in the patient's blood sugar, so he could adjust the treatment of her diabetes. Her diabetes had led to frequent emergencies and puzzling episodes in the past few days, and he had ordered regular blood sugars drawn, a meticulous I&O chart, and careful recording of the food she actually ate. In her chart, he was finding erratic patterns of blood draws, big gaps in the I&O chart, and records of what the patient was served but not what she ate. He could not prescribe treatment with these records, and the patient's insurance company would not be likely to approve a longer stay in order to collect this information all over again. He picked up the phone and called the office of the Director of Nursing.

"Dr. Goldstein, I am dismayed by your staff's shoddy charting. I want to meet with you to review the data on one of my patients immediately."

Shirley Goldstein was alarmed by the call. Dr. Raj was known as a patient, understanding physician. Something must be seriously wrong to make him so agitated. When she saw the chart he brought with him, she could see why. "First of all," she said, "I will see if the documentation exists elsewhere. Second, this is as unacceptable to me as it is to you. In 1 hour, I will let you know what I have found and what is being done to rectify this. This is totally unacceptable."

Dr. Goldstein marched down to the unit on the 7th floor where the patient was being treated. It was a very unwelcome visit for Ramona Hernandez, the charge nurse on duty that day. Ramona was aware of deficits in the quality of the charting, so much so that she reviewed the patients' charts at the end of each of her shifts to assure that the documentation was complete and accurate. She knew which nurses and nursing assistants were the problem

charters, and she had been thinking about how to approach the problem. Unfortunately, other charge nurses let the charting slide, and when the nurses and nursing assistant were reporting to them, they often failed to chart accurately or even at all. The matter of charting was getting an inconsistent message from management. Dr. Goldstein pointed out each deficit in the charting, and Ramona wasn't surprised by any of it. "How could this happen, Ramona? Why didn't you report your concerns to your supervisor?"

Just then, one of the nurses burst into the nursing station. "Sorry to interrupt—we have a concern in room 14A, Emily Gillespie. She's unresponsive, and her breathing is shallow. We just pulled some blood work, and it's not good." Ramona went with the nurse, and Dr. Goldstein went looking for the unit's nursing supervisor, Harvey Wing. She found him in his office having an early lunch. "Come with me," she told him.

By the time they arrived in 14A, Dr. Raj was already there, making adjustments to the IV. He just gave Dr. Goldstein a look and went about trying to stabilize the patient. Dr. Goldstein motioned for Harvey to follow her out into the hallway. "We're going to have another discussion about the ABCs of charting," she told him, "and this will be our last discussion."

QUESTIONS FOR THOUGHT AND REFLECTION

1. Who is affected by poor charting?
2. What decisions depended on the quality of the charting?
3. How is charting affecting this hospital's operations? What functions are affected?
4. How do you think the conversation went between Dr. Goldstein and Harvey Wing?
5. What do you think Dr. Goldstein will tell Dr. Raj?

⭐ EXPERIENTIAL EXERCISES

1. Review the policies that govern record keeping at your place of employment.
2. What is the role of electronic record keeping at your institution?
3. Identify a particularly effective piece of patient documentation.
4. Ask colleagues how good or bad record keeping helped or hindered their practice.

◎ CROSS CURRENTS WITH OTHER SOFT SKILLS

THINKING CRITICALLY: Record keeping should be an occasion to think analytically about the data you have collected and its implications. (pp. 320-325)
WRITING, GRAMMAR, AND SPELLING: Your record keeping should reflect correctness and professionalism. (pp. 249-257)
TAKING ACCOUNTABILITY: In the end, no one can document your observations and care except you, and your patients and colleagues depend on you to do it consistently and accurately. (pp. 333-336)

Financial Literacy

Managing Your Money

The safest way to double your money is to fold it over and put it in your pocket.

—Kin Hubbard

LEARNING OBJECTIVE 5: MANAGING OUR MONEY

- Explain the difference between gross and net income and the types of deductions that affect gross income.
- Plan for your retirement and describe the most common pension plans.
- Establish a personal budget.
- Describe ways to build a good credit record and explain how your credit record is used.
- Discuss differences in types of student loans.
- Explain the process for making a loan decision.
- Describe smart strategies for buying a car.
- Detail a solid plan for getting out of debt.

Take Control—It's Your Money

"Where does the money go?"

Have you ever asked yourself that? Sure you have; we *all* have! Next to love and romance, money—both loving it and losing it—may be the most popular theme for songs, from early blues to jazz to rock and rap. Everybody wants more money, and everybody wonders where it goes.

How Do You Handle Your Money—and Why?

You can probably find the answers in how you grew up: We get many of our financial habits from our families and their financial situations, our ethnic or religious communities, and the larger national culture. Media and social media—advertising and themes in magazines, TV, movies, podcasts, blogs—also influence how we handle money. For example, did you know that the most successful romantic comedies center on characters with above-average incomes?

So, how does all of this affect us?

Often, all these beautiful images, ads, and movies leave us dissatisfied with our lives. They cause us to think that we need more than we really do (which, we might note, is precisely their purpose). The idea that more money does not buy more happiness happens to be true. Wanting more than we have money to pay for leads to all kinds of problems—money problems, to be sure, but money problems are the cause of so many more, and bigger, problems.

Do you have trouble managing your money? Do you find yourself worrying over a shortage of money at the end of each month? Take heart: You *can* take control.

⟵ JOURNALING 10-6

- Who or what do you think has been the greatest influence on how you handle money? Try to identify (a) one event and (b) one individual (or group), then describe the effect each has had on you.
- What would you most like to change—not about events beyond your control but instead about your own behavior, your own response to money?

What's in Your Paycheck?

To begin to talk about money management, let's look at your first paycheck. Say you are starting fresh with your first job in your new career. The first time you get that crisp ink-scented paycheck (or receipt, if your employer automatically deposits your wages into your bank account), you may be surprised to discover that what you'll take home each month is not quite what you expected.

Keep in mind that your gross salary includes everything before removal of employee benefits, Social Security, some state and federal taxes, and more (Figure 10-9); after these are taken from each month's salary, the amount remaining, signed over to you in a paycheck, is called your net salary. All of these **deductions** from the gross salary benefit us in one way or another, some more obviously than others. (In other words, although our taxes go to build our roads and provide other services, they're not quite as direct as money that goes into our savings plans at work.)

Withholding Taxes

When you first get a job, you will fill out a Form W-4, the Employee's Withholding Allowance Certificate. This form helps you avoid having too much or too little federal income tax withheld from your pay.

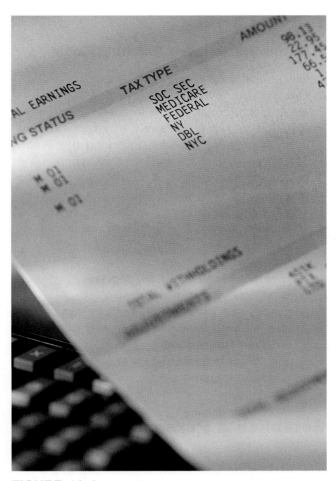

FIGURE 10-9 Itemization of deductions from a typical paycheck (Copyright © thinkstock.com).

But how do you know what to have withheld on your W-4? To answer that, let's look more closely at how tax withholding works:

Every pay cycle, a certain amount is removed from your paycheck as a means of contributing, a little at a time, to the state (in some states) and federal income tax you'll pay at the end of the year. In the case of federal tax, you have some control over how much you want deducted. For example, if you have children and you claim them when you fill out your new-employee forms, less money will be taken from each paycheck. This will help you cover the costs of raising your children. The disadvantage is that you may wind up owing taxes at the end of the year. In other words, have too little withheld, and at the end of the year you'll owe the government money.

For this reason, some parents decide not to claim a child tax credit on the Form 4-W (though they'll claim their children later when they pay their taxes). This means that more money is withheld all year long, and at the end of the year, instead of owing,

they'll be more likely to get a refund. But be careful: This is no bonus, and it is not "free money." If you have too much money withheld from your check, thinking that you're playing it safe, just remember: Sure, you'll get any excess back as a refund at the end of the year, but you could also come up short before then and wish that you had the money in hand. The other disadvantage of withholding more than you end up owing is that all year long, as that money is being withheld until refund time, you're losing the interest you could have been making on it by putting it into savings.

Employee Benefits

Of all the things that make up your total salary (aside from your take-home pay), the most valuable by far are employee benefits. When you are choosing a job or company, weighing employee benefits against net income is another savvy way to save money wisely. Benefits may differ widely from one company to the next; when you receive a copy of the employee benefits package, read it carefully so you know what you are entitled to. Typical employee benefits include:

* Paid vacation days
* Personal days (either paid or unpaid; sometimes called sick leave)
* Maternity/paternity leave (paid or unpaid)
* Education or training reimbursement
* Health insurance
* Pension plan

In some cases, you may have a choice of several insurance plans. The smaller the business you work for, though, the fewer benefits your employer may be able to afford. If this is the case, look for socially rewarding benefits of working for a smaller business.

Planning for Retirement

Finally, you have probably heard that it is never too early to start planning for your retirement. Your employer may be large enough to offer you some sort of retirement or pension plan, but you must take most or all of the responsibility. Whole books on retirement planning are available, but let's look at a few very basic options to get you started on your journey.

A pension plan is a retirement fund sponsored by an employer. These plans generally fall into one of two categories: Either your employer contributes a fixed amount of money to your retirement plan each year or your employer bases its contribution to your account on the company's profits for that year, meaning that it may be as much as 15 percent of your salary in a great year or very little to nothing in a rough year.

In other pension plans, your employer makes a contribution when you put money in. For instance, if you put in a dollar, your employer may put in 25 cents. Some even match your own contributions (up to a certain limit). The more you contribute, the more your employer does. But you do have to contribute: If you put in nothing, that's exactly what your employer puts in.

Another option is a 401(k) plan, which enables you to delay paying taxes on the money you save for retirement. (This is called a tax deferment.) When you retire, you'll receive regular fixed payments from that total amount saved, on which you'll need to pay taxes.

Regardless of what your company provides, you're going to need to establish your own retirement plan as well. These plans include:

* The personal 401(k) plan, a retirement savings account that you set up for yourself instead of through a company, which lets you defer paying taxes on it while you're saving
* The IRA, or Individual Retirement Account
* The annuity, a fund to which you contribute that pays a fixed sum of money to you each year after you retire
* Investments such as stocks and bonds

It is beyond the scope of this text to advise you on which plan might be best for you. Instead, take advantage of the many great online resources for designing your own plan. See Box 10-8 for a list of some tools to get you started, then consider paying a visit to a financial advisor. Once you've decided which plan is best for you, you can usually set it up on your own. After that, it's up to you how much you want to involve yourself in monitoring markets and other developments, but as a rule it's smart to reevaluate your retirement plan on a yearly basis to ensure that it's still the right plan for you.

JOURNALING 10-7

- When you think about saving for retirement, what kind of lifestyle do you imagine is realistic after you stop working? How does this compare with what you'd like to have or do after retirement?
- What types of savings or investment avenues do you think would be easiest for you to stick with and contribute to over the years to save for retirement?

BOX 10-8

Online Retirement Planning Tools

Online calculation tools are a great way to start creating your own savings, investment, or retirement plan. Experiment with these free online resources to get an idea of the possibilities and what might best suit you. Exploring these and other free (and even fun!) informational online resources is a great way to pinpoint the best retirement plan for you.

The Official Website of the U.S. Social Security Administration: Retirement Planner
http://www.ssa.gov/retire2/

Retirement Planner at CNN Money
http://cgi.money.cnn.com/tools/retirementplanner/retirementplanner.jsp

A Step-by-Step Guide to Painlessly Plan and Vet Your Retirement
http://lifehacker.com/5814716/ten-tools-that-do-the-retirement-planning-for-you

Establish a Personal Budget

Once you have a regular paycheck (and maybe some benefits) coming in, it's easy for someone to tell you, "Just save your money," but that's not particularly helpful if you don't have the proper tools. A few simple strategies are all you need to start taking control. And because it's your money, why wouldn't you want to take control? (We'll be talking about tackling debt a little later in this chapter.)

Step 1: Keep Track

The first step to financial responsibility is simply becoming aware of where your money goes. Start keeping track. Carry a small notebook with you and write down how you spend your money over the course of each day. Don't judge or second-guess yourself; just keep track. Don't think of any spending as right or wrong, for now. You want to look back at this record and see what you value. After the necessities—rent, food, utilities, medications, gas or bus money, occasional clothing items, and, in some cases child care—we all like to have a little something left for fun. So keep track of that as well, without second-guessing what you want. The goal here is to find out where you want to conserve and where it's worth it to spend. (More on that later.)

Step 2: Take Stock

At the end of a week or two, stop and make your first assessment. Are you getting an idea of where your money goes? Most Americans spend an average of 25 to 30 percent of their income on housing and 8 to 12 percent on utilities. Food runs 10 to 15 percent for most of us, and transportation or gas money is roughly 15 to 20 percent. Generally the poorer you are, the more you'll spend on health care and health insurance, usually 7 to 10 percent. Education, for most of us, becomes a matter of student loans—an expense that is deferred until later, but then watch out! The wrong student loan can cost a fortune later in added-up interest. For now, though, let's look at balancing your current budget.

After the first week or two of tracking your spending, how does your spending compare with some of the general figures given above? And what, then, about your "fun money"? How much did you spend on entertainment? For most people, this runs around 5% of overall income.

Step 3: Create a One-Month Balance Sheet

In this next phase, continue keeping track of your spending patterns; it's a great habit to get into, and after a while it becomes second nature. Now you can start establishing your budget. There are many systems for doing this, including good software packages.

Assuming that you have a job of some kind or some other source of income, this step will be easier if you use one payday as your start date. On the day you receive your main check for the month, draw four columns on a sheet of paper. Title the first column "Date," the second "Money Available," the third "Expenses," and the fourth "Balance." As you list how much money you have at the top of that second column, date it. (Don't count money you don't want to tap into—for instance, any money you have saved. Include only the money you want as part of your monthly budget.)

Next, as you purchase or pay for something, put a date by each of those expenditures in column three.

Step 4: Do the Math

At the end of the first month, add up all of the numbers under "Expenses" and subtract the total from the "Money Available" column. This is your balance— what you have left after one month's spending.

Step 5: Analyze Your Spending Patterns

How did you do? The first goal (1) is to cover all necessities (food, housing, utilities, health, and transportation). Once those have been taken care of, you want enough left over for (2) emergencies, (3) entertainment and incidentals (replacing a clothing item, paying for a small repair, etc.), and finally, (4) savings (Figure 10-10). (**Note:** You might think that savings should come before entertainment and incidentals, but this is rarely practical. Every human being genuinely needs a little fun on a regular basis, rather than having all of our fun when we are retired, and sometimes this costs money—and then there are inevitable, unavoidable, and necessary incidentals.) *Proportion and amounts are what count:* Obviously, you should try to put much more toward savings and retirement than you spend on entertainment and incidental needs! For a while, until you are established in your career, some of these goals can be difficult to fulfill; savings, in particular, may be tough to accomplish for a while, but you'll want to begin a savings plan eventually. (You don't want to work forever, do you?)

So let's conduct a little analysis. This is where you really get to know yourself—moneywise, that is. Are you coming up short every month? Can that be corrected? Often it can. It just means making choices.

FIGURE 10-10 Estimate what you need to cover monthly expenses, then subtract that from your net salary for the month. Make saving for emergencies, retirement, entertainment, and incidental expenses your priorities for the balance (Copyright © thinkstock.com).

Step 6: Make Choices

If you are tempted to overspend, stop and make choices. Most of the time if you have a reasonable income, even if it is not very high, you can manage to do *something* for fun. Would you rather buy this book or that CD? Do you want the mocha latte with your best friend, or would you rather chip in on the pizza party later? Often we really can do any *one* thing we like—we just can't afford to do them all!

Also, learn to separate wants from needs. Do you really need the name-brand shampoo, or is there a plain-label product that's just as good, at least in the short term? Have you tried the store-brand milk instead of the brand-name one you grew up with? Do you need the multicolored note pens for class, or will the cheap multipack do? Slowing down to make choices not only saves you money but also gives you a nice feeling of being in control: You don't need everything you see or happen to like (Figure 10-11)!

? WHAT IF?

- *What if you had to choose between two different social events because doing both would cost too much? How would you establish your priorities?*
- *What do you do when a good friend or close family member wants you to do something special with him or her but in your heart you know you just can't afford it?*
- *If a utility bill seemed too high to you, what might you do about it?*

FIGURE 10-11 Making choices not only saves you money but also gives you a nice feeling of being in control: You *don't* need everything you see! (Copyright © thinkstock.com)

Step 7: Look Ahead to Set Your Financial Goals

Financial goal-setting, both short and long term, can't be started soon enough. In the short term, write down your more immediate money goals: Do you need to save for books for next semester? For a prescription refill? Or can you afford to start setting money aside for a smartphone? Set your priorities. In the long term, you will want to start building an emergency cushion, something you can fall back on if you should lose your job or have an accident. At first, this will be a slow grower, but eventually you'll want to take the advice of many financial advisors and build an emergency fund deep enough to help you get by for six to nine months if you were to lose your income.

Step 8: Open an Account and Follow Your Game Plan

Remember that little notebook of expenses and the one-month ledger you used to analyze your money habits? That's called a balance sheet, and you get one with every checkbook when you establish a checking account. If at all possible, open a checking account as soon as you can; free accounts are available, but others carry nominal fees or require a minimum balance. This is a smart, easy, inexpensive way to keep track of your income and spending, as well as that all-important final column we talked about: the balance, what you have left at the end of each month. The bigger your balance (while meeting your needs and priorities), the better. Keep in mind, though, that a checking account is not the same as a savings account. A savings account offers interest earnings to inspire you to *keep* your money *in* the account, not just manage it.

Managing Money in the Workplace

By now you may feel fairly savvy about handling personal finances. You've learned what to expect to see in your paycheck (or direct deposit pay notice) and its itemized deductions. But suppose, then, that on your first day of work you learn that you will have some financial responsibilities in the workplace! Don't panic! Learning a few simple terms will give you a working knowledge of workplace money management.

An employee's financial responsibilities will differ greatly not only from workplace to workplace but also from one job to the next. You're already aware of the purpose of a balance sheet. Other documents you may encounter are expense logs and transaction receipts. An expense log is used to help a company keep track of what everyone is spending money on, from a bag of coffee or box of rubber bands to booking a conference room. A transaction receipt is just what it sounds like: a receipt that you will give to a client when a payment is made.

As in other professions, financial responsibilities in the health care field may vary greatly from position to position, and they generally include on-the-job training. These responsibilities might include the preferred ways of logging expenses, keeping inventory of office or clinic supplies, carrying out paperwork and authorization procedures properly, and following accounting's rules within your group or department.

What Is Credit—and Do You Need It?

In grade school you may have learned that William Shakespeare wrote, "Neither a borrower nor a lender be." This is still a good way to keep friendships free of drama, but eventually, to function in today's larger economy, you're going to need to establish good credit. No doubt you've heard that expression; nearly everyone now has a credit report. But what is credit? And do you really need it?

◐ JOURNALING 10-8

- What do you think of when you hear the term "bad credit"? What do you think it means? How do you think bad credit happens?
- Do you know what your own credit score is? How does one get "good" credit?

Credit, in short, is your financial reputation. It's important because it tells others whether they can trust you to repay your loans. Your credit report is created and kept by a company called a credit bureau, which studies patterns in your borrowing history to produce a profile of your performance and generates a credit score.

Your credit score is made up of your payment history (e.g., utilities, rent, car payments), the types of credit you have (e.g., loans or credit cards), and how many times someone such as a credit card company

or prospective lender has asked for your credit score. Making a lot of applications for credit cards, for example, can negatively affect your score.

Who Checks Your Credit Score?

You may not have asked to have a credit history or credit score, but because most of us have one whether we like it or not, it's important to carefully manage any loans you have taken out and to honor the terms of your contracts (e.g., paying your utilities, being a good renter, etc.). Banks and lenders are not the only agencies looking at your credit score. Insurance companies now assess your credit before deciding whether to insure you, and good credit is frequently required for approval for employment or for leasing an apartment (Figure 10-12).

How Do You Establish Good Credit?

The first step is to get a job to prove that you can handle bills. For most people, the first "creditor" is either a utility company or rental agency (sometimes, at least the first time, co-signed with someone who does have a good credit record). By paying utilities and rent fully on time, you can establish the beginnings of a good credit record. Another strategy, slightly more risky, is to establish good credit with a credit card company. This works fine as long as you keep your spending under tight control. The purpose, remember, is to establish a good reputation for paying back a small loan. If you keep your first purchases small and promptly pay them back in full, opening a credit card account can be a fairly fast and easy way to prove that you're responsible and start establishing good credit.

FIGURE 10-12 Good credit is often required for approval for employment or for leasing an apartment (Copyright © thinkstock.com).

Credit Card Pitfalls

Useful though they may be, credit cards can also be financially dangerous if you use them excessively or let yourself depend on them. Fees and interest charged over time can add up fast and will put you in debt, exactly what you are trying to avoid. And the longer you take to pay something off, the more it can end up costing you—we're talking thousands of dollars, in many cases. So it's important to purchase something small and manageable, something you know that you can pay off promptly without any financial stress. You want to establish credit, but it doesn't take much to do that. Once you've demonstrated your reliability, ease off the credit card use. Use the card enough to keep it active (it doesn't take much), but make sure to pay each expenditure back promptly. A good rule of thumb when you're starting out is to ensure that you can be debt free if you need to, as far as your credit cards are concerned, at the end of every month.

Of course, once you've taken out a car or home loan, credit cards become less necessary in establishing or maintaining your credit. Once they've established good credit, many people destroy their credit cards. Others are able to discipline themselves to keep one only for genuine emergencies so they can avoid creating debt. Though it can be challenging to carry out some forms of business, such as purchasing airline tickets, without a credit card, it can be done.

? WHAT IF?

- *What if you had just one credit card that you tried to keep for emergencies? What, for you, would that mean?*

Personal Loans—Safety Net or Danger Zone?

Student Loans

You are likely familiar with student loans, but these loans vary widely, and some are much safer than others in terms of accumulating less debt.

Federal student loans. Depending on your situation, several kinds of federal education loans are available to you as a student. The terms of these loans are subject to change and include limits on the amount you may borrow. They tend to be low-interest loans for people who can demonstrate significant financial

need. (Interest is a fee in excess of the loan amount and is a way to pay for the loan service itself.) Some federal loans don't cover all school expenses, so supplemental loans are available to students or parents to cover these additional costs.

Some federal loans offer a deferment, which means that your repayment is postponed until you graduate, with no accruing (accumulating) interest charged to you during that time. In some cases, you may be eligible to apply for "forbearance," in which repayment is postponed but interest still accrues. Most federal student loans require complete repayment within 10 years, but there are usually a variety of repayment plans to choose from.

Private loans. Students who do not qualify for federal education loans may be eligible for private loans. These loans, which carry higher interest rates than federal loans do, include institutional loans (given directly by the school itself to its students) and private and state loans, which help students who do not qualify for federal assistance or whose other loans are not enough to cover the cost of their education. Although it's always important to read the terms of something as important as a loan, it's crucial in the case of private or institutional loans because of higher or complex interest rates. Remember, too: The longer the loan's payback period, the more interest you'll pay over time.

Consolidation loans. These loans can sound pretty good—especially if you have credit card debts *and* student loans—because they enable you to combine two or more existing loans to create a new loan with a fixed interest rate (one that doesn't go up over time while you're paying it back). In addition, a consolidation loan usually gives you a much longer period, often 30 years, in which to pay back the loan. However, always use caution when considering a consolidation loan. Read the fine print to see what might be required from you for collateral (something the lender will keep if you bail out), as well as how much more interest you might be paying over such an extended period.

Student loans, like any other type of credit, are a source of individual debt—not a good way to start out your professional life. It's important to pay student loans back to save your credit score. Before you sign anything, be sure to ask about options offered by the lender to someone struggling to pay back a loan. Defaulting on a loan is not always allowed and can ruin your credit for decades. Also remember that student loans cannot be wiped away in bankruptcy.

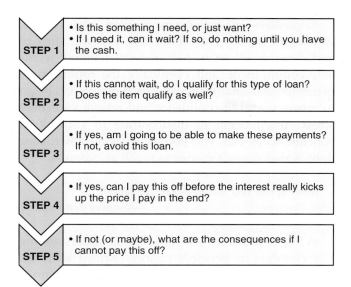

STEP 1	• Is this something I need, or just want? • If I need it, can it wait? If so, do nothing until you have the cash.
STEP 2	• If this cannot wait, do I qualify for this type of loan? Does the item qualify as well?
STEP 3	• If yes, am I going to be able to make these payments? If not, avoid this loan.
STEP 4	• If yes, can I pay this off before the interest really kicks up the price I pay in the end?
STEP 5	• If not (or maybe), what are the consequences if I cannot pay this off?

FIGURE 10-13 The Five-Step Decision Chain.

FIGURE 10-14 A good used car costs a lot less than a new car, and buying one also saves you from the depreciation in value to which a new car is subject the moment you drive it off the lot (Copyright © thinkstock.com).

The Five-Step Decision Chain

As a rule, it's wisest not to borrow money unless, or until, you really need to. Before taking on any kind of loan, ask yourself a few key questions, such as those listed in the Five-Step Decision Chain (Figure 10-13).

A Word About Car Loans

So what types of loans are worthwhile when you're just starting out? Well, if you're just starting out, it's probably going to be quite a while before you borrow money for a home. (This type of loan is called a mortgage.) But some people need a car for work. If you don't have access to good public transportation, a car loan *may* become your first, or next, big loan—but you may be able to avoid this. So when is it appropriate to apply for a car loan? You can figure this out with a few steps:

1. **Calculate** carefully how much you can afford to pay for a car. Be sure to take into account related expenses such as gas, oil, insurance, maintenance, and parking.
2. **Consider a cash-only purchase of a good used car first.** Not only does a used car cost a lot less than a new one, but a new car depreciates rapidly in value the moment you drive it off the lot. Buying a reliable used car saves you from that significant loss (Figure 10-14).
3. **If you decide you do need to take out a loan,** either apply for preapproval at a credit union (which usually offers the lowest possible rates) or see whether your current bank offers discounted loans

for existing customers. Once you have this information, compare these rates with the dealer's rates before choosing.
4. **Whether you pay cash or take out a loan,** once you think you have found your car, invest in a prepurchase inspection by a reputable mechanic to get feedback on the car's condition.
5. **Finally, if you do take out a car loan,** pay it back as soon as possible, but be careful: Check to ensure that there is no penalty for paying back too soon and, if there is such a penalty, weigh it against the interest you're being charged on the payment plan.

Lending Money

Many of us have done it: lent money to a friend or relative. However, you may know someone who habitually borrows large sums but never seems quite able to pay you back. Such people may need help learning to budget. They may also be a little too comfortable being in financial trouble. Lending too much in these situations can put you—not the borrower—at risk if it means that you, in turn, become unable to pay your own bills because you are waiting for someone else to pay you. At that point, the borrower has also become your greatest credit risk. Lending money can be the compassionate and moral thing to do; just judge wisely before you do it.

Get Out—and Stay Out—of Debt

All of this is about establishing good credit. But what if you are already in debt? Go back to that balance sheet we talked about. Sit down and make a plan for paying off your debts, a little at a time.

* Begin by weighing your income against those necessary expenses we talked about earlier, then look at your balance.
* From that information, assign what you can to paying back each of your debts as you can. Don't let yourself be discouraged if you can't pay much; most creditors are willing to work with someone who is trying and paying at least a minimal amount.
* Be sure to talk with your creditors. Explain your situation and express an honest desire to pay them back.
* In the case of debt such as child support, once you have work you can request that a portion be automatically removed from each paycheck to contribute to the support of your child; this withholding is called *garnishment* of your wages. In some cases, when a partner neglects to do this, the courts have done it for him or her. Not only will you look more responsible if you initiate payments yourself first, you will also make a much better impression on your employer.

Regardless of the payment plan you choose, commit to a plan that you know you can stick to and don't dwell on it. Just make a genuine, workable commitment, and eventually the routine payments (even if small) you make each month will begin to renew your self-confidence and relieve your debt stress. You'll begin to demonstrate to yourself in concrete ways that, yes, you *are* working down your debt. Speed doesn't matter as much as progress.

Never spend your money before you have it.
—Thomas Jefferson

A big step toward job readiness is understanding key concepts in personal finance. Armed with the skills and tools needed to create and maintain a budget, save money, and build both your savings and your credit record, you will be well equipped to take on the challenges of becoming an independent professional. Financial responsibility is only intimidating if you've never tried it before. Once you start taking control of your money and planning your financial future, you'll feel more empowered and self-confident.

CASE STUDY 10-5
Getting Off the Tightrope

Ava doesn't have enough money to pay for the books for her dental assisting classes, and there just doesn't seem to be enough time to figure out how. She picked up Chinese food last night before collecting her daughter from the babysitter, and now she sits down at the kitchen table with a bowl of fried rice and calls her friend Brigitte to borrow money.

"Again?" Brigitte says. "Honey, I just don't know."

Ava calls her brother Jonah and asks him.

After a long pause, Jonah sighs. "This time I'm charging you interest if you don't pay me back this month. I'm getting tired of this."

Ava's tired of it, too. She complains to her mother, who says, "That's just the way life is. There's just never enough money for a person to get by." She asks whether Ava has any cigarettes, and Ava ends up handing over half of her last pack.

Later, Ava picks up the money from Jonah, who says, "I'm serious, girl. You need to start budgeting your money."

"That's easy to say," she says, "but I'm not sure where to start."

"With that," he says, gently tapping her hand, which holds a cigarette. Smiling sadly, Ava drops the cigarette and tamps it out. "Smoking," she says, "is the only pleasure I have."

"Change that," he replies.

Jonah helps Ava set up a budget. He also reminds her of her assets and how to use them to encourage herself. For instance, because she's so sociable, funny, and warm, Ava has held the same job as a front office medical assistant for two years. Her boss and co-workers like her. She's smart and attractive. She's getting good grades in night school.

"Stop and appreciate what you have going for you once in a while," Jonah says. "Sometimes we spend money just to feel better about ourselves. If you remind yourself how good you're doing, it can curb your urge to spend for the sake of spending. You'll think, 'Yeah, I don't really need that to feel good about me.'"

Ava complains that because she's going to school and has a young daughter, plus home responsibilities, it's difficult for her to plan.

"I get that," Jonah says. "I used to struggle with budgeting." He has a job in construction that pays pretty well, but he also has a wife, three children, a mortgage, and his youngest child has asthma that is not covered by his health insurance because it's a preexisting condition. These expenses eat up most of Jonah's extra money.

"But I've taken some steps to save," he tells Ava. "For one thing, Natasha and I gave up smoking together. And instead of picking up noodles on the way home, we make our own! You can buy frozen veggies or chicken already cut up and just throw them over a bowl of rice or noodles a lot cheaper than you can get it at a restaurant. And we just drink tap water instead of bottled. Figure out where your money goes—there must be something you can cut out."

Over the next month, Ava keeps a diary, tracking what she spends each week against what she has left in the bank or at home.

"Just doing this makes me feel more in control," she tells Brigitte. "I've never bothered to keep track before," she says.

"So what are you doing differently now?" Brigitte asks.

"Well, making my own coffee and packing more lunches," Ava says. "I actually like brown-bagging it. And Snickers—"

"What about your Snickers? They're your guilty pleasure."

"Well, I stopped getting them out of the vending machine at school," Ava says. "They're a lot cheaper if I buy a bag of little ones and take two with me in my backpack. And two little ones instead of one vending machine size bar means I'm saving a *few* calories."

Brigitte laughs. "Multi-savings!"

Ava says, "You know, Mom's always said budgets are a waste of time, and I used to agree with her. It was, like, what was the point? I'm broke. But now I can see where my money is going, and some of the stuff I put down money for? I don't even really like it."

"Like what?" Brigitte asks.

"Drive-through breakfast biscuits. They're hard and nasty—I was just buying them because they were convenient."

"What do you eat now instead?"

"Toast. I love toast … with peanut butter!"

Brigitte blinks at Ava. She's trying not to laugh.

By the end of the month, Ava is saving enough that she not only pays Jonah back but also finds that she's still got a little money left over.

QUESTIONS FOR THOUGHT AND REFLECTION

1. Why do you think Ava lacked confidence in her ability to save?
2. What is the main advantage Ava has gained from keeping track of what she spends?
3. Are there any secondary advantages to Ava's budgeting?
4. What were the root causes of Ava's money management problems?

Down a Dark Road

Sophie has big plans. She has a new job as a surgical technologist and wants to take her little boy, Jack, on a biking trip—but first she has to buy the bikes, one for each of them. On her first day of work, Ms. Underwood, the human resources coordinator, has Sophie fill out a Form W-4, among other papers.

"What's this?" Sophie says.

"It's a form that lets you control how much income tax is withheld from your paycheck each month," Ms. Underwood tells her. "Do you have any kids? You can have us take out less for taxes so you have more money to use for them every month."

"What if I keep too much?" Sophie asks.

"You may have to pay the rest at the end of the year when you do your income taxes."

"Yikes," Sophie says. "Who wants that?"

"Well," Ms. Underwood says, "some people prefer it that way. They may need access to as much for their day-to-day expenses as they can get, because they have kids, and they just deal with whatever they owe when the time comes."

"What if I pay too much?" Sophie asks.

Ms. Underwood smiles again. "No problem! You'll get it back as a refund."

"Now *that's* smart!" Sophie says. "Take out the maximum!"

"Well, it's not really fr—"

"Sign me up!" Sophie says. "Take out the max! Next question!"

Ms. Underwood shrugs, then continues: "Okay, we have a nice 401(k) plan here at work. I'm sure you'd like to take advantage of that?"

"What is it?"

"A retirement plan. If you put just a little something in, the company will match—"

"Retirement?" Sophie laughs. "Are you kidding? I'm only 27! I'm kind of young to start taking money out for retirement, especially with a little boy to raise."

"Well …" says Ms. Underwood.

"Anything else?" Sophie asks.

"No," Ms. Underwood says, shuffling through Sophie's documents. "No, it looks like you've filled out everything else just fine."

"Great!" Sophie stands. "Thanks for your help."

"You're welcome!" Ms. Underwood says. "And welcome to the team! I hope you like it here."

Sophie looks out the window as she pulls on her jacket. "It's gorgeous out there today, isn't it? I think this weekend I'll take my son to the amusement park."

"Oh, that's nice. I used to take my kids there once a year."

"Once a year?" Sophie says. "Oh, I hope I take Jack there more than that. Look at all the money I'll be taking home every month—$2500!"

"$2500? Well, not exactly. That's your *gross*—"

Sophie interrupts: "Ms. Underwood, I hope you have a fabulous weekend! I just got an inspiration!"

Within an hour, Sophie is at her father's house.

"You want how much—$600?" he says. "Sophie, that's a lot of money!"

"But I have a new job, Dad—I'm getting $2500 a month."

Her father is skeptical: "I'm retired, Sophie, on a low fixed income." He turns to face her. "How soon would you pay me back?"

"At the end of the month, Dad, seriously. I'll get $2500, and I'll pay you back out of that before I even spend the first dime."

He studies her a moment.

"Please, Dad? It's for your grandson. He's a good kid. He deserves this."

"All right," he mumbles with a tired smile. "Come back tomorrow, and I'll have it for you."

By the next weekend, Sophie has used the loan to surprise nine-year-old Jack: two beautiful new bikes, along with new helmets, gloves, and knee pads.

"Wow, Mom!" Jack exclaims. "Oh man! Mom, you're the best!"

"And that's not all, Jackie boy," says Sophie. "You and I are going camping with our new bikes out at the state park. We're going to hit those bike trails Saturday *and* Sunday!"

Jack is thrilled. So is Sophie.

Over the next three weeks, Sophie sits up at night paying bills and counting out her money till the end of the month. She's not sure she's going to make it. At the end of the month, she rips open her pay envelope—and suddenly realizes that she can't pay her father back yet. She sees the "$2500" up in the corner of her pay stub, but then there are all those deductions. Under "Net Pay" she sees that she's fallen far short of what she expected.

But things just get tighter. Sophie's miscalculation and her failure to plan ahead and set some goals are both catching up with her. After six months, she borrows more money from her father.

"Sophie," he says. "We're both going to sink if you keep this up. Let's sit down together Friday night and compare our budgets."

On Friday night Sophie and her father sit down to go over their budgets and make a plan to help them both pull out of this.

"Here's the deal," Dad says. "That $600 has sort of put me in trouble with utilities, honey. Now, if you don't have enough saved by the end of the year, I have an idea. I know it's possible to withdraw early from your 401(k) in case of true hardship—"

"Dad—"

"—and your old man not being able to pay for his diabetes medications by then, and you running into deep trouble like you are now … well, I think you can get what's called a hardship withdrawal—"

"Dad—"

"I saw from the papers you brought home when you got the job that your 401(k) plan will allow that—"

"Dad!"

He looks up. "What is it?"

"Dad, I didn't join the 401(k) plan."

"What? Why not?"

"I'm too young!"

"Oh, Sophie!" He rubs his face distractedly. "That's a real bargain, Sophie. A guaranteed double-your-money kind of offer."

"I know, Dad, but I'm young. I have other priorities."

"Oh, geez." He looks around the kitchen, worried. "Oh geez. Okay."

Dad looks at his daughter. He tries to smile. "Okay. Okay, that's fine. This will work. Let's move on. Now, how much are you putting away each month in savings?"

Sophie turns red. "Well. I'd have to look at my pay stubs."

"Oh?" her dad says. "You're in the company savings plan."

"Kind of!" she brightens up.

"What do you mean, 'Kind of'? Sophie, you have a kid. We talked about the company savings plans, and you said you'd—"

"Dad. I've got this," she reassures him. "I'm saving."

"Good. How?"

"I'm having the maximum withheld from my check each month. At the end of this year I'll be able to pay you back!"

"From your savings account?"

"No, something better, goofball. A big fat refund check!"

"That's it? That's your savings plan?"

"Dad," Sophie says. "It's free money."

"Oh geez," her father says.

QUESTIONS FOR THOUGHT AND REFLECTION

1. How would you help Sophie understand that a refund check is not "free money"?

2. What are *two* disadvantages of not applying for a child tax credit and instead withholding the maximum amount?

3. What would have been a smarter way to use the excess amount Sophie expects to get back as a refund? How could it have made a bigger difference in her situation now?

4. Describe what potential savings Sophie has lost out on by not contributing to a 401(k) plan this year. Use real numbers as examples of what she's lost.

⭐ EXPERIENTIAL EXERCISE

1. Interview three people you know who seem to be doing a pretty good job of saving, investing, or saving for retirement. Make a chart showing (1) what's worked best for each of these people; (2) what one thing each learned that has helped the most in saving; and (3) the one thing each wishes he or she hadn't done.

2. Test out one or two of the investment tools in Box 10-8. Which was most helpful, and why? What, if anything, do you feel is missing from this tool?

3. Identify someone who has used a professional financial advisor. Find out (1) at what stage in the person's financial planning he or she consulted the professional and (2) whether the person felt that it was worth the investment.

4. You've probably received emails or seen Internet ads that offer to give you your credit score right now for free. Try to find your own credit score. How easy is it? Can this information be obtained for free, or would you have to pay money to really find out?

5. Most lending agencies can give you a brochure or breakdown sheet that outlines the terms of their loans. Choose something fairly expensive that you'd like to have, then investigate how and where you would purchase each item on credit or through a loan. Looking at the terms and conditions for the loan and how much it might end up costing in the long run, apply the Five-Step Decision Chain set forth in the text. Is the purchase worth taking out a loan at this time?

🔄 CROSS CURRENTS WITH OTHER SOFT SKILLS

SETTING GOALS AND PLANNING ACTIONS: You've already acquired some strategic tools for (1) how to establish good credit, (2) how to save for the future in general, (3) how to get out of debt if you're in it, and even (4) how to plan for your retirement. The task now is to set your goals: Which of these four aspects of money management is most pertinent to your situation right now? Choose a reasonable, realistic goal that takes your financial needs into account, then set down your plan of action. (pp. 286-291)

TAKING ACCOUNTABILITY: Establishing good credit does more than give you some borrowing power when you really need it. Remember: Landlords and employers alike now routinely run credit checks to see how reliable an applicant is. Taking responsibility for your financial obligations and your spending behaviors affects much more than just your financial bottom line. (pp. 333-336)

Bibliography

"How the Poor, the Middle Class, and the Rich Spend Their Money." *Money* at NPR.org: http://www.npr.org/sections/money/2012/08/01/157664524/how-the-poor-the-middle-class-and-the-rich-spend-their-money.

CHAPTER 11

Enhancing Your Promotability

- Learn how to form a positive relationship with your manager.
- Develop strategies for handling difficult conversations with your manager.
- Understand the benefits of taking a accountability for your actions.
- Identify what teams you belong to.
- List ways you can maximize your role on your teams.
- Explain the benefits of joining a professional organization.
- Place research in the context of your practice.

Great things await you in your future, but you will have to work for them. Fortunately, there are actions you can take to help advance yourself and your career. In this chapter, we address the importance of developing a positive working relationship with your supervisor. You can start by establishing a record of personal accomplishments and by taking personal accountability not only for your work but also for your success. Expand this notion by thinking not just in terms of your own accomplishments but in terms of those of the entire team. Health care is a team sport, and you want to distinguish yourself as a contributing member of every team you are part of. Finally, to excel in your career, you need to play an active role in your particular profession.

There is no shortcut to anywhere worth going.

—Beverly Sills

Thinking Critically

Begin challenging your own assumptions.
Your assumptions are your windows on the world.
Scrub them off every once in awhile, or the light won't come in.

—Alan Alda

LEARNING OBJECTIVE 1: THINKING CRITICALLY

- Recognize the value of critical thinking and how it can advance your career.
- Challenge yourself to gather in-depth information and learn as much as possible about your profession.
- Train yourself to observe critically.

- Develop focus, objectivity, inference, and selectiveness when approaching all situations.
- Identify the problem, issue, concern, or question being discussed or considered in any given situation.
- Understand why you are thinking about the problem; what accomplishment will it help you with? In health care, this answer involves knowing what to believe or do in many situations.
- Take notice of your own ideas about an issue, and how they change your thinking compared to another person's view. Strive to be fair-minded.
- Become a problem solver using the steps to critical thinking.

Thinking critically is a skill acquired through attention to detail and intellectual reasoning. To develop critical thinking skills, we must have a solid foundation in the basics of our chosen profession. Critical thinkers stick to intellectual standards and remain logical and fair. They are clear and concise when speaking, reading, writing, and listening. Critical thinking involves thinking through all possible outcomes, each with their possible courses of action, like a game of chess. When you have critical thinking skills, you are able to work independently and to know what is required or expected of you, without being told. You are not task-oriented; you have become a self-starter.

In health care, critical thinking is essential. It is the "thinking on your feet" skill that is required in many situations relating to patient care. Critical thinking is knowing what to believe or do in any given scenario. This way of thinking can help to reduce confusion and stress in the workplace by giving you clarity and confidence, thus increasing your value as a team member.

As a student, you emerge from school armed with a diploma and a well of knowledge, only to find out that the facts you were taught in school do not always apply in the world of work. In school, you learn how to prepare for examinations by studying facts and mastering skills. The problem is that, while you learned rote facts, you may not have been given an opportunity to apply those facts to health care scenarios and develop the critical thinking skills that will bridge the gap between textbook and patient. This section is designed to help you develop critical thinking skills you can use to find fulfillment in the workplace. Learning all you can about your profession is the first step; critical thinking is knowledge-based!

Review Box 11-1 for the six steps of critical thinking. Reflect on these steps as you read this section.

BOX 11-1

The Six Steps of Critical Thinking

1. Gather—Collect all the information you can.
2. Understand—Formulate ideas about what the information means.
3. Apply—Use the knowledge in a real situation.
4. Analyze—Break down the ideas into ordered parts; break down relevant facts and discard irrelevant facts.
5. Synthesize—Put the parts back together to form a whole, or combine the many into one.
6. Evaluate—Come to a conclusion about what you have heard or read. Always do this *last* to avoid snap judgments.

? WHAT IF?

What if a friend or classmate was struggling with the tasks assigned to her at an extern site you both share, and was constantly relying on you for instruction?

How can you help your classmate to think tasks through for herself and then decide how to perform them?

Will you be able to observe and focus effectively if she depends on you for information? Will her uncertainty help you to learn as well?

Will a prospective employer view you and you classmate differently, even though your education was the same? What is the difference between critical thinkers versus task-oriented performers?

The Power of Observation

Being observant is a habit that can be developed with practice and mindfulness. In the workplace, employees who are observant are more easily trained, perform their jobs better, and are more productive while working. It is easy to see why employers value the observant employee.

In the fields of observation, chance favors only the prepared mind.

—Louis Pasteur

Concentration

Develop the skill of observation by testing yourself each day. Practice the following skills: focusing, noticing, and remembering. Find someone around you,

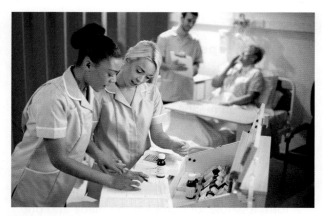

FIGURE 11-1 A new hospital worker learns proper medicine dispensing procedures while observing a coworker (Copyright © istock.com).

inspect a photo, or listen to an overheard conversation. *Focus* on details that stand out for some reason or another, and then *notice* why the details are interesting or strange. Take your time with each section of this activity to ensure you do not stop observing too soon. When you are training your brain to observe, speed is not a factor. You are more likely to make a good observation and *remember* as you concentrate more thoroughly on the object of your examination.

The power of observation is used by employees to develop effective relationships with their co-workers (Figure 11-1). You are likely to emulate others in the same position in the work environment to find the appropriate level of assertiveness, humor, and familiarity with others in the work environment. Choose a person in your work environment that you respect. Observe their qualities and how they deal with different patients and professional situations. Watching others who are successful is a key step toward developing your own critical thinking.

In Focus

Are you focus-challenged? Even if you think you are not, the hectic pace of health care and the urgency of certain medical situations may confound your ability to narrow your attention. Learning to focus on the matter at hand requires good observational, concentration, and communication skills. You may have to become skilled at silent signals to keep others from interrupting your concentration. Try avoiding eye contact with others outside of your focus until you have completed the task at hand. Avoid interrupting others, and observe how other successful co-workers

keep their focus. After an issue has been identified and the key features noted, your focus may then be diverted. Thus, your focus of attention can zoom in, and zoom out, depending on where you need to place your attention at any given moment.

Logical and Reasoned Thinking

As a health care professional, you are a scientist, committed to reasoning and the scientific method of inquiry. Although intuition will develop after a long time in practice, the decision you make and the outcomes you pursue must be based on logic and sound thinking.

Maintaining Objectivity

Education and reading are the best tools to open up your mind to possibilities beyond those you have already encountered in your own life. Learning about many different scenarios in school may have helped to broaden the way you think. How do you use this broader thinking to keep your main objective in mind? First, grasp onto facts, rather than subjective impressions. Don't allow personal bias to make decisions before all the facts are known. Practice removing your automated mental shortcut shoes at the door and let your mind be free of stereotyping and preconceived ideas at work. If you are "barefoot" in your thinking, you will watch where you step and become more selective before reaching a conclusion.

Inference

Inference, which improves over time, is the ability to draw on past experiences to guide you through current issues and situations. In contrast with biased thinking, inference draws on successful resolutions to past problems and does not narrow to only one incident. It may combine many past events to help solve today's issue. Using a prior situation and its outcome is helpful to problem solving. It will give you a basis for what to do and what not to do in health care.

As a new employee, you may be unfocused and overwhelmed by the many inputs and trivial details you encounter. As your experience grows, so will your confidence, objectivity, and organization skills. Employers value inference and experience. As a new employee, you should highlight your willingness to learn and be shaped and molded by the new input. An employer will value you when you build on each day to infer the routine for the days ahead.

Problem Solving

Critical thinkers solve problems more quickly than those who have rote memorization of facts (Figure 11-2). In health care, this paid problem solving is invaluable. Start small to develop problem solving skills. Watch for issues that arise during a normal day and silently come up with possible solutions to the problems. Do your solutions match the outcomes you observe? If not, can you draw parallels between the solution used and your logic? Where are they different? Practice considering acceptable outcomes to train your brain into a better resolution station.

Learning to think critically in health care will require some effort at first. Each day, we must be diligent about observing, focusing, maintaining objectivity, and building on past experiences. The benefit to putting in the time at the start of your career lies in fewer mistakes, greater confidence, higher salary, and above all quality patient care—the goal of any health care worker. Still, mistakes are also a part of how we learn. Keep your focus when dealing with new situations, and base your actions on solid concepts you have learned. Trust yourself with the basics. Confidence in problem solving will build on successes you achieve daily in your career.

Decision Making

In many health care situations, the decisions we make can change or save a life. Learning to trust our problem solving skills is the first step in making good decisions. Once the problem has been identified, use all relevant information to make a decision, and try to filter out irrelevant or unimportant facts. Choose the most likely solutions and then assess the risks of each outcome if you were to choose that solution. This process of elimination is a hallmark of your critical thinking.

When your co-workers begin to trust your decision-making skills, you are given more responsibility and respect, which translates into good performance reviews and increases in income. This, in turn, increases the level of critical thinking that becomes part of your work reputation. Your co-workers will not feel they have to "carry you" when times are busy or rushed, and you will gain a new confidence that is bound to show.

FIGURE 11-2 A paramedic and a firefighter rely on critical thinking skills while administering proper emergency care to a crash victim (Copyright © istock.com).

Knowing a great deal is not the same as being smart; intelligence is not information alone but also judgment, the manner in which information is collected and used.

—Carl Sagan

CASE STUDY 11-1
A Thought Bubble

Sara was a night shift nurse at the local hospital and nearing the end of a long night on her floor. Her feet were aching. As she entered her last patient's room, all that was on her mind was a hot bubble bath. The patient's wife began speaking as soon as she entered the room.

"Please … my husband … his color is so bad … the last nurse said it was the narcotic and not to worry, but …" said Mrs. Walsh.

Sara pulled up Mr. Walsh's chart on the monitor and read the last entry, then assessed the patient. She was alarmed at the bluish tinge around the patient's mouth and nail beds, and at the difficulty she had rousing him for a few words. She entered the note that the patient was recovering from surgery, and that the previous nurse had felt the wife was a bit of a worry wart. Sara knew the strong narcotic he was on for pain could make him groggy, and looking at the history she found nothing to indicate a breathing problem. Sara decided to alert the physician on call, but was afraid the doctor would ridicule her for waking him and mistaking narcotic suppression for a pulmonary problem. She also knew she would not be leaving on time today.

The doctor arrived in 15 minutes, and Mr. Walsh was found to be suffering from an embolism that required immediate treatment. The doctor gave Sara high praise for her observation skills, and Mrs. Walsh gave Sara a great big hug. Mr. Walsh sent a gratitude card after leaving the hospital when his wife described Sara's diligence.

QUESTIONS FOR THOUGHT AND REFLECTION

1. Why do you think Sara was more successful at treating Mr. Walsh than the nurse before her?
2. What are the factors that were against her decision to call the physician? For her decision?
3. If you were Sara, would you have done the same thing? List the critical thinking steps you would take.
4. How will the physician and other co-workers feel about Sara after this situation?
5. What if Sara, had given in to the desire to just go home and soak in the tub? How will the patient and the physician be changed by Sara's actions?

Down a Dark Road

Amanda was thrilled to be hired by the dentist near her house after completing her externship with a dentist many miles away. The commute was going to be much shorter, and she was really looking forward to making some new friends in her new office. The practice was owned by a dentist husband and wife team, and there were two other dental assistants already on staff.

Amanda was nervous and excited on her first day—she couldn't keep the smile from her face. She greeted her new co-workers and shadowed Doreen, the assistant who had been with the practice for 20 years. After the first procedure, Amanda was feeling confused. Doreen did not do anything the way that Amanda had been taught in school, and her externship office had seemed much more modern. She recalled her dental assisting instructor saying something about modern verses older techniques, but she couldn't recall what her instructor had said to do when faced with a co-worker stuck in outdated practices. Amanda worried about offending Doreen, but after watching her

disinfect a room she could not help but blurt out, "That's not how we did it in school." Amanda then proceeded to list facts she had been taught.

Amanda felt better that she had said what was on her mind, but she noticed that Doreen began moving faster and Amanda was unable to follow each step. That afternoon, Amanda knew she might have made a critical error in judgment when Doreen pushed her to "do it your way." Amanda quickly discovered that the supplies needed to perform a procedure as she had been instructed were not present in the office. Instead of doing it her way, she was unable to do it at all.

QUESTIONS FOR THOUGHT AND REFLECTION

1. What was Amanda's critical error in judgment?
2. If you were Amanda, what would you have done? List your answers in terms of critical thinking steps.
3. What should Amanda do to show that she might still be the right person for the job?

1. Observe students around you on exam day. Spend a few minutes noticing nervous behaviors. At the next exam, see if those behaviors are the same, or if some have begun to master their test taking jitters. What can you focus, notice, and remember?
2. Train your brain: find a focus or memory game on the internet, or try a few puzzles with more than 250 pieces to see what you enjoy. Keeping the mind active helps to train thought.
3. Enhance your knowledge of your chosen profession by tracing the pattern of something tiny that contributes to a whole, such as a drop of blood in the circulatory system or a bacterium in the mouth. Focus on what interests you to keep your attention fresh.

CROSS CURRENTS WITH OTHER SOFT SKILLS

ADOPTING A POSITIVE MENTAL ATTITUDE: Your attitude can cloud your thinking and affect your ability to think critically. (pp. 2-11)

READING AND SPEAKING BODY LANGUAGE: Your inferences and observations are based in large part on the body language of others. Note that in health care, body language is often substituted for spoken word to keep out of the patient's earshot. (pp. 277-284)

FOLLOWING RULES AND REGULATIONS: Any critical thinking decision should be made with the rules and regulations of the facility in the forefront. (pp. 291-297)

VOWING TO BE DRUG FREE AND UNIMPAIRED: This is the most essential step to allow critical thinking to be effective. (pp. 197-203)

Talking to Your Manager or Supervisor

LEARNING OBJECTIVE 2: TALKING TO YOUR MANAGER OR SUPERVISOR

- Have a strategy for developing a positive relationship with your boss.
- Handle difficult conversations with your manager.
- Develop solutions to problems.
- Use your supervisor as an advisor and source of feedback.

- Manage the performance evaluation process.
- Deal effectively with a difficult boss.

> *To avoid criticism, say nothing, do nothing, and be nothing.*
> —Aristotle

One of your most important tasks on your first day at work is to begin building a positive relationship with your supervisor. Your supervisor is extremely important to your success, as you are to hers. Only your clinical competence, hard work, and attitude are more important. As you manage your workload, your effectiveness will reflect positively on her. In turn, gaining experience on a successful team makes *you* look good.

Managing Up

Many new employees are intimidated by anybody who is in a position higher than theirs. They are shy, insecure, or fearful around their supervisor, and they seek to avoid rather than engage their manager. This is a mistake that can set their careers back. Your boss is just another person with responsibilities and pressures, just like you. Your boss wants to quickly feel she can depend on you. Consciously overcome any fears and plan to have frequent positive interactions with your supervisor.

> *And the day came when the risk it took to remain tight inside the bud was more painful than the risk it took to blossom.*
> —Anais Nin

← JOURNALING 11-3

Describe the perfect boss. Consider how you would want to use him or her as an asset. Include his or her role and influence in your organization, communication style, and how he or she could motivate you to give your highest performance.

Bring Solutions to Your Supervisor

Pretend you are a supervisor. Two employees knock on your door at the same time and want to talk about the same issue. Which one are you more eager to listen to? Employee A or Employee B?

Employee A: "We have a big problem."

Employee B: "I think I see a way we can avoid facing a big mess next month."

When you bring a problem to your manager, make sure to include solutions. While your manager gets paid to find solutions and make good decisions, that doesn't mean she is a dumping ground for your problems. Consider the following questions when you encounter a problem at work: Is this a problem you can solve yourself? Are you authorized and empowered to solve this problem? If you are unsure, ask your supervisor for clarification. Otherwise, solve it.

Your manager wants you to communicate with him about the problems you encounter, but he will value you very highly if you simply let him know what the problem was and what you did about it. If you are seen as a problem-solver, you will be empowered and maybe even promoted to solve more of them. You also empower your boss, freeing him up to concentrate on problems that only he can deal with. Even then, you can still make his job easier by presenting a problem in as helpful a way as possible, employing these three tactics:

* Bring the problem to your manager's attention as soon as you become aware of it. Many problems can be easily dealt with early but become difficult if action is delayed.
* Gather as many facts about the problem as you can. If you are unclear on the facts, investigate their accuracy before you inform your supervisor. Revising the facts later can be difficult and damaging when a solution built on false information has to be reversed.
* Be objective, not emotional.

By being thoughtful and creative, you can become your manager's partner and advisor in solving workplace problems, instead of being part of the problem yourself.

Seek Your Manager's Guidance

Your manager is there to offer you training, guidance, feedback, criticism, and encouragement. Rather than waiting for your manager to bestow these blessings on you, it will be easier for your manager if you seek them out, to help guide you in making better decisions, getting more work done, and achieving the mission of your employer. In Figure 11-3, a health professional seeks guidance from his supervisor.

Supervisors differ in their personalities and work styles. Some are highly focused on work, and your relationship with this supervisor will be solely based on work issues. Many other supervisors are more relationship oriented. They feel that the best way to work is to motivate their team, and they strive to develop relationships with the people on their team. Still others are creative types who are always seeking new,

FIGURE 11-3 A health professional interacting with his supervisor. (From Proctor DB, Adams AP: *Kinn's the medical assistant: an applied learning approach*, ed 12, St Louis, 2014, Elsevier.)

better, and more innovative ways to work. Finally, process types are sticklers for detail and seek smooth operations. Your response to your supervisor depends a lot on the supervisor's preferred style. Work to develop compatibility with your boss's work style, so you can approach her more effectively.

In addition, you should observe the habits and preferences of your boss. What is the best time to approach him with your ideas and suggestions? When will he be most receptive? Is he a morning person, or does he spring to life later in the afternoon? Is he more formal, preferring meetings and appointments to discuss issues? Or is he more informal, receptive to hallway conversations? Pay particular attention to your manager's communication style and preferences. Does he prefer verbal communication, emails, or both? How should you use email to communicate with your boss, and what issues should you copy him on? Some supervisors want highly detailed emails so they have a written resource they can use later. Others prefer short messages such as reminders or questions. And still others want to be emailed only when they are not available personally. If you are uncertain about your manager's communication preferences, ask him. It is important to approach this matter correctly.

JOURNALING 11-4

Describe aspects of your supervisor's personal style. How focused is he or she on work and relationships? What are his or her most receptive times of the day or week? What is his or her preferred communication style? Does he or she have any other traits or preferences that will help you relate to him or her?

When your manager asks you to do something specific, and you are able to do so, you show respect for your boss when you drop everything to complete the request. Often, the manager's request is an urgent matter anyway, such as attending to a patient in need. If, however, you are unable to comply with the request immediately, you will gain your boss's respect by explaining the circumstances that prevent you from performing the new task immediately. In fact, you may even ask for guidance. "If I do the guided tour for the Deputy Mayor this afternoon, I won't be able to get our monthly newsletter to the printer today. Can you guide me on my priorities here?" You compliment your manager by asking for her advice. In no case should you ever promise to do something you can't complete by its deadline or commit to conflicting tasks.

Conversations with Your Boss

Your manager's time is valuable, but you and your work are important as well. Plan to speak with your boss when you need guidance, when you have something important to communicate, when your needs are not being met, or when you have ideas and solutions to problems. Think about your conversations before you have them. Visualize and anticipate them. Imagine what could go right or go wrong. When you plan for a successful outcome to a conversation, you will more likely get one.

To help establish rapport with your boss, mirror her body language, as you learned in Chapter 9. Proper body language helps people bond and treat each other as professionals engaged in a business discussion. Smile if it is appropriate. Make small talk at the beginning, but keep it short. Get to the point, and state the purpose of your conversation clearly. As in all conversations, practice active listening skills, as you learned in Chapter 9. The more your manager talks, the more you will learn, and the better the questions you can ask.

Be appreciative of your manager's time, but be sure you clearly understand any directions you receive or promises you make. Ask questions to be sure you understand. If necessary, summarize your understanding verbally or in a follow-up email. Always inform your supervisor of actions you took in response to your conversation. Clarity and follow-up are two qualities all managers prize in their employees. Box 11-2 reviews some of the most common mistakes people make when communicating with supervisors.

 WHAT IF?

What if you need to clarify your supervisor's directions, but you feel your question is "dumb"? What would you do?

Seek Feedback and Even Criticism from Your Supervisor

Brace yourself. How would you react if your supervisor said one of the following statements to you:

* "I know you don't mean it to be, but it feels disrespectful to those who are speaking when you tap on the table during our meetings."
* "Do you realize that sometimes you cut patients off during intake interviews?"

Nobody likes to be criticized, but comments like these are actually meant to help an employee perform better at work and face greater success. Constructive criticism is part of your supervisor's job and can be the most important gift your boss can give you. You can react more constructively yourself if you think of it not as criticism but as insightful feedback. No one is perfect, and none of us can see ourselves with the clarity with which others see us. If your boss is kind enough to make you aware of some of these problems, she is doing you a huge favor by giving you an opportunity to correct a problem that would otherwise plague your career and baffle you for years. You can take your positive response to feedback one step further by showing your supervisor you care enough to not wait for feedback but to seek it out by asking, "I've been reviewing the way I do this. Is there anything you'd like me to do differently?"

 WHAT IF?

What if your boss was angry with you and told you that you were a poor communicator because you should have disclosed a problem to her that has now blind-sided her and created an even more difficult problem?

Your Performance Evaluation

At regular intervals, usually annually (and sometimes more often if you're a new employee), you can expect to receive a formal performance evaluation from your supervisor. This evaluation covers the entire period since the last evaluation, and it becomes part of your file in Human Resources. Sometimes the performance evaluation is used to determine pay raises. Regardless of whatever salary implications it may or may not carry, the performance evaluation is a major opportunity for you and your supervisor to agree on your strengths and weaknesses and decide what developmental and learning goals you will work on in the coming review period. Of course, this periodic evaluation is not the only time you should solicit feedback from your boss. Between reviews, refer to your practice's performance evaluation form as a reminder of growth opportunities. See Figure 11-4 for a sample evaluation.

It's natural for you to feel a bit nervous before your annual performance evaluation, but keep in mind that it is not an easy time for managers. First of all, they may have many performance evaluations to perform, and they have a deadline to complete them all. Often, doing quality performance evaluations is one of their own developmental goals. Moreover, they probably don't have a detailed file of your performance and all your achievements over the past year.

Employee Performance Evaluation Form

Employee name: _____   Date: _____

Position: _____   Hire date: _____

Description of responsibilities:

_____

_____

_____

Performance on a scale of 1 to 10, with 10 being outstanding/exceptional performance and 1 being poor/below expectations.

Professional performance	Self-appraisal rating	Manager rating
1. Knowledge of office procedures		
2. Patient awareness and communication		
3. Adhering to office policies		
4. Judgment and ability to recognize/solve problems		
5. Administrative/organization/working within system		
6. Quality of work		
7. Productivity/results		
8. Willingness to learn/grasp of instruction		

FIGURE 11-4 A performance evaluation form.

Instead, what they do have are general impressions and a fading memory of recent events. On top of that, conducting the performance evaluation itself is usually an anxiety-provoking event for your manager. Is the evaluation accurate and fair? Will there be a disagreement or conflict? Will a disappointing evaluation lower the employee's motivation rather than raise it? Performance evaluations are a high-stress time for everyone involved.

You can help, and actually raise your profile in your supervisor's eyes, by preparing on your own evaluation. First, start a file of your accomplishments, including dates and details; keep track of aspects or skills you'd like to improve. Then, a week or two before performance evaluations are due, and before your manager has a chance to write yours, compose a "self-evaluation" and give it to your supervisor. Tell her that you hope her general impressions of your performance are in agreement with your own assessment. Be as objective as you can be in your self-evaluation. Your honest self-evaluation is certainly an opportunity to cast yourself in a positive light and show initiative. Your manager might have forgotten events that happened months ago, but she will be impressed when you remind her of them in your detailed evaluation, a document that will also reflect positively on her when her boss reviews it.

In the event that your manager strongly disagrees with your self-evaluation, at least you will know that you are not on the same page as your boss regarding your performance, and the ensuing discussion gives you a chance to work to improve your performance, regain your supervisor's confidence, and take specific actions to ensure that your work is visible and appreciated.

Continual Feedback and Improvement

Your goal in seeking regular feedback is to keep a pulse on your supervisor's opinion of you and your performance, and learn how you can do an even better job (Figure 11-5). By learning about general concerns on your boss's mind, you can identify opportunities where you may be in a position to help him. But in seeking continuous feedback, you do not want to be seen as an insecure person constantly seeking praise and reassurance: continuous means regular, not constant.

So how often is enough? It is certainly appropriate to make an appointment with your manager every several months to review your progress on your developmental goals for the year and to offer

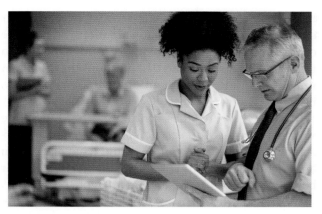

FIGURE 11-5 A medical professional receives feedback (Copyright © istock.com).

solutions for any problems you're facing, such as the need for training, a proposed reorganization of work, an arbitration plan, and so on.

What if You Have a Difficult Boss?

Bosses are not perfect. Because they are human, they can be difficult—too aggressive, too passive, indecisive, rude, unappreciative, grumpy, arrogant, demanding, controlling, harassing, unpredictable, bullying, demeaning, intimidating, micromanaging, incompetent, antagonistic, and even abusive. You do not usually get to pick your boss. You hope for a good one, but there are tactics you can pursue if you have a bad one.

Approaches to Dealing with Your Manager's Difficult Behavior

Instead of suffering and venting, think about how to handle the situation. Ask yourself some of the following objective questions:

* What is driving my boss's behavior? Why is she acting like that?
* Is this a temporary behavior, or a personality problem?
* Am I a target, or is everyone treated this way?
* Am I doing anything to contribute to my boss's bad behavior?
* Based on what I know about my boss, is there anything I can do to improve the situation?

First of all, some supervisors are not really qualified to be in a leadership role. They may have done their previous job well and been promoted beyond their abilities. They may have come from another employer with high recommendations, when the other company was only trying to get rid of the person themselves. They may have connections that got them hired or promoted without regard to merit. Few, however, will see themselves as bad managers.

Based on the realities confronting you, there are several strategies you can pursue. First, try to understand what motivates your boss, and what makes him angry or difficult. If you understand what makes your boss tick, you can at least avoid antagonizing him.

Whatever you do, maintain two things: the quality of your work and an upbeat attitude. Both are under your personal control. Nothing makes a bad boss worse than employees who are sullen, unproductive, insubordinate, uncooperative, lazy, disagreeable, or untrustworthy. These reactive strategies are totally unproductive. Control these impulses and try to choose productive strategies. Never embarrass, publicly confront, or threaten a bad boss, as this will only bring out the very worst in her.

One perhaps counterintuitive strategy might be to ignore your boss's behavior, and act as if it was normal. Thank her when appropriate. Praise him when appropriate. Do a good job, and let your boss know what you have accomplished. If necessary, share the credit for your success with your boss. Otherwise, fly below the radar and try not to be a target. Don't call attention to yourself, unless it is positive attention that will reflect favorably on your boss.

> *The higher a monkey gets up the tree, the more rear end he's got showing.*
>
> —Louis Harris

If your boss demands unreasonable performance, explain what you will have to do to attain an unreasonable goal, including stopping the things you are already accomplishing. Refuse to do anything you feel is unethical. Doing so will seldom cost you your job, and it will often mark you as someone your boss should not trifle with. Other strategies for dealing with a difficult supervisor appear in Box 11-3.

Above all, stay calm, especially when your supervisor is being emotional.

In addition to this low-profile strategy, try to see the bigger picture. If you like the employer but not your boss, the quality of your employer means that your boss will not last forever. You may want to impress someone senior to your boss by volunteering for a task force, discussing an operations issue with them, or finding some common ground or interest with them. Your bad boss may steer clear of someone

---

BOX 11-3

Tips for Dealing Positively with a Demanding or Difficult Supervisor

- As always, first seek to understand the supervisor's difficult behavior.
- Be politely assertive, not attacking or threatening. Acting intimidated will invite more of the same bad treatment.
- In private, provide your boss with feedback following this structure: "When you _____, it makes me feel _____.
- When being criticized, ask for details. Explain that you want the details so you can improve next time. Details require the supervisor to be more thoughtful.
- Control your emotions and choose your response carefully.
- To protect yourself and preserve details, document any instance in which your boss engages in any dishonest, unethical, or abusive behavior.
- Refuse to do anything dishonest, unethical, or abusive.
- Don't do anything rash that could jeopardize your career, no matter what the provocation.
- If all else fails, consult with your Human Resources Department, which exists in part to help employees deal with difficult bosses. However, you should exhaust all other remedies before taking the matter to HR.

---

who seems to have a positive relationship with *his* boss. You may want to seek a transfer to a better boss or wait your bad boss out, maybe even positioning yourself to replace him or her.

If you are the target of abuse, however, and you don't think your employer or senior management team members will do anything about it, you should consider looking elsewhere, without giving up your present employment until you are offered a new position. Just as patients judge your employer through you, you judge your employer through your boss. Employees seek jobs based on their impression of the employer, but they leave them based on their relationship with their supervisor. In the face of abuse, work is too important, and life is too short.

Coping with Change and Stress

Before you give up, however, keep in mind that often a manager's bad behavior is just a reflection of how they behave when they are stressed. Recognize that stress accompanies management. Some supervisors are better at dealing with stress than others. One of the best ways you can support your boss and help him deal with his stress is to help him manage change. If change is tough on employees, it's even harder on your manager. He will inevitably encounter people with negative mindsets who want to resist or sabotage the change. Don't be one of those people. Many times, your manager did not choose the change; he simply is responsible for implementing it. Your support will make him see you as an ally during challenging times.

How can you support your manager during a time of change? Visualize. Rely on your own grit and support systems. Disagree with those who resist the change. Help people see the positive side. Suggest ways your boss can make the change seem more positive. Even if you don't like change yourself, you must recognize that change, sometimes rapid, is inevitable. Change is an accelerating reality of the 21st century. You have to accept this and get used to it, and accept that one of your boss's main roles is to be an agent of change. You want to be an ally in this endeavor.

CASE STUDY 11-2
Dr. Jekyll and Mr. Hyde

Everybody who worked in Dr. Ray Brazos's pediatric practice marveled at how he could be the beloved, kindly, gentle doctor his patients loved while treating his employees so disrespectfully.

"Look at this *Newsweek*. It's from last summer. Do you think my patients want to read last summer's news?" Just then, Brenda, one of the medical assistants, arrived. "Nice of you to join us today, Miss Flores," he said. "You're visiting Starbucks on my time," he said, pointing at her coffee.

"Actually, I'm right on time," she said, annoyed with herself for sounding defensive.

"Good. Get to work," said Dr. Brazos, stalking down the hallway to his office.

Brenda followed him. "I need to speak to you," she said.

"Make an appointment," he said brusquely.

"Actually, I make your appointments, and I have the next fifteen minutes of your time."

"What's on your mind?"

"I've only been here two months, but you have a lot more no-shows than other offices where I've worked."

"I do?"

"Yes. It's a waste, and totally unnecessary. There are ways you can reduce the number."

"Don't you call patients the day before?"

"Yes, but we can also call them the morning of the appointment to remind them again. Many say they forget."

"They do?"

"Yes. If you call them again in the morning, and they can't come, at least they can tell us, and we can book somebody else when they call. Instead of having patients just come in and wait until you have a break, we could schedule them into the cancellations."

"That's a good idea."

"We could also tell the kids they'll get a sucker. They'll nag their parents or at least remind them."

"Those ideas sound great, Brenda. Please share them with the rest of the staff and begin implementing them immediately."

QUESTIONS FOR THOUGHT AND REFLECTION

1. Was Brenda successful in looking past Dr. Brazos's obnoxious behavior?
2. What solution did she offer Dr. Brazos?
3. Did the relationship between Dr. Brazos and Brenda Flores change today?

Down a Dark Road

Saul could see Sue circling outside of his office again. He didn't know what to do with her. "Don't you have some work to do?" he called to her.

"I'm way ahead of schedule," she said with a big smile, although Saul didn't know what that meant, since the waiting room was full of patients. She sat down in the chair in front of Saul's desk. "I don't know if you know or not," she said, "but our medical records committee is making great progress. We have already identified the five market-leading software systems, and we're putting together a pilot, a sample of the data, to run through each system."

"Yes, I know," said Saul. "I get regular updates from Rachel."

"I wouldn't be surprised. She's great for reports. But it took me four hours to compile the test data, the information we're using for the pilots, to test the software. The vendors gave us samples."

"I know all that, Sue."

"The samples limit the number of records we can enter, but I compiled the maximum number. I just wanted to be sure you were up to date, because the software samples expire at the end of the month, and we really need to get going."

"So you think we're behind schedule?" said Saul.

"Oh no, ahead of schedule," said Sue. "I've already got the data entered and everything."

"Well, that's good."

"I do what I can. I try to contribute."

"OK," said Saul with a wan smile. "Back to work," and he waved her out.

At lunch, Sue sat with the boys from the ambulance service. "This Rachel is driving me nuts," she said as she sat down. "Just because she's in charge of this electronic medical records adoption committee, she's giving Saul minute-by-minute reports, and she doesn't give me an ounce of credit, even though I'm doing nine-tenths of the work. If this place ever gets electronic medical records, they'll have me to thank for it, but Saul just says he gets reports from Rachel. That girl is driving me nuts."

"Why don't you talk to her about it?" said Alex, immediately regretting his question.

"Like she talks to me. I'm shunned. I don't have a speaking relationship with one single medical assistant here, and that's fine with me. They all drive me nuts. I swear, Saul does the worst job in the world of hiring these people. He's clueless. If I didn't keep him informed, he wouldn't know half of what's going on.

Back on the unit, Sue ran into Rachel in the hallway and put on a big smile. "I got that data all compiled now," she told Rachel.

"You already told me," said Rachel.

Sue lost the smile and headed toward Saul's office again, peeking through the glass. He waved her in.

"What now?" he asked.

"Well, I'm just a little bit concerned," she said. "I think I'm being cut out of the loop here," she said. "I just ran into Rachel, and I'm not sure she understands the importance of compiling the test data. I mean, did she mention me in her report?"

"I don't really remember, Sue."

"I didn't think so. Saul, without that test data, this project is going nowhere. Nowhere! Are you sure Rachel is the right one for this job?"

"I'm confident in Rachel," said Saul.

"Well, I wouldn't want to doubt your confidence in her, Saul, but I would keep a close eye on her if I were you."

"I tell you what, Sue. I want you to get back to work now, and I don't want to see you in this office until Friday at the earliest."

QUESTIONS FOR THOUGHT AND REFLECTION

1. Is Sue seeking feedback on her work?
2. Is Sue making good use of her supervisor's time?
3. What kind of a working relationship does Sue have with her peers?
4. What is Saul's opinion of Sue?
5. Is Sue contributing valuable work on the medical records committee?
6. In your opinion, is Saul an effective manager?

EXPERIENTIAL EXERCISES

1. Think about teachers you have had as if they were your boss at work. Which ones were the best and the worst? Why?
2. Would your parents make good bosses?
3. Identify the strengths and weaknesses of five managers you see on television.
4. Write a self-evaluation.
5. Ask someone you know who is in a supervisory position to describe their ideal employee.

CROSS CURRENTS WITH OTHER SOFT SKILLS

THINKING CRITICALLY: Thinking skills are what managers are paid to have. You can interact with your supervisor more effectively by thinking critically, too. (pp. 320-325)

SPEAKING PROFESSIONALLY IN YOUR WORKPLACE: How you speak matters as much as what you say. (pp. 244-249)

LISTENING ACTIVELY: In your communications with your manager, listening is paramount. (pp. 263-269)

READING AND SPEAKING BODY LANGUAGE: You put yourself and your boss at ease by mirroring her body language. (pp. 277-284)

Taking Accountability

I've missed more than 9,000 shots in my career. I've lost almost 300 games. Twenty-six times, I've been trusted to take the game-winning shot and missed. I've failed over and over and over again in my life. And that is why I succeed.

—Michael Jordan

LEARNING OBJECTIVE 3: TAKING ACCOUNTABILITY

- Understand why accountability is a choice.
- Develop methods to assert more personal accountability at work.
- Take ownership.
- Never say "It's not my job."
- Know what your personal best is.

Health professions are "high trust" professions.

Accountability is a choice. There are plenty of people to blame when things go wrong. There are plenty of people responsible for shortcomings. You can even blame your own shortcomings on someone else if you are desperate enough to assign blame outside of yourself. Should it be a comfort to know that, no matter how much you fall down on the job, there are plenty of people to blame for it? No. Because in the end, you always know; and in the end, even subtle lies will be unearthed. The only genuine comfort in any mistake is the freedom of transparency—taking accountability, both in your life and your work.

All right. You can't take accountability for everything that happens to you—take the weather, for starters. And you can't actually do someone else's job for them. Even the most responsible and accountable people in the whole world can't control everything. And who wants to be a control freak anyway? Nevertheless, accountability is a choice. And when it comes to what you can control—yourself—the choice is yours.

JOURNALING 11-5

Consider a negative situation you had no personal control over. Using questions beginning with "What" or "How," and using "I," ask yourself what would have given you more control and accountability.

Accountability 101

Learning, Changing, Growing

When something goes wrong, what does true accountability look like?

* Being annoyed with yourself for not taking ownership earlier.
* Regretting not admitting up front that you needed more training before taking on a failed task.
* Being annoyed with yourself because you depended on someone who wasn't dependable.
* Learning a lesson from how events unfolded.
* Recognizing the benefit in an event turning out a certain way and using it as an opportunity to practice your accountability skills.

If you experience any of these feelings or ask any of these questions, you are taking ownership, learning, and advancing to a higher level of accountability.

Taking accountability is not an easy thing. Just as when you have to act ethically, behaving with accountability is a heavy responsibility that involves difficult decisions and extra effort.

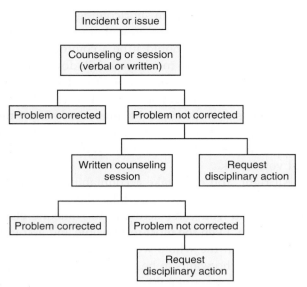

FIGURE 11-6 Disciplinary action relating to accountability.

Taking Ownership

Ownership is all or nothing. Blaming and pointing fingers is not ownership. Complaining and whining is not ownership. Making excuses is not ownership. Ownership is difficult because it puts you at the very center of the outcome. If you make a mistake, it will show. If you fail, it goes to your account. Other problems may arise. This is when you must decide what you are made of. Taking ownership means focusing on solutions rather than problems. The focus is always on what's next. "What about this?" "Let's try this." Ownership means devising solutions, and owners who create solutions are known as leaders.

Figure 11-6 displays a chart showing how to take ownership of issues at work.

"It's Not My Job"

Certainly, there will be times when a task is not your job. Instead of refusing to pitch in, ask, "How can I help?" Sometimes it is a matter of referring the person to the co-worker whose job it *is*. In these cases, introduce the patient to the co-worker if you can; don't blow them off with vague directions. On many occasions, you might help the patient in the short term while you are arranging for them to get help from the person who manages the issues they are concerned about. Of the many things you can do to help, listening actively may be the best thing you can do to fully understand the patient, treat them with respect and kindness, and get them the help they need, even if that involves a co-worker.

Always remember that a patient's opinion of your entire facility depends almost exclusively on their interaction with you. Be helpful—whether it is your job or not.

Trust, and Be Worthy of Trust

It is a pleasure to work in an organization characterized by trust. Nobody who is worthy of trust needs to be micromanaged. Workers need not be suspicious of one another's motives. The dual poisons of gossip and cynicism are virtually absent. But this happy state of affairs, a trusting organization, only comes about when everyone takes personal accountability for being trustworthy.

The first step is to always tell the truth, even when it is difficult, embarrassing, or inconvenient. Being polite or wanting to spare someone's feelings are not excuses for avoiding the truth. Truth takes courage, but the benefit is that others will trust you.

Never talk about someone behind their back, especially if you have criticism to offer. Instead, always bring concerns directly to that individual. Backstabbing never solves problems, and it marks you as untrustworthy. For example, if you have concerns about someone else's ability, should you stand on the sidelines and let the disaster unfold? Never! Instead, you can be honest but supportive at the same time. Depending on the situation, you might do any one of the following: volunteer to help, express your concerns to someone in a position of authority, support additional training for this individual, or find someone with the skills and experience necessary to handle the situation more successfully.

In the same vein, when someone complains to you about a third party behind their back, direct the person to the third party. Say you are uncomfortable with the conversation and feel the issue should be discussed with the person being talked about so something can be done about it. Collaborating with a co-worker to arrive at the right solution is great example of coaching.

Gossip is highly destructive. Like blame, it creates problems, not solutions. Box 11-4 suggests some ways you can respond to and, over time, eliminate gossip.

WHAT IF?

What if you are being talked about negatively behind your back?

BOX 11-4

How to Avoid Getting Involved with Gossip

- Assume that everything you say about a co-worker will be repeated.
- When gossip starts and you are there:
  - Say something positive about the person being gossiped about.
  - Change the subject.
  - Leave.
- Remember: You want as many alliances as possible at work, and no enemies.

- Just because others gossip doesn't mean you have to.
- If you have a concern about a co-worker, address it directly with him or her.
- When you gossip, you open a process that can spin out of control.
- People who gossip become the topic of gossip.

Do Your Best

Your best is by definition always a reach, a stretch. It requires your unique talents and abilities, from your personality to your clinical skills. When your best becomes a daily goal, you have created a high standard of accountability. It will make life easier in the long run because you don't have to worry about criticism when you deliver your very best, or take it personally. Instead, you have satisfied the only critic that really matters: yourself.

CASE STUDY 11-3
Rumor and Redemption

A friend of Grace's tipped her off. "Cathy tells me you're having a relationship with Dr. Anderson." Grace looked shocked, and her friend burst into laughter. "I knew it wasn't true," she said. "But that's what Cathy said."

Grace went looking for Cathy. When she saw her, Cathy turned around as soon as she caught a glimpse of the look on Grace's face. Grace had to run to catch up with her.

"Cathy, I've heard that you think I'm having a relationship with Dr. Anderson."

"Who said I said that?"

"That doesn't matter. I heard it, and I'm asking you if you said that."

At this point, Cathy paused for too long of a time.

"Well, I might have said something like that. I saw you two holding hands in the parking lot."

"Oh, is that so? You saw me holding hands with Dr. Anderson?"

"Yes, I did," said Cathy, her confidence coming back.

"Well, you're right, Cathy. It's true that we were holding hands. I was telling Dr. Anderson that my niece was diagnosed with leukemia. He expressed his concern and support by grasping my hand. Do you really think you had enough information to say something that would damage my reputation?"

Cathy was speechless.

"I really don't know Dr. Anderson very well. I can tell you he seems like a very kind, sympathetic man. How do you think this rumor you started will affect him?"

"I—I—I don't know," she said.

Grace looked at her watch. "It's 2:00. Tomorrow afternoon at this time, I am going to ask Dr. Anderson if you apologized to him."

QUESTIONS FOR THOUGHT AND REFLECTION

1. Should Grace have told Cathy how she found out about the rumor?
2. Did Grace owe Cathy an explanation for why she was holding hands with Dr. Anderson?
3. Did Cathy have a reasonable basis for starting this rumor?
4. Do you think Cathy will apologize to Dr. Anderson?
5. Will Cathy start any other rumors about Grace?

Martina got the job of her dreams when she graduated from her LPN program. They wouldn't let her pour meds until she passed her NCLEX-PN licensing exam, but she knew the exam was a done deal. She graduated from her program, so she should be able to pass the exam if the school did its job.

To her surprise, however, she failed. She was horrified. What happened?

Her supervisor at work, Ms. Forbes, said she could keep her job for now, but she would have to work as a nursing assistant and her pay would be cut. That's why she went to school for the LPN in the first place, to move up from nursing assistant, and make more money. As soon as she got off work that afternoon, she drove right over to the school and marched herself into the office of her advisor, Professor Ott.

"How could this happen?" Martina demanded to know. "What kind of school is this? I paid good money to go here, and now I'm back to where I started."

"Let's have a look at your test scores, Martina," said Professor Ott in a soft voice.

"I don't need to look at my test scores," shouted Martina. "I passed, right? I graduated, right?"

"Your scores were adequate for your courses, Martina," Professor Ott pressed on. "But you did poorly on the NCLEX practice exam. Don't you remember us talking about that?"

"So what? I graduated. That's all that counts."

"I told you that research shows you need to practice 4000 to 5000 questions, get 70% right, and read all the rationales for the right and wrong answers."

"That's ridiculous. Does the research know that I have to work for a living? Does the research think I have time for 5000 questions? I went to school here, and you didn't teach me right."

QUESTIONS FOR THOUGHT AND REFLECTION

1. Does Martina take accountability for her NCLEX-PN results?
2. Who is to blame for Martina's failure?
3. What role is emotion playing in Martina's behavior?
4. Is it ridiculous to do 5000 practice questions if you passed all the courses?

⊛ EXPERIENTIAL EXERCISES

1. Play the "Blame Game." In your mind, blame someone else for three bad things that happened to you this week. Ask yourself whether this activity produces any solutions to the problems. Ask yourself if you could have improved the situation if you took more accountability for the outcome. How would you feel about yourself if you took more accountability?
2. Examine the last test you took. Can you hold yourself accountable for those results?
3. Have you ever gotten away with anything? How did that make you feel?
4. Have you ever been treated unfairly? Is there some way you can hold yourself accountable for that?

⊘ CROSS CURRENTS WITH OTHER SOFT SKILLS

BUILDING SELF-ESTEEM: Want to feel great about yourself? Take accountability. (pp. 350-356)

ADOPTING A POSITIVE MENTAL ATTITUDE: Taking accountability reflects that positive attitude you want to be known for. (pp. 2-11)

Contributing as a Member of the Team

I am a member of a team, and I rely on the team, I defer to it and sacrifice for it, because the team, not the individual, is the ultimate champion.

—Mia Hamm

LEARNING OBJECTIVE 4: CONTRIBUTING AS A MEMBER OF THE TEAM

- Define *team*.
- Clearly understand the roles of team members.
- Describe the benefits of teams in health care settings.
- Know what it means to be a team player.
- Observe the purpose of meetings.
- Describe five problems that teams could encounter.

The effective delivery of health care is a team-based activity. It calls for the expertise of multiple professionals, who must work together to produce positive outcomes. Teams are built on trust. Each team member must feel comfortable that every other team member will do their part. That, in fact, is the magic of teams: everyone wants to do their best, because the team depends on them.

Aspects of a Team

A group is not a team. Teams have special characteristics, including a unified purpose with common incremental goals, as well as an internal structure and specific expectations for each member. In fact, in the health care field, you are likely to become a member of multiple teams. For example, you could be a member of a particular doctor's or dentist's team, but also be a member of a team of assistants while belonging to a subteam with a specific function, such as maintaining the facility.

Let's examine some of the key characteristics of a team.

Team Purpose

The purpose of a team is to accomplish specific tasks and goals. You will likely be a member of one or more permanent teams. You may be on the team that supports a doctor. You may be on a team that performs a specific function, like providing emergency care, dispensing medication, improving patients' communication skills, providing diagnostic images, or providing a range of massage or rehabilitation services. You may also be on a team with the other members of your health profession. As a dental assistant, you and your fellow dental assistants may jointly manage the reception area, the supply room, or cover shifts for each other. As a physical therapist, you may join your fellow physical therapists in planning or reviewing care for a specific patient, evaluating and purchasing equipment, or assisting and consulting one another. These are the kinds of permanent teams that function every day at work. Few health professionals operate in solitude or isolation.

Other teams may be temporary and have a specific goal to achieve. Once the goal has been achieved, the team dissolves. Often, these are called committees, or ad hoc teams. Such teams could include recruitment groups for new employees, planning teams for accreditation visits, teams that review the hospital formulary, or teams that plan the holiday party. In every case, though, the team has been formed for a specific purpose, and the purpose is achieved by meeting criteria everyone approves and agrees with.

Team Goals, Responsibilities, and Rewards

The goals of the team need to be clear to everyone. Moreover, everyone needs to agree when the goals have been achieved. What are the desired outcomes? Providing effective patient care? Maintaining smooth operations? Creating a document? Planning a successful event?

 WHAT IF?

What if you are asked to join a team? What information will you want? What questions will you ask?

Sometimes, a team gets a specific reward, like a bonus, a plaque, or public recognition. More often, though, the reward is a job well done. If you serve on a team that accomplishes great things, and your contribution is visible, your career will prosper. As much as individual contributions, your contributions to a team can be meaningful and lead to promotions, increases in pay, and career success.

Team Structure, Leadership, and Size

Research shows that teams function best when they are made up of five to twelve people. Fewer than five members makes it impossible to spread the work effectively. Having more than twelve members causes communication problems and destroys the idea of everyone being individually responsible to everyone else.

A team is ideally structured so that the members' varying talents can be optimally combined to accomplish particular goals. Therefore, it is important to understand and define the expected contributions of each team member. As an individual, are you there to lead, take notes, do research, write a report, or contribute ideas? To succeed as a team member, you must know exactly why you were picked for this team and what you are expected to contribute.

Finally, every team has to have a leader. The leader combines, organizes, and leverages all the members' special skills and expertise to accomplish a challenging and important goal. However, teams are organizationally flat groups where everyone is important. In fact, teams allow health care organizations to function without steep hierarchies because the real work is being done by teams of people who are treated equally and held accountable by one another (Figure 11-7). Teams take excess costs out of health care and make each team member a significant contributor to the success of the organization.

FIGURE 11-7 Teamwork is essential in health care. Members of the surgical team on rely on each other during procedures, just as teams of technicians, aides and others work together to provide before and aftercare (Copyright © istock.com).

FIGURE 11-8 Team discussion. (From Proctor DB, Adams AP: Kinn's the medical assistant: an applied learning approach, ed 12, St Louis, 2014, Elsevier.)

Benefits of Teams

Let's face it. The workload in health care is heavy, almost crushing at times in some settings. Establishing teams is an efficient way to manage a demanding workload because they allow for specialization. Patients who encounter teams are handled methodically. Someone checks them in and starts to collect data, including insurance, medical history, and vital signs. They may be sent to specialists in imaging, lab work, or other diagnostic tests. Next, they are examined by nurses, physicians, and other professionals. Finally, the treatment program is prescribed, which could involve nursing assistants, pharmacists, physical and occupational therapists, and counselors or social workers. Health care is too complex to be delivered by any one person.

Expertise

There are more than 100 health professions, each with its own skill set, body of knowledge, and role. You already know how long it took and how difficult it was to master the skills and knowledge of your own particular profession. Health professionals are experts in one aspect of health care. Your expertise is needed, and you and your patients need the expertise of your colleagues in other health professions.

➤ JOURNALING 11-6

Consider a team you are part of. What, exactly, is the expertise you bring to this team? Record your expertise in the form of skills and knowledge. Be as broad and specific as you can be.

Because of the varying types of expertise represented on a team, there has to be a clear role for everybody, and everybody has to contribute. Everybody matters, giving every team member a sense of equality on the team. Differences in status disappear as the work of the team becomes a mosaic of everyone's talents. This is one reason that team work can be a pleasure and produce positive feelings about work.

Social Connection

An often overlooked benefit of teams is the social connection it offers to its members. This is a double benefit, because it is the social connection that team members feel that leads to the sense of trust. Trust and a sense of responsibility to the team prompts team members to go to extra lengths to perform and not let their team members down. You can see from the body language in Figure 11-8 the bonding that goes into a fun and effective team.

Requirements of Teams and Being a Team Player

Teams don't function all by themselves. They need not only identified goals, a reliable internal structure, multiple expertise, and mutual trust among members, but established, predictable processes. These processes usually involve meetings as well as assignments between meetings. Many times, teamwork is governed by documents the team has created to facilitate its work. Some examples of these documents appear in Box 11-5.

Team Meetings

Many teams have regularly scheduled meetings. A team may hold staff meetings every Monday or once a month. Regular meetings ensure that the work conducted in the background is accomplished. Teams function like deadlines that require a personal report to one's peers. That is powerful motivation!

Part of your commitment and responsibility as a team member is to attend meetings, be on time, and be prepared. Usually, an agenda is circulated ahead of time, and reports and discussions are on the agenda. If an agenda item requires your expertise, always be prepared to lead the discussion, provide any needed information, and seek contributions and ideas from others. Further, you should be prepared to offer your ideas and input for all other agenda items. Meetings that are more formal may involve motions, votes, and recorded notes. You should learn the ground rules at your first meeting and prepare accordingly for subsequent meetings.

Other teams may have occasional and even emergency meetings. A team planning a holiday party might meet three or four times at odd intervals. In health care, however, emergency meetings are fairly common. If a traumatic or disruptive event has happened on a unit or in an office, the staff may hold a meeting to collect their wits, share information, and develop a planned response to the situation. Many times, a leader may call a meeting to make an announcement. Perhaps someone is leaving or joining the team, or a major policy or event is announced. Often, the purpose of having the meeting is not so much to make the announcement but to prevent the spread of gossip or process people's feelings about the

announcement. At these meetings, thoughtful questions are always welcome because they are questions likely to be on the minds of others, and questions give leaders an opportunity to read the group and plan their responses better.

Finally, there are regular meetings in health care such as the shift change meeting, a case presentation, or admission or discharge meetings. These kinds of regular meetings ensure the continuity of quality care. Their importance should not be overlooked just because they are routine. Often, these clinical exchanges of information involve a shifting constellation of team members. Every person who interacts with or cares for patients has something important to contribute to these meetings.

Teamwork

Teams are the preferred work method in health care because a team can accomplish so much more together than its individuals working separately. It can be fun and rewarding to be part of a team and see so much good work get done so quickly. A team working a shift together in a health care facility can take pride in the progress they make in moving a group of five, fifteen, or twenty patients toward recovering their health. A team at work in a dental office or pharmacy can really appreciate how much gets done in a day by working together.

None of us is as smart as all of us.

—Ken Blanchard

Problems Experienced by Teams

Naturally, your job is to do your part, cheerfully and collaboratively. Unfortunately, teams can and will experience problems from time to time. Use some of the conflict resolution and communication skills you've mastered from earlier chapters to resolve these problems.

Distrust

When someone on the team has proven themselves to be untrustworthy, the work of the team can be severely compromised. Often, the work of one team member depends on the work another team member can accomplish. Of course, even the most committed individuals slip up from time to time. No one's perfect. At other times, however, you might have a team member who doesn't really want to be there, or who isn't committed to the team's mission. When that happens, they are sure to drag their feet. In severe cases, sabotage and bad team behavior may manifest itself in communication. A team member may omit key data, falsify data, or offer misleading information. Such behavior, if deliberate, can be dangerous to your patients, and in that case the team member should be immediately released from the team. The best way to prevent this from happening when setting up a team is to ensure that everyone supports its mission, and replace those who can't or won't support the team's goals from the beginning.

Even if you have everyone's commitment from the start, teams and their goals often need to change. Although lots of us don't like change, for the most part, our initial commitment to a team and its mission is enough to help us adjust and remain a team player. Sometimes, however, a team member may be unable or unwilling to adapt to the change. Just one person resistant to change can sabotage its successful implementation. This person may have good reasons for resisting the change, but if, after considering the person's opinion, the rest of the team still supports the change and the conflict still exists, it is usually better for everyone to replace someone who's resistant with someone who can support the new goals and be a team player.

Conflict

Conflict is not necessarily a problem for teams. Constructive disagreement leads to discussion that improves outcomes. However, any conflict that is purely interpersonal takes away from accomplishing the mission of the team. When working together on a team, people must agree to put their differences aside and work together to achieve the team's goals. Interpersonal conflict can take place elsewhere, but teamwork is not the place for it.

Lack of Commitment, Lack of Accountability, and Loss of Focus on Results

All team members must uphold their responsibilities and contributions to the team. Anyone not holding up their end will soon be apparent to everyone else. If you ever find yourself lacking commitment to your team, failing to take accountability, or find yourself not caring about the outcomes, ask yourself if you are in the right job or if you are getting burned out. Then take steps to resolve the problem right away. You have personal control over how seriously you live up to your commitments to your team.

The name on the front of the shirt is more important than the name on the back.

—Anonymous

CASE STUDY 11-4
The Wine Tasting

Rachel was honored to be chosen to lead an ad hoc team to select an electronic medical records system for her hospital. She had been involved with a similar effort at her previous employer, and her experience with electronic medical systems was one of the reasons she was hired.

Her manager, Saul Bremer, gave her the authority to run the task force as she saw fit, giving her the goal of evaluating and recommending a new medical records software system by the end of November, so it could be purchased and implemented early in the new fiscal year. He appointed task force members from throughout the hospital, encompassing many different departments and functions, so there would be broad acceptance of the recommendation. He

asked Rachel to give him weekly reports by email, so he would have a record of her progress. But he said he would also meet with her each Friday to discuss the team's progress in more detail.

Since Rachel was fairly new, and since the task force members did not all know each other, she planned a social event for their first meeting. She was also concerned about the leadership challenges involved with the large size of the 12-person team. She wanted everyone to feel fully engaged with the team's mission. She had a small team-building budget, and she thought a wine tasting would be fun. She had a lot of knowledge about wines, and thought her wine expertise might translate to the leadership style she wanted to establish. She rented a function room at the Bella Vina restaurant, which she knew had a good wine list. She met with the wine steward there ahead of time to plan the event. She thought it would be fun to set up tastings of three different vintage years for three different wines, so her people could appreciate the differences in grape qualities from one year to another.

The event included appetizers and took place on a Friday evening from 5:00 to 7:00. Rachel arrived before her team so she could greet and introduce herself to everyone individually. She already knew everyone's department and position, but she asked everyone the same few questions to get to know them better—where they went to school, if they had children, and how long they had lived in Omaha. At the very least, she would find people who knew their way around the city much better than she did.

One man from IT, Chet, explained that he was good at "stress-testing" software, so Rachel put him in charge of that and paired him with two clinicians to tap their knowledge and educate them about stress-testing. An older woman from medical records, Velma, had been with the hospital for several decades, and she was skeptical about the changes electronic medical records would bring. In Rachel's mind, any system they chose would have to pass the "Velma Test."

After a couple of rounds of appetizers, the three wine stations were mixing up the group and everyone was getting along well.

Rachel noticed that one team member, Sue, was off to herself, so Rachel approached her. Rachel learned that Sue didn't know too many people on the team. "I'm good at data processing," Sue volunteered.

"That's great, Sue. We're lucky to have your talent on the team," said Rachel.

QUESTIONS FOR REVIEW AND REFLECTION

1. Has this team bonded effectively?
2. Do you think Rachel's boss is managing her effectively?
3. What did Rachel learn about her team at the wine tasting?
4. Was Rachel effective in establishing her leadership on the team?
5. How do you think Rachel will manage Sue?
6. Would you be happy to be a member of this team?
7. Do you think the team will achieve its goals and a positive outcome?

Down a Dark Road

Gary from accounting was rotated into the leadership role of the team responsible for keeping the policy manual updated. The team had representation from all different departments, and each person served for three months as the leader before leaving the team and being replaced by a new member, just to keep things fresh and provide everyone with a leadership opportunity. Gary called the team's next meeting for a Monday morning at 8:00.

"Oh, boy," said Della to her friend Evelyn, who was also on the committee. "Can you believe he called a meeting for 8:00? I'm still listening to my alarm at that hour." Evelyn laughed. She represented the nursing staff on the team, and Della was the administrative medical assistant for one of the orthopedic surgery units.

Della made it to the meeting on time, but she wasn't too happy about it.

Gary passed out the agenda. "You received this by email, but I made hard copies for everyone. Let's get started." The first thing on the agenda was reporting and filing lab results. Della's expertise would come in handy.

"Have you reviewed the current procedure on this?" Gary asked her.

"Hmmm, I am now."

Gary took a deep breath and waited patiently, with the rest of the team, while Della read over the procedure.

"Well, it looks OK, except we don't use paper charts anymore." She looked at Gary. "You can't exactly staple a lab report to an electronic record, now can you?"

"You can link it. Della, that is exactly why we're revising this procedure. Didn't you read the meeting announcement?"

"The one that said we're meeting at 8:00? I'm here, aren't I?"

"Maybe you should have actually opened the message," said Gary.

Della crossed her arms. She had had just about enough from this guy.

QUESTIONS FOR THOUGHT AND REFLECTION

1. Did Della understand the goal of her team?
2. Did the time of the meeting or Gary's personality have anything to do with the team's work?
3. Is Della living up to commitment to the team and sharing her expertise?
4. What is Della's role on the team? How is she functioning in that role?

1. Identify all the teams you are a part of.
2. Plan a modest activity that would help the members on one of your teams get to know each other better.
3. Think of a team you are a member of, whether it is a bowling group, a PTA, a church group, or a book club. Who leads these teams? What are the responsibilities of the members to one another?

CROSS CURRENTS WITH OTHER SOFT SKILLS

BEING DEPENDABLE: Your team members count on you, and you on them. (pp. 35-38)

BUILDING TRUST: Trust is the basis for team function. (pp. 212-218)

DEALING WITH DIFFICULT PEOPLE: Unfortunately, being a member of a team forces you to confront difficult people, since you must work effectively with everyone on your team. (pp. 231-238)

READING AND SPEAKING BODY LANGUAGE: Team settings require you to transmit and receive a full range of communication to get the team's work done. (pp. 277-284)

Committing to Your Profession

Your work is to discover your work and then with all your heart to give yourself to it.

—Buddha

LEARNING OBJECTIVE 5: COMMITTING TO YOUR PROFESSION

- Know the local, state, and national professional societies for your profession.
- Understand the benefits of society or association membership.
- Develop a networking plan within your profession.
- Know the journals, magazines, and blogs that support your profession.
- Access new research being performed and published in your profession.
- Leverage the resources of your profession to improve the quality of your work.

Through your education, you have joined a great profession. You have satisfied the criteria to graduate, obtained licensure or certification, and readied yourself to be hired in your chosen profession. Now, you should realize that your profession has a whole infrastructure to support it, and you can tap into that infrastructure by making a commitment to your profession.

One or more professional societies and numerous journals and publications support your profession. If you don't already know what they are, you should learn about as many organizations and publications as you can. If there are multiple options, you should determine which best meets your needs and even consider joining multiple organizations or subscribing to multiple publications.

Your Professional Society

For a cost typically under $200, you can join your professional society. The annual membership cost is usually a small price to pay for the benefits you receive. Professional societies and associations try very hard to create an attractive value proposition for their members, far above the membership cost. Some of these benefits are monetary, such as discounts, magazines, or continuing education. But the intangible benefits are probably more valuable to you. For instance, a professional society keeps you up to date about what's going on in your profession, emerging trends, specialties, regulations, and opportunities. Your knowledge about these issues and trends makes you a more valuable employee at work. A list of typical association membership benefits appears in Box 11-6.

Moreover, national professional societies and associations typically have state and local chapters or affiliates. Sometimes, membership in the state or local chapters comes with the membership fee for the national organization; other times, a small additional fee is required. However, most of the benefits of the national organization can be accessed through your local affiliate, including meetings and networking. Plus, local branches are much easier and less expensive.

JOURNALING 11-7

Imagine you are going to attend a national convention in your profession. Write down all the experiences and benefits you would like to gain from such an experience. Be expansive. Pick a city in your imagination, and think about the travel experience as well as the professional and networking experience.

Certification, Recertification, and Continuing Education

One of the main functions of professional associations is to offer and manage continuing education, certification, recertification, or specialty certification. Most health professions require both certification and continuing education to maintain certification. Your association handles certification and either offers continuing education (CE) or endorses others who offer it, or both. Usually, when you seek recertification, you have to submit proof that you took the required amount of continuing education units. CE units can be obtained through classroom courses, online courses, and meeting attendance. Since regulations vary by profession, you should make sure you know your requirements and the agencies or associations that manage your certification.

 WHAT IF?

What if you wanted to get a specialty certification in your field? Do you know what they are, and which one would appeal to you? Do you know where to get information about obtaining this certification? What would the certification mean to your career?

Conventions and Professional Meetings

One of the pleasures and rewards of being a health professional is an opportunity to attend meetings in your profession. Most professional societies put on an annual convention, and many offer smaller meetings devoted to specialties and subspecialties. Usually, there are state, regional, and local meetings available too, which may be a good place for you to start.

A meeting usually involves a modest registration fee that allows you to attend the meeting and all its functions, such as keynote speeches, awards ceremonies, educational sessions, continuing education credit, exhibit halls, and social events. You will also have to pay any travel, lodging, dining, and personal recreation or entertainment costs. A national convention certainly requires some advance planning and budgeting.

When you arrive at a convention with your proof of registration, you usually receive a badge that permits access to all the events. At big conventions, a wide range of educational classes and seminars are scheduled simultaneously, so you will have to plan ahead and choose those of greatest interest to you. Typically, between sessions you can visit an exhibit hall featuring hundreds of vendors, manufacturers, publishers, recruiters, and agencies related to your profession. There you may explore jobs in your profession, learn about the latest research, inspect new medical equipment, and preview emerging laws and regulations that affect your practice. Medical equipment manufacturers may offer you training on their new equipment right at their booth, and you may be able to get sample issues of journals and other literature. Your badge also gives you access to all the celebratory events, such as speeches and banquets.

Political campaign activities are a key part of any convention, as elections for new leaders and officers are frequently timed to occur after an annual convention so members can get to know the candidates. You may have an opportunity to vote right at the convention, and you can even get involved in a campaign, if you like. Not as glamorous, but just as important, new rules and regulations of practice are also debated, voted on, and enacted. Issues to vote on can range from best practices to specialty certification requirements. When you leave a professional convention, you'll feel that you have brought yourself completely up to date with the state of the art in your profession, if you have used your time wisely. While most people have a lot of fun at conventions, they are also usually exhausted by the time they get home!

FIGURE 11-9 Two conference participants greet each other during a networking event (Copyright © istock.com).

State, local, and specialty conventions and meetings may not have all the glitz and trappings of a national meeting, but they are much less expensive and often just as informative and gratifying as national meetings. The issues will be closer to home, in that the emerging rules may affect your local practice, and the educational events may be highly relevant to your particular practice's interests. You will meet colleagues living in your area and learn more about the relationship between your local chapter and its national organization.

Professional Networking

Just as you may have "summer friends" from your summer vacations, you can develop "convention friends" if you attend your society conventions regularly. One of the most valuable activities any health professional can pursue is networking (Figure 11-9). You already have interesting and talented co-workers at work, many of whom you count as friends. Networking takes the pleasures of socialization and friendship to a broader level. When you attend professional activities outside of your workplace, whether a convention or just volunteering at a community center, you have a chance to meet new colleagues, learn, gain influence, and make friends that could last a lifetime.

Now more than ever, networking is an extremely important part of your professional life. If you have a strong network, you can get answers to and opinions on clinical issues, discuss the important issues in your profession, seek information, and even look for new jobs, consulting engagements, and career specialization paths.

You may want to establish your professional presence or "personal brand" on a professional social media site like LinkedIn. It is free and easy to do. You simply complete a profile on yourself that includes your educational and work experience. Typically, you can include a photograph of yourself, list your personal mission statement, say what your interests and hobbies are, and even join groups of individuals with common interests. Once your profile is online, others can search for you and you can search for others as well. The idea is to facilitate networking. For instance, if you are attending a convention in an unfamiliar city, you can locate and contact local professionals there who may be able to recommend restaurants or local attractions. If you are looking for a job, you may be able to leverage your contacts to refer you to others with information about open positions. You can raise questions and issues and start or participate in discussions.

Publications and Research

Medical knowledge is exploding. Research is funded by billions of dollars annually supplied by government agencies such as the National Institutes of Health, and foundations such as the March of Dimes. In your profession, the findings are reported constantly by the journals and books supporting your profession. Journals can be expensive, but they may also be available in local, university, or hospital libraries. If you locate a journal that speaks directly to your areas of interest, you should consider subscribing to it. Journals are priced for individual and institutional customers. Whereas an institutional subscription, which may be accessed by dozens of readers, could cost hundreds of dollars, an individual subscription usually costs in the $50 to $100 range. These days, subscriptions usually include electronic access to searchable archives of past issues, making your subscription more valuable. Thousands of scientific and health-related journals are published around the world, almost all of them in English.

The Internet offers a wealth of resources for practice in your profession. Sites range from government agencies to organizations and foundations to research labs and facilities. You might find additional sources, like blogs or Twitter feeds, by searching the names of leaders in your field. Bookmark these sites as you come across them, adding them to a professional folder you keep in your web browser. Then, make a schedule to review them occasionally, so you can benefit from the information they offer.

Lifelong learning is the norm in the health professions. Knowledge is constantly being outdated and replaced by new knowledge. Create a plan to ensure that your learning is continually updated by taking advantage of all the resources covered in this chapter. The more successful you are at maintaining current knowledge of your profession, the more valuable you will be to your employer and to your patients or clients. Moreover, committing yourself to your profession positions you for advancement, promotions, success, and personal satisfaction in your career.

CASE STUDY 11-5
Network Chicago

Rinda Khalif was a speech pathologist in search of a new job. Her husband, Ayman, a pathologist, had just been recruited to a new position in Chicago, and they would be moving there at the end of the summer with their two preschool-age children, Randy and Joe. Neither Ayman nor Rinda was familiar with Chicago, and they didn't know anybody there. Rinda just knew they would love Chicago, but she was worried about finding a job in a new city.

Rinda subscribed to the *Chicago Tribune* online and registered with the Human Resources Department at the hospital where Ayman would work. She created an attractive resume, and she applied for jobs she saw. Despite her efforts she felt frustrated because it was like she was starting all over. She decided to be more proactive and utilize her own professional network.

She wrote emails to her professional contacts, explaining her situation and asking them to keep her in mind if they became aware of any openings. She didn't expect this to help much, but she wanted to cast a wide net. As she was doing this, she became aware that three of her contacts actually did live and work in the Chicago area. She had been introduced to them at separate functions at last year's convention of the American Speech-Language-Hearing Association (ASHA) in Philadelphia. She called them all to reintroduce herself and explained what she was looking for. They all agreed to help her and said they would make some inquiries on her behalf. More importantly, they shared information about the area where the medical center was and told her some good neighborhoods and school systems to explore there. She sent them her resume electronically and in the mail, and she hoped they would become friends after the move to Chicago.

That experience reminded her of the ASHA Web site. She went there, entered "jobs" in the search box, and a whole world of job resources opened up to her. There was a searchable job database that yielded seven positions she hadn't discovered previously. There was a career fair scheduled later in the month in a nearby city that might prove useful. There were classified ads in *The Leader*, the biweekly magazine she received in connection with her ASHA membership, which she had completely overlooked. Both the Web site and *The Leader* had ads for recruiters and jobs. These resources greatly expanded Rinda's opportunities.

Rinda even turned to LinkedIn. She updated her profile there and was active on the site. As she researched her prospective contacts, she found that three of them had mutual contacts. Another contact worked for the Chicago Public Schools Human Resources Department. First, she called the friends she had in common with the three LinkedIn contacts. What did they know about the Chicago people? What could they tell her? Could she use their names when she called them?

Then she began calling the LinkedIn contacts, using phone numbers provided by her friends, who had all said she could use their names. Rinda planned each call, carefully choosing the words she would use to explain her relationship to them, and state the purpose of her call. She was ready in case she ran into voice-mail to be clear and concise, and left her name and number twice, speaking clearly and slowly. She actually got through to one of the Chicago Public Schools contacts who confirmed that Rinda's LinkedIn connection was the person to contact. So Rinda wrote an email to the HR contact, attached her resume, and requested a telephone appointment. The HR person responded within an hour and proposed a time when they could talk by phone.

The telephone conversation went well and they arranged for a day of interviews in Chicago for the week after next.

QUESTIONS FOR THOUGHT AND REFLECTION

1. In what ways did Rinda leverage her network to find a job? What else could she have done?
2. How did Rinda's membership in ASHA and her attendance at their meetings help her uncover this opportunity?
3. What if Rinda had not uncovered the Chicago Public Schools opportunity by herself?
4. How will Rinda's networking efforts help her after she moves to Chicago?
5. Do you think health professionals have better networking and job search opportunities than other professionals?

Down a Dark Road

Caitlyn Day had gotten funding from her new employer to attend a regional meeting of the American Association of Professional Coders (AAPC). It was held nearby in Nashville and she had been to the Gaylord Opryland Hotel facility many times on family vacations. The registration fee was only $325 for almost three days of education and fun events. Specifically, Caitlyn's employer wanted her to learn more about the upcoming ICD-10 implementation, any changes to ICD-9, and what to expect from Health Care Reform. Caitlyn's employer asked her to make a presentation to the coding staff when she got back. Caitlyn also had some personal goals. She wanted to get an update on what was going on at the AAPC, and she wanted to learn more about specialty certifications. She also wanted to start establishing her professional network.

The first night featured a big networking reception that featured a sundae buffet. It was a lot of fun, and Caitlyn made friends with some young women from Knoxville. When the reception was over, they hit the bars for country music and dancing. It was after midnight by the time Caitlyn found her room and collapsed into the bed.

The maid's knock on the door woke her up. What time was it? Almost 10:00? She had missed the "State of the AAPC" breakfast session and the ICD-9 update. Caitlyn sobered up quickly, showered and dressed, and found the next available session, on coding for reimbursement for conditions related to childhood obesity, which, much to her relief, was a focus at her practice. She took copious notes. Later sessions bored her though, and she could barely keep awake. At the afternoon break, she ran into the girls from Knoxville again. Even though she knew she shouldn't, she found herself agreeing to meet them at 7:00 for drinks and dancing again.

Before she went out, she checked the following day's events in the program. The Health Care Reform panel was at 9:00, which she thought wouldn't be too early. There was nothing else that interested her until the exhibit hall opened at noon. Caitlyn laid out the clothes she would wear the next day. She had hoped to meet more people than just her new Knoxville friends, but she couldn't think of a way to gracefully excuse herself.

The next day, she barely made the exhibit opening at noon. She had no idea what she was going to say about ICD-9 and Health Care Reform, since she had missed both sessions. She wondered how she could turn her childhood obesity notes into a respectable presentation. She spent the next hour collecting as many magnets, pens, key fobs, and other give-aways she could scrounge from the vendors' booths. She filled up a whole canvas bag. At least she could pass this stuff out when she gave her presentation, whatever that would be.

QUESTIONS FOR THOUGHT AND REFLECTION

1. Did Caitlyn set goals for the regional meeting? Were they the right ones?
2. Was it a bad decision for Caitlyn to go out with her new friends the first night?
3. Where did Caitlyn falter in her planning?
4. Will the souvenirs make up for a poor presentation? What do you think of Caitlyn's thought processes?
5. How do you imagine Caitlyn's presentation went? Could she just switch the topic to childhood obesity? What would you do in her shoes? Will her employer be sending Caitlyn to any more conferences?

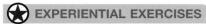 **EXPERIENTIAL EXERCISES**

1. Identify an influential person in your profession and reach out to him or her via the person's online profile.
2. Familiarize yourself with all the associations and journals that support your profession.
3. Plan to attend a local professional meeting.
4. Create a personal networking plan.
5. Find five sources of continuing education credit in your field.
6. Bookmark governmental sites related to your professions.
7. Sign up to follow a blog or Twitter feed in your area of interest.
8. Buy a pin online that signifies your profession.

 CROSS CURRENTS WITH OTHER SOFT SKILLS

SETTING GOALS AND PLANNING ACTIONS: Connecting with your profession requires appropriate goals and careful planning. (pp. 286-291)

EXUDING OPTIMISM, ENTHUSIASM, AND POSITIVITY: Connecting with your profession is a forward-looking, career-developing move. (pp. 380-384)

EMOTIONAL SKILLS— MANAGING YOUR EMOTIONS

Building Personal Emotional Strengths

Building Self-Esteem

Don't let anyone speak for you, and don't rely on others to fight for you.

—Michelle Obama

LEARNING OBJECTIVE 1: BUILDING SELF-ESTEEM

- Define *self-esteem*.
- Set goals to increase your self-esteem.
- Make your self-talk more positive.
- Bring more positive things into your life.
- Learn to like yourself better.

Everyone Struggles with Self-Esteem

Everyone struggles with self-esteem. Does that surprise you? It might not if you think about it for a minute. Nobody has a precisely accurate view of their self-worth. Everyone's self-esteem fluctuates in response to moment-by-moment events, perceptions, self-talk, and feedback. Our self-esteem gets a shake-up every time we experience change, especially on the job, whether it is an extremely challenging patient, a new piece of medical equipment or software, or a different supervisor. No one brings all the skills and experiences to the change that will make us as comfortable as we will eventually become. Just when we get used to a change, and begin to manage or deal with it effectively, everything changes again. Fortunately, your co-workers are in the same boat when change happens at work.

We all judge ourselves compared to others, even if we know we shouldn't. This process is automatic, and our self-esteem has been under construction since we were babies. It was both built and battered by the messages we received from members of our household and friends, bolstered by achievements and bashed by failures, and influenced by all kinds of feedback, including grades, relationships, and brush-offs.

> *Being saddled with low self-esteem is like being prejudiced against yourself. Only you can place a value, high or low, on the way you view yourself. No one can make you feel inferior without your consent.*
>
> —Eleanor Roosevelt

Characteristics and Benefits of Self-Esteem

How do you know if you have strong self-esteem? Most of us go through our daily lives without really evaluating the role our self-esteem contributes to our success and well-being. Yet, our self-esteem is always evolving, quietly processing our experiences, perceptions and misperceptions, self-talk, and interactions with others. In truth, our self-esteem is shaped not so much by what happens to us but by how we interpret what happens to us.

> *It ain't what they call you, it's what you answer to.*
>
> —W.C. Fields

 WHAT IF?

What if a patient yells at you for something that isn't your fault? How would you respond?

Fortunately, self-esteem is largely under your personal control. By bringing your self-esteem out of the darkness and into the light of day, you can mold it to become a healthier, more confident, and more effective human being. In fact, your work performance is a great opportunity for building and molding your self-esteem. Use the opportunity of a new job to become more like the person you really want and deserve to be.

For one thing, you can learn to abandon the practices mentioned in Box 12-1 that result in low self-esteem.

How to Build Self-Esteem

Your self-esteem is based on your interpretation of yourself. It may have first evolved from childhood experiences that were beyond your control, but you're in charge now. You don't have to live with low self-esteem because you are in control of your own thoughts. You can choose how you view yourself. Even if you have a healthy amount of self-esteem, you can increase it even more.

Make the Right Comparisons; Set the Right Goals

The absolute worst thing you can do is compare yourself to others. There are always going to be people out there who are better than you in some ways. So what? No one can be best at everything. In the same vein, you are going to be better at some things than others. Comparisons with other people are very flimsy platforms for self-esteem.

Rather than comparing yourself with others, compare your present self with your former self. Are you getting better? Do you have a plan to improve your life and circumstances so that you have a brighter future? Instead of trying to impress or seek the approval of others, try to impress yourself. You are the person who cares most about you anyway.

> *There is nothing noble about being superior to some other man. The true nobility is in being superior to your previous self.*
>
> —Hindu proverb

As you learned in Chapter 10, setting realistic goals is the path to a better life and improved self-esteem. If you know what you want to achieve in life, and you feel you are working on a plan to achieve those goals, your self-esteem will rise. Visualize a future full of meaning, success, and satisfaction. Imagine it as richly as you can, using all your senses to think about all the areas of your life. Do not let past failures and disappointments interfere with your opinion of yourself. Those mistakes are over and should be used as learning opportunities. Move on. If you embrace the present—the only place where you can be effective—and take actions that move you closer to the future that you envision and desire, you will have positive self-esteem.

Edit Your Self-Talk

You know your self-talk, that inner chatterbox that just won't keep quiet? Is your self-talk supportive, or critical? If your self-talk kicks you when you're down, or if you are harsher with yourself than you would be with others, improve it by changing your beliefs about yourself. Recast your beliefs. Beliefs, including those about yourself, are learned, so choose positive beliefs. Reframe and recast negative beliefs into positive ones.

Like any habit, self-talk can be changed if necessary. The first step is to notice what you are telling yourself and start looking for patterns.

← JOURNALING 12-1

Notice your negative self-talk. Maybe you doubt your ability in some area, or you have reprimanded yourself for something you did or thought. Record this negative self-talk and then list reasons to counteract it.

If you are giving yourself positive self-talk, that's great. Keep it up. If you detect a strain of negative self-talk, however, cut it out immediately. Say "Stop!" out loud or silently to yourself. This is called *thought-stopping,* and it forces you to recognize and interrupt bad self-talk. Now that you have interrupted your negative self-talk, you can analyze it and change it.

Reword your negative self-talk to make it less powerful. Just as you would call pain "discomfort" to help

lessen the severity when speaking to a patient, soften the words you use in your own self-talk. If you make a mistake and start silently criticizing yourself, just tell yourself that you made a mistake. That way, you simply acknowledge making a mistake. You will have moved your self-talk from being negative to being neutral.

Turning a negative self-assessment into a neutral one is important. To take things a step further, see if you can turn it into a bit of positive self-talk. "I made a mistake, and I'm going to learn from this mistake so I don't make it again." Look for the positive side of a negative situation.

❓ WHAT IF?

What if you catch yourself engaging in negative self-talk? Convert that negative message into a neutral or positive one.

How you feel is determined mostly by what you are consciously thinking and talking to yourself about. In other words, your self-talk determines your mood.

> *People become what they think about most of the time.*
>
> —Earl Nightingale

Know Yourself, Love Yourself

Is it wrong to love yourself? Do you *deserve* to be happy and successful? Do you give yourself permission to celebrate your accomplishments?

Certainly, self-love can have an ugly side if it veers toward narcissism or arrogance. A strong sense of self-esteem is always best when tempered with humility and modesty. However, never be afraid to give yourself the gift of love. How can the love you give to others be meaningful and genuine if you can't extend it to yourself? Recognize your strengths and give yourself credit for them. Develop them and keep track of your achievements (Figure 12-1).

What about your weaknesses? We all have limitations. We can all work to minimize the effects of these limitations, but in doing so, we have to accept them and move on. Let's concentrate on our strengths and learn to laugh at our limitations. Most importantly, don't invent limitations through negative self-talk and false beliefs.

> *You yourself, as much as anybody in the entire universe, deserve your love and affection.*
>
> —Buddha

FIGURE 12-1 A confident medical professional gives a presentation (Copyright © istock.com).

Build the Positive into Your Daily Life

Nurturing your self-esteem is a daily struggle. You are constantly being evaluated, challenged, and offered feedback you may not even want. Pursuing actions every day that support your positive self-esteem will help you accept and process criticism.

For starters, make it a point to associate with positive people. Humans need social interaction and acceptance, and you can make this an extremely positive part of your daily life if you choose who you spend your time with. Avoid the "Debbie Downers" out there by surrounding yourself with positive people.

When you are alone, take time to make yourself feel good. Meditate. Practice yoga. Detach yourself from your daily stressors, even it means stepping into a quiet room or taking some deep breaths. The more you know how to protect yourself from stress, the better you will feel about yourself.

Project confidence with your body language. To *feel* confident, *act as if* you are confident. A confident mindset is the strongest pathway to actually achieving healthy self-esteem.

Finally, accept praise and criticism with a simple "Thank you." Even those who criticize you are giving you something to think about. They might be off base, but simply smile, thank them, and say you will give some thought to the help they are offering. When you receive a compliment, a simple thank you acknowledges the kind comment. Put the praise in your gratitude journal.

JOURNALING 12-2

Make a section of your journal a "gratitude journal." At the end of every day, describe an instance that you are grateful for.

Challenge Yourself

Nobody improves without challenging themselves. We must all challenge ourselves to become better people. When you accomplish something challenging, you raise your self-esteem. Think about playing a sport. If you play against someone who is much worse than you, you won't get better. By the same token, if you play against someone who is better than you, you will improve your game. This philosophy applies to any activity or role. You learn best from those who are more advanced than you, so seek these people out when you want to improve your abilities and your self-esteem.

Once your efforts to improve your self-esteem start to pay off, begin developing skills to layer on top of your confidence. Assertiveness, for example, is a great skill to expand. Being assertive is not the same as being aggressive or defensive. Rather, it is simply sticking up for yourself, for others, and for the issues you care about. Of course, there is a proper time and place for asserting yourself. You should defend yourself when something is at stake, such as your self-esteem. You should also use assertiveness to defend the policies and rules of your workplace, the safety and professionalism of your practice, and the standards of behavior you expect from co-workers and clients.

Fear is one enemy of self-esteem. Although some fears are real, most are irrational. Consider ways you could increase your self-esteem at work if you weren't being held back by fears. To test a fear, challenge it. Most fears, when challenged, disappear or at least recede. If you fear approaching strangers, you will usually find that new people are not as scary as you thought if you challenge your fear. Perhaps you fear public speaking, a particular medical procedure, or aggressive co-workers. Once you identify a fear that is holding you back, make a plan to confront the fear and master the behavior. You will be more effective at your job and possess a solid level of positive self-esteem. When you step outside of your comfort zone, it will feel a little dangerous at first, but persist. "Fake it until you make it," and soon your comfort zone will open up.

Make Positive Connections

Asking for help is not a sign of weakness. Rather, needing help and not asking for it is weak. Health professionals are usually eager to share their expertise when asked. When you ask for help, you receive assistance with your immediate problem and strengthen a relationship with your co-worker.

Relationships are a source of self-esteem. Attend as many social events with co-workers as you can. Treat meetings as an opportunity to strengthen relationships. Meet co-workers you don't already know and try to engage in some activity with them. Try to connect with your patients using a smile, body language, eye contact, and active listening. By helping others, you receive help in the form of recognition, acknowledgement, respect, appreciation, and gratitude—all great things for building self-esteem.

CASE STUDY 12-1
The Diploma

Christine Sarkasian had been working as a professional coder on cardiology units for three years. She had already earned her Certified Professional Coder® (CPC®) certification, and she had a goal of making a yearly salary of at least $50,000 within two years. She had advanced knowledge of cardiac coding, and she thought she would try for the Certified Cardiology Coder (CCC™) Credential. She submitted the required two letters of recommendation and signed up for a test site. As an American Academy of Professional Coders (AAPC) member, the fee was $245 and included one retake.

The exam didn't go as well as Christine had anticipated. The 150 multiple choice questions covered many situations she had never encountered before and she had to guess on several of them.

The week-long wait for her score was excruciating. Christine had told many of her colleagues, friends, and family members that she was going for the CCC Credential. Finally, she went online and learned that she had failed.

At first, she was angry. How could she fail the exam with all of her experience? How was she going to tell her friends and colleagues? Christine started beating herself up about her score. "I'm just stupid," she told herself. "I'm not worth it." That night, she had trouble sleeping.

When she awoke, she felt better. She called up her friend Marsha who was an instructor with a CPC-I certification and taught at the college Christine had attended. "You should have called me *before* you took that test," Marsha said. "That exam is super hard. I could have given you some prep tips."

"I didn't prep at all," Christine said. "I'm so stupid."

"It was a mistake not to prep, but you're not stupid," Marsha said. "You just made an error in judgment."

After speaking with Marsha, Christine put together a plan for retaking the exam. She asked her colleague, Dr. Bachmann, for help with her cardiac catheterization procedures. He agreed to help her devise a study plan. Christine registered for online practice exams at the AAPC site. With her membership, she could register for less than $30. Plus, the practice exams included rationales, and she could take them as often as she wanted. She asked colleagues about their CCC exam experiences.

After four weeks, Christine took advantage of the exam retake. She figured out that she had two minutes and fifteen seconds to answer each question. She left the test site that afternoon feeling confident about her effort.

Thanks to all of her hard work, Christine passed the exam. Ten days after taking it, she received the certificate diploma and had it framed.

QUESTIONS FOR THOUGHT AND REFLECTION

1. Could Christine have succumbed to low self-esteem? What indicates that possibility?
2. Christine was able to move on despite being upset. What does that indicate?
3. How did Christine's conversation with Marsha help her?
4. What else could Christine have done to prepare for the retake?

Down a Dark Road

Ava had been a surgical technologist for two years, but she had never had trouble like this. She had been hauled into a meeting of the surgical oncology team for a review of a recent surgery that had gone wrong. The patient had lung cancer, but developed sepsis shortly after the lobectomy, and now he was in a coma and not expected to live.

"For one thing, Ava, we don't seem to have the patient's informed consent for the surgery on file," said Dr. Hector, his face a pale shade of purple. "You did get the informed consent, didn't you?"

"Yes. You initialed it," she said.

"Then where is it?" he thundered. "And stop chewing that gum!"

Ava muttered that she would look for it. She was bad at filing. She hated it. But it must be somewhere in the stack on her desk.

"It's only a matter of time before lawyers are sifting through that chart. Mr. Longoria won't be signing another one, so I want that consent form in the chart immediately." He waved her out of the room.

Ava found the consent. "What an idiot I am," she thought to herself. "I'm making problems for myself." She put the consent in Mr. Longoria's chart and went to let the doctors know.

"Great. Now, what about the infection? What can you tell us about your autoclaving of the instruments?"

Ava's heart sunk. She thought she had properly sterilized the instruments, but it seemed now as though they were blaming her. "I don't know."

"You don't know, or you didn't sterilize them properly?"

"I think I did."

"You think you did," Dr. Hector snarled at her. "I can hear that in court now. 'I think I did.'" He waved her out again.

Ava went home angry at herself and the doctors. She flopped on the bed. All that time to become a surg tech, and for what? From now on, it was just a paycheck to her.

QUESTIONS FOR THOUGHT AND DISCUSSION

1. Did Ava defend herself against the bullying she was getting?
2. Do you think this story would have been different if Ava had put the informed consent in the patient's chart?
3. What could Ava have done to better protect her self-esteem?
4. How do you think Ava will behave when she returns to work?

⭐ EXPERIENTIAL EXERCISES

1. Review the journal you have kept for this book and look for evidence of your self-esteem.
2. Pick out a positive self-affirmation you can always use silently to yourself when your self-esteem is challenged.
3. Make a list of your "greatest hits," the things you have accomplished in your life that you are most proud of.
4. Make a list of all your weaknesses. Now, cross out all of those that don't really hold you back. If there are any left uncrossed, make a plan to correct them to the level that they stop holding you back. Then, return to your strengths.
5. Wear a rubber band around your wrist. Whenever you notice that your self-talk is negative, snap the rubber band against the inside of your wrist.

🔄 CROSS CURRENTS WITH OTHER SOFT SKILLS

ADOPTING A POSITIVE MENTAL ATTITUDE: When you choose to be positive and enthusiastic, your self-esteem rises. (pp. 2-11)

MANAGING STRESS: Many of the strategies and techniques you use to manage stress can contribute to your healthy self-esteem. (pp. 203-210)

SHOWING EMPATHY, SENSITIVITY, AND CARING: Paradoxically, when your focus is on others, you are being kind to yourself. (pp. 218-222)

READING AND SPEAKING BODY LANGUAGE: Let your body language project confidence to the outside world, and your inner world will follow. (pp. 277-284)

SETTING GOALS AND PLANNING ACTIONS: When you are working on your personal achievements, you are strengthening your self-esteem. (pp. 286-291)

Controlling Anxiety

LEARNING OBJECTIVE 2:
CONTROLLING ANXIETY

- Explain anxiety.
- Manage internal thought processes.
- Manage interactions with individuals at work.
- Identify and manage irrational anxiety-provoking thoughts.
- Effectively follow through on behaviors that produce positive outcomes.

Anxiety is a thin stream of fear trickling through the mind. If encouraged, it cuts a stream through which all other thoughts are drained.

—Arthur Somers Roche

WHAT IF?

What if your entire life were anxiety-free? You didn't worry about the bills being paid, the children being safe, getting in a car accident, not graduating, or not having a job. What would you feel like? Why do you think people choose to worry?

In contrast, what if your day was filled with anxious thoughts about everything at work? What physical symptoms do you think this would manifest if you continued being anxious from one moment to the next?

What Is Anxiety?

Anxiety is the feeling you get when your well-being is threatened. You or a loved one could be in physical danger. Perhaps something is challenging your self-esteem. Maybe your status is being threatened because you are criticized in public. Maybe you had a falling out with a friend that threatens the relationship. Maybe you are being micromanaged at work, and it feels as if you've lost control of your time and activities. Maybe you are treated unfairly. When you have something to fear or lose, anxiety can dominate your feelings.

Anxiety occurs on a continuum from mild to debilitating. Mild anxiety can actually improve your performance by motivating you and helping you to concentrate on the activity that has raised your feelings of anxiety (Figure 12-2). For instance, you may be extra careful when taking blood from someone who intimidates you. You may focus intently on your job when you are assisting a dentist you may not know very well. Anxiety like this can still be uncomfortable,

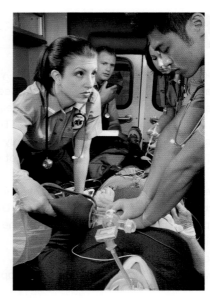

FIGURE 12-2 Emergency Medical Technicians quickly and efficiently respond to the immediate medical needs of an injured man (Copyright © istock.com).

but it can help improve your performance by forcing you to plan and concentrate.

Most anxiety associated with work is temporary. It may be triggered by a past negative experience such as losing a job or observing a negative treatment outcome. The more anxiety you experience, the more poorly you may perform, which can create additional anxiety. For that reason, the smartest strategy is to nip your anxiety in the bud.

When anxiety goes beyond mild, however, it impairs performance. Anxiety triggers the stress response, discussed in Chapter 5. It clouds your thinking process, creates rapid, shallow breathing, raises your heart rate, and imposes a sense of panic. More severe is chronic anxiety, which is a constant and general feeling of dread about everything, and phobias, which are anxieties in response to specific triggers such as spiders (arachnophobia) or closed spaces (claustrophobia). If you suffer from chronic anxiety or phobias, you should seek treatment.

How Irrational Thoughts Form Misbeliefs

When anxiety is not addressed in the moment, it can leave you with an irrational bias that affects your professional behavior. For example, a medical assistant may avoid screaming children due to a stressful interaction. He may develop an unfounded belief, such as, "I'm not good with children. I always make them cry." However, the health professional didn't necessarily cause the outburst and it doesn't mean that the same reaction will happen every time. Always take time to challenge the original negative thought before it develops into a bias.

Sometimes, when a profound incident occurs, we develop stories to justify why we perceived the event as negative instead of neutral. For example, almost every medical office assistant will encounter a patient who is upset about a billing error sooner or later. One will handle the situation and not attach any meaning to it, but another one might avoid handling any future billing questions, because he or she thinks, "I always mess up patients' accounts. Someone who is better at math should handle billing questions."

For example, suppose a patient vomited after a dental assistant took x-rays of his teeth. The assistant may believe that she caused the patient to gag and vomit, and therefore is not good at taking x-rays. This, in turn, causes her to avoid taking x-rays of patients, which creates hardships for her co-workers.

Avoidance limits your usefulness on the job and creates obstacles to your progress.

◐ JOURNALING 12-3

Write about something or someone you avoid at work because of a past negative experience. What thoughts and feelings did you choose to associate with this event or person? What story did you create to justify avoiding future encounters? Rewrite the story with a new, positive, and realistic outcome.

Controlling Anxiety

Learning how to effectively manage your anxiety is crucial to your overall and day-to-day success at work. It is important to catch anxious thinking early, before it evolves into fearful behavior. To do so, you will have to be skilled in identifying your anxious-negative thoughts on a regular basis, then employing the following strategies to conquer them. You cannot always control external events, especially those causing anxiety, but you can almost always control your internal responses to external events.

We cannot direct the wind, but we can adjust our sails.
—Bertha Calloway

Choose Your Thoughts

Believe it or not, you get to choose your thoughts. You stand at the gate of your mind and you get to determine what passes through, and what is cast down. When you guard the door of your thinking, you can refute some of the thoughts that do not align with reality. For example, let's say you're administering an IV for a patient in the hospital and you think, "What if I give the patient the wrong medication?" In that moment, if you are aware of the thought, you can stop and refute the thought by checking the medication order before it develops into fear. You do this by:

1. Identifying the concerning thought so that it breaks through to your awareness.
2. Analyzing whether it is a logical thought.
3. Refuting the thought or challenging its validity.
4. Carrying out the action you intended before the fearful or anxious thought intruded on you.

Refuting or challenging an anxious thought is not about being in denial. It is really about examining the content of your thoughts and determining whether they are rational and proportional to the situation.

Cognitive psychology offers effective approaches you can use to alleviate your anxiety. Using cognitive psychology, you realize that the reality you experience is based on your thinking, your thoughts, and your interpretation of events and circumstances. When you challenge irrational thoughts that are provoking anxiety, you can replace them with rational thoughts that tend to drain the anxiety out of the situation. Box 12-2 offers a series of rational thoughts you can use to substitute for irrational thoughts.

BOX 12-2

Some Rational Beliefs that Can Help Alleviate Anxiety

Self-approval is more important that the approval of others.
Mistakes and failures are not negative if I can learn from them.
Other people are not perfect; they will make mistakes.
Not everything has to go my way.
Events may be outside of my control, but I can control my response to them.
Problems will get worse if I ignore them.
The past is over with; I must live in the present and plan for the future.
Uncontrolled emotions are usually an unproductive response to my problems.
Problems have solutions, usually many of them.

Do you harbor irrational beliefs? For example, it is irrational to think that everything is directed at you personally. List as many as you can think of. Then, refute each of them.

Conquer Your Avoidance Behaviors

To avoid avoidance, you must have enough courage to take a small step toward your fear and pass through it. For example, the dental assistant who is anxious about taking x-rays can use a process called "gradual exposure" to combat the feared stimulus (taking x-rays) until it no longer produces anxiety. She can start by developing the films for another assistant who has taken x-rays and then mount the films. Next, when she is confident that she can complete this task, she can move to setting up the films and film holders for the other assistant and seat the patient. Then, she can hand the other assistant the film holder for placement in the patient's mouth. This process will provide enough positive experiences to nullify the "all or nothing" thinking developed by the negative experience and allow for full resolution of the anxiety.

Learn to Relax

Relaxation is a learned behavior; it is knowledge you should have in your battle against anxiety. Many techniques, such as deep breathing, are simple and require little time. Others strategies, such as recomposing yourself in private, as shown in Figure 12-3, require a more focused approach. Other relaxation strategies appear in Box 12-3.

Let Yourself Off the Hook

We can be amazingly hard on ourselves. Negative self-talk, low self-esteem, anxiety, uncontrolled emotions, impatience, intolerance, and even self-hatred are common ways we beat ourselves up. If you are your own worst enemy, bring yourself immediate peace of mind simply by recognizing how hard you have been on yourself. Next, try to be kind to yourself. You are compassionate toward your patients. Why not be compassionate toward yourself?

Anxiety and Your Health

Finally, use your own health as strong motivation for controlling anxiety. Remember that anxiety can cause

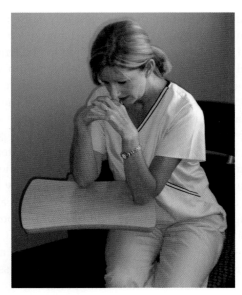

FIGURE 12-3 Health professional regaining her composure.

BOX 12-3

Relaxation and Other Antianxiety Techniques

- Hypnosis
- Yoga
- Meditation
- Intensely visualized peaceful settings
- Deep breathing
- Mantras and affirmations
- Progressive muscle relaxation
- White noise

---

physical symptoms including shortness of breath, stomach pains, nausea, muscular tension, shakiness, and dizziness. Many of these symptoms can interrupt a normal work day and even cause biochemical changes in the body, which can create illness. If anxiety becomes chronic or severe, you may need medication and mental health care to eradicate it. It's much easier to prevent out-of-control anxiety than to address it once it's out of control.

Heavy thoughts bring on physical maladies; when the soul is oppressed, so is the body.

—Martin Luther

As a last thought, think of some remedies for anxiety that you developed as a child. Children possess great wisdom, as the antianxiety techniques listed in Box 12-4 demonstrate.

CASE STUDY 12-2
The King Exception

Martha had been a dental assistant for about five years. She knew the clinical side well, but she was too timid for the front office.

In order to be more assertive, she decided to work the front office one day. She was assisting a patient, Mr. King, with an outstanding balance on his account when she decided to test out her assertiveness. She presented the longtime patient with his statement and requested payment in full. Mr. King was used to being billed, but Martha wasn't aware of that arrangement, stating, "This is the policy."

Mr. King fumbled for a credit card and slammed it on the counter. "Here! Put the entire balance on this." Martha did so, thanked him, and gave him his receipt. Mr. King grabbed it angrily and walked out, muttering, "You can cancel my next appointment...I won't be returning."

Martha was all shook up. She hadn't intended to make the patient angry. She was just trying to be assertive, but it backfired. Dr. Singh would be infuriated. She should have had a better grasp of the policy before trying to enforce it. She could lose her job over this, and—"Stop!" she said out loud.

"Stop what?" asked Muriel, Martha's co-worker, startled.

"I was talking to myself," Martha said. "I didn't mean to say it out loud."

"Well, what are you stopping?" Muriel asked.

"You know, Mr. King canceled his next appointment and left in a huff because I made him pay his bill in full."

"Ahh, he's a pain in the neck," Muriel said. "He insists on being billed. I should have told you that."

Martha felt a little better, but she still wanted to discuss it with Dr. Singh. "Oh, he is a hothead, that one," Dr. Singh said, "but we can bill him."

So Martha called Mr. King that afternoon to explain the misunderstanding.

"Mr. King, I made a mistake in taking your credit card," she said. "You were absolutely right. You are to be billed. I have already refunded your card."

"Yeah? What happened to your policy," he said sarcastically.

"I'm new at the front desk," she told him cheerfully. "It was my mistake."

"I guess anyone can make a mistake," grumbled Mr. King.

"Can I confirm your next appointment, on May 7?"

"Yeah, I'll be there," Mr. King said.

QUESTIONS FOR THOUGHT AND REFLECTION

1. Describe the anxiety symptoms that Martha was experiencing.
2. How did she manage to control her anxiety?
3. What did Martha learn about herself?

Down a Dark Road

Kathy and Charlene were dental assistants at a busy cosmetic practice in an upscale area. Kathy was the assistant for the owner, Dr. Cromwell, and Charlene was the assistant of the associate dentist, Dr. Gerald. Charlene was new to the practice, but she and Kathy were already not getting along. Kathy just did not like Charlene, and Charlene did not care. Charlene knew that both dentists appreciated her hard work, and this seemed to make Kathy jealous. Kathy took her time when she worked, but Charlene moved quickly and efficiently. It didn't help that both dentists always spoke highly of Charlene and didn't say much about Kathy even though she had been there longer.

As time passed, both assistants avoided each other. After a few months, Kathy left her keys on Dr. Cromwell's desk one day with a short note: "You think Charlene is so great. You can have her. I quit."

The following Monday, everyone found out that Kathy quit without notice. Charlene felt it was because of her. She suddenly felt anxious. She never expected Kathy to quit. Her anxiety escalated throughout the day as she ran between the two dentists, trying to assist them both. She felt oddly responsible for the office drama.

Charlene's thoughts continued to take shape in a negative direction. She formed and accepted thoughts such as "I can't get along with anyone. She quit because of me. I'm going to get fired because of what happened." She found herself perspiring and dropping instruments. As soon as she made one mistake, more cascaded.

"Calm down, Charlene," said Dr. Cromwell. "Everything is fine."

Still, she couldn't calm down. It seemed to her that people stopped talking when she arrived, as if they were talking about her. She just wanted to be a dental assistant, not the center of a work crisis. Maybe she wasn't cut out to be a dental assistant.

That night, she lay awake in bed. How was she ever going to get through Tuesday?

QUESTIONS FOR THOUGHT AND REFLECTION

1. Do you think Kathy quit because of Charlene?
2. Is it productive for Charlene to play negative thoughts in her head?
3. Is the anxiety that Charlene is experiencing proportionate to the situation?
4. What is an instance of positive self-talk that Charlene could use to neutralize her negative self-talk?
5. Anxiety usually occurs in relation to someone or something. When Charlene experienced anxiety, do you think she was anxious about losing her job or causing someone else to quit?

⊛ EXPERIENTIAL EXERCISES

1. The next time you feel anxious, see if deep breathing makes you feel better.
2. Identify a traumatic or profound past incident that still makes you feel anxious today when you think of it; what can you do to lower or eliminate the anxiety it still causes you?
3. List tasks or duties at work that you like to avoid or that make you feel anxious.
4. How do you relax?
5. How did you handle anxiety when you were a child?

CROSS CURRENTS WITH OTHER SOFT SKILLS

MANAGING YOUR TIME AND ORGANIZING YOUR LIFE: This eliminates a major source of anxiety in everyone's life. (pp. 11-18)

MANAGING AND RESOLVING CONFLICT: Conflict will not go away by itself; it will cause anxiety until it is satisfactorily resolved. (pp. 224-231)

FOLLOWING RULES AND REGULATIONS: Knowing what is expected and what is permissible helps alleviate anxiety. (pp. 291-297)

Practicing Patience

How poor are they that have not patience! What wound did ever heal but by degrees?

—William Shakespeare

- See patience in its long-term context.
- List the dangers of impatience.
- Learn to be slow and methodical.
- Identify your impatience triggers.
- Describe flow.
- Relate patience to emotions.

Anxiety is the enemy of patience. Conversely, patience is a remedy for anxiety. Patience is enduring provocation, delay, or annoyance. It is a positive that can be chosen.

As communication has become instantaneous, we are sometimes expected to be in two places at once and produce or perform at increasingly faster rates. Everyone wants immediate results—that is, instant gratification.

Patience and Long-term Gratification

Instant gratification is a 21st-century trap because most of the finest things in life take time and patience: health, education, meaningful relationships, raising children, rising in your field, developing your skills, wealth, maturity.

With impatience, we risk missing out on the fun and meaningful parts of life and work. Being stretched too thin might result in depression, anxiety, and anhedonia, which is the inability to experience pleasure.

Patience is the only real pathway to the big things that matter. Fortunately, patience can be learned and made a habit. Developing patience can be a slow process. It is a difficult, step-by-step approach to attaining things that matter.

How to Gain Patience

If you want to cultivate patience, you have to make a few sacrifices that seem to be at odds with the times we live in.

Go Slow for the Flow

Go slow. We are encouraged to get things done quickly. It may be a paradox, but going slow is often the best way to go fast. If you slow down, you don't make mistakes as easily and you don't have to do as many tasks over again. Making a little extra time now, when things are not rushed, can make a big difference later, when things are hectic. For instance, take a few minutes to clean up examination rooms or dental stations after seeing a patient so they will be ready when someone else is rushed in. Many activities in health care require precision. You want to go slow when you are calibrating an IV drip, mixing dental cement, or positioning a patient for a radiograph. Making deliberate decisions and movements are often standard best practices in the health care field.

Under ideal circumstances, health professionals report a state of "flow," described by psychologist Mihaly Csikszentmihaly as a state of total involvement with your work, where time seems to disappear and you merge with your work. It is a state of intense concentration which you can learn to establish by developing deep patience. The health professional in Figure 12-4 is engrossed in her conversation with a nursing home patient. With practice, almost any activity can lend itself to the flow state.

Keep Big Goals and Rewards in Mind

Focus on the big, long-term things like goals, relationships, and health. Whenever you feel that you may lose patience, consider the long-term reward of your activity. Take yourself out of the moment as much as possible, and tell yourself that only small steps can add up to big achievements.

FIGURE 12-4 Health professional spending time with a nursing home patient (Copyright © istock.com).

BOX 12-5

Tips for Maintaining Patience

- Avoid staring at clocks.
- Savor an empty moment; they are hard to come by.
- Practice yoga.
- Breathe deeply.
- Reflect before acting or reacting.
- Be nonjudgmental.
- See waiting as a positive experience.

Maintain Your Cool

Keep on hand an arsenal of techniques to help you maintain your cool. When challenged by something you cannot change, accept it and let it go. Empty your mind. Meditate to regain your patience and better judgment.

More patience techniques appear in Box 12-5. Chief among these techniques is deep breathing. Take a deep breath from your diaphragm. You should be able to see your abdomen expand as you fill your lungs with oxygen. Inhale slowly, and then exhale even more slowly. Take your mind off whatever is making you feel impatient and focus just on your breath. After several breaths, you will be able to reassert your patience, and choose a rational, healthy response to whatever is provoking you.

In addition to deep breathing, adopt some simple activities you enjoy as a stopgap against impatience. Sometimes it's a matter of physically removing yourself from the irritation you are experiencing. Exercise or take a drive if you have the time. If time is limited, just step outside or look out a window. A change of scenery often takes your mind away from your impatience and helps you restore equilibrium.

Start Small and Build Patience

Patience is a sign of respect. Whether you are patient with elderly people or children, people with communication disorders, or with a friend's tedious concerns, you will be seen as a person who is respectful. People who give respect, get respect.

Health care workers often need great reserves of patience. Some work will be tedious but necessary. On other occasions, you may have to spend a lot of time with patients in nursing homes, psychiatric facilities, or surgical units. You have to build up your patience reserve. Start small. Exercise patience in a line, in traffic, or in a meeting. Build the patience demanded for the important things in life and work.

Delays, waiting, and unexpected events are all part of life. Don't get too attached to your original plans. Be ready to make new ones when the need to do so arises.

? WHAT IF?

What if your day doesn't go as planned? How can you handle this in a positive way?

Guard Against Impatience Triggers

Identify the triggers that make you impatient, such as crying children, crashed computers, thoughtless co-workers, or unscheduled interruptions. Anticipating triggers before they occur will help you remind yourself that you have a choice in how you react.

← JOURNALING 12-5

List the people, places, situations, circumstances, and times that cause you to lose your patience. This will help you become aware of these triggers. Next, list tips to help you remain patient when faced with these triggers.

Ultimate Benefits of Patience

One of the great benefits of patience is that it is often your best defense against impatient people. Waiting patients and clients are often the most impatient people. Their lives are often highly scheduled, and being anxious about a delayed appointment or their condition can stress them out further. Meet impatient clients with patience. Take time to smile. Make eye contact. Use your body language. Listen actively without interrupting. Speak calmly and softly. Offer to help in any way you can. Patience often begets patience.

Finally, too many people end up wondering, "Where did the time go?" Nobody wants to look back and find they have filled their time with trivial arguments and excessive attention to everyday hassles. You want all your small moments and little efforts to add up to satisfaction and goal achievement. Patience is the pathway to meaning.

You can't always get what you want. But if you try some time, you just might find you get what you need.

—Mick Jagger

CASE STUDY 12-3
The Foot Lady

Jaime Claxon was much loved by the patients, their families, and her co-workers at the Whiteside County Nursing Home, where she worked five evenings a week. She was known as the "Foot Lady" because she gave the best foot massages.

The day started winding down at the beginning of Jaime's shift. Dinner started as early as 4:00. Baths and personal care took place shortly after. By seven or eight o'clock, the place was quiet. Some patients were in bed. Others watched TV, talked, or played games. At this time, the staff members' main job was to spend time and talk with their patients. Jaime used her foot massages to make this time the best part of her patients' day.

Jaime had assembled a collection of supplies in an old-fashioned shoeshine box: clippers, files, lotions, creams, and aromatic ointments. Every patient, whether they were able to talk with Jaime or could not communicate at all, enjoyed visits from the Foot Lady. She took her time, examining each foot, each nail bed, each callous. "I know their feet better than their faces," she joked to the staff.

Between patients, Jaime was a virtual model of hand-washing best practices, washing her hands using a fingernail brush.

Even the staff received the special treatment on their birthdays. Lydia Hodges, the Director of Nursing, said she looked forward to her birthday every year only because of Jaime's foot care.

One afternoon, Dr. Cronin was reviewing charts in the nursing station. He came in twice a week as a matter of routine, and more often if there was a medical issue. "You know, Jaime," he said, "we could have a podiatrist come in and charge Medicare for it. It would raise some revenue."

Lydia spoke up. "I think the patients would notice the difference. We'd have a revolt on our hands."

QUESTIONS FOR THOUGHT AND REFLECTION

1. What benefits did Jaime enjoy from her highly developed sense of patience?
2. What observations can you make linking patience to human connections?
3. What made Jaime special?

Down a Dark Road

When Axel became a physical therapy assistant, he worked for a man named Orville Chance who ran the small practice in central New Jersey. Orville encouraged Axel to get his Bachelor's degree in Physical Therapy. "You have talent," Orville told him, "but you won't get anywhere without a college degree." So Axel took some courses and continued to work part time at the Jersey practice.

Axel earned a Master's degree, and he might have pursued a doctorate if he had not been offered a chance to buy the Jersey practice. By then, Orville was going through a divorce, and his children were always in trouble. Axel had to manage a lot of the day-to-day responsibilities of the practice. It turned out that Axel had a talent for the business side of the practice. He negotiated contracts for referrals and became a preferred provider for area hospitals and practices. Soon, he opened up a second branch in

Brunswick and bought a third practice in Atlantic City. He was so busy that he had to hire managers for his second and third locations, and he needed Orville to step up to the plate and manage the original practice.

Orville wasn't doing well. He was losing weight and looking haggard. Axel barely had time to notice. He asked Orville about his health, but Orville just said he was OK.

"Good," said Axel, "because you're missing too much work. I don't have time to manage this practice."

Increasingly, Axel worked out of his car. One day he called the original practice, and Penny, the receptionist, was whispering in the phone.

"What? I can't hear you. What?" He was getting annoyed. It was something about Orville, something she had to whisper about. So he changed directions and drove to the practice. He found Orville sitting in the parking lot, smoking a cigarette.

"What's going on, Orville?" Axel demanded to know. "You smoke now? Outside a PT practice?"

"At least I'm smoking outside," said Orville, not really looking at him.

"I don't need sarcasm, Orville. You're behind on the billing. There's constant turnover here. What's going on?"

"I have a lot on my mind," shrugged Orville.

"A lot on your mind? You don't have the luxury of checking out. There's too much work to do here," Axel said.

Orville just blew smoke.

"I'm not putting up with this, Orville. I've carried you too long. You've got to either step up or move on."

Orville said nothing.

Axel went inside. The first person he saw was Tony. "You're in charge here," he told Tony and brushed past him. He went to the front desk. "Penny, make sure that Orville's health insurance is paid up. We'll carry him for a year. Pay him $100 a week until you hear from me."

Over the years, Axel built more than twenty practices. Orville disappeared and the checks started coming back in the mail. Whenever Axel reflected on his goals and accomplishments, he always left the same goal unchanged at the bottom of his portfolio: "More patience with Orville."

QUESTIONS FOR THOUGHT AND REFLECTION

1. Why did Axel lose patience with Orville?
2. What happened to Axel's friendship with Orville? Was Axel a good friend?
3. How did Axel's friendship with Orville fit into his long-term goals?
4. How did Axel feel about Orville in the end?

⭐ EXPERIENTIAL EXERCISES

1. Take some deep breaths the next time you are annoyed or irked. How did that feel?
2. The next time you are waiting in a line, try to focus on something else besides how fast the line is moving and why it is moving so slowly. See if by concentrating on something the line seems to go faster. You can do the same thing when you are stuck in traffic.
3. Empty your mind of all thoughts for one minute. Practice this twice a day for ten days.
4. Try some new activity that takes concentration, like sewing, ice skating, or a musical instrument. Go slow. Challenge yourself to be exact.
5. Do something you like and that you're good at. See if you can experience a state of flow.

🌀 CROSS CURRENTS WITH OTHER SOFT SKILLS

MANAGING STRESS: Learning to become patient can actually be a tool to combat stress. (pp. 203-210)

SHOWING EMPATHY, SENSITIVITY, AND CARING: How does patience as a learned skill complement patient care? (pp. 218-222)

LISTENING ACTIVELY: Is listening thoughtfully possible without patience? (pp. 263-269)

SETTING GOALS AND PLANNING ACTIONS: Goals can only be achieved little by little, working patiently every day. (pp. 286-291)

Strengthening Resilience

Inside of a ring or out, ain't nothing wrong with going down. It's staying down that's wrong.

—Muhammad Ali

LEARNING OBJECTIVE 4: STRENGTHENING RESILIENCE

- Understand the relationship between stress and resilience.
- Understand the relationship between resilience and problem solving.
- Describe the internal locus of control.
- Understand the relationship between resilience and optimism.

Resilience is the upside of stress. It is the ability to bounce back when you are knocked down.

← JOURNALING 12-6

Record three crises or stressors you have encountered in the past month. Then, briefly describe anything positive that could or did come from these stressors.

Choose Your Response to Life's Lemons

The human body goes into the stress response only when it *perceives* a stressor. If you can prevent the

BOX 12-6

Resilient Responses to Common Stressors

Instead of	Try
Black-and-white thinking	Looking for the shades of gray in a situation
Responding emotionally	Striving for objectivity and neutrality
Judging yourself harshly	Being kind and reflective toward yourself
Resolving issues as good or bad, right or wrong	Experiencing the anxiety and nuance of reality
Seeking certainty in an uncertain world	Accepting uncertainty and doing what you can

FIGURE 12-5 Locus of control.

perception of stress, even in the face of an objective threat, you can prevent the physiological stress response and simultaneously respond much more resiliently to the stressor. This chapter has offered you an arsenal of tools for reframing the threat such as seeking the bright side of a problem or viewing it in a larger context. Ask yourself, "Will this still matter in 24 hours? Is this just one more obstacle along the way? Is this stressful event perhaps a minor occurrence in a larger plan you believe in?"

As with anxiety, many stressors can be addressed using straightforward analysis. Do you see any patterns in the stressor? Has this happened before? Do you already know how this turns out, or do you already have strategies for dealing with this? Box 12-6 suggests some irrational responses to stress, coupled with more rational thoughts. For instance, if you receive a poor score on a test, you probably already know you could have done more to prepare. Now you can use the poor score as a lesson to turn things around by preparing more for the next test.

A stressor is usually just a problem. The sooner you switch to problem-solving mode, the less the stressor will overcome you in any way.

When I knew better, I did better.

—Maya Angelou

Resilient people have what is called an "internal locus of control" as seen in Figure 12-5. They feel that, ultimately, they have control over their life. They do not believe that they have to give themselves up to external circumstances they don't like. They might move to Arizona if they can't stand the winter. They might decide to get divorced after trying everything to make it work. They will change jobs if they are abused. How do people change their locus of control?

First, they recognize that there is always a choice. It may take awhile to implement the choice, or it might be a hard choice to make, but it exists. If you don't think you have a choice, brainstorm. Write down all your possible choices, no matter how ridiculous. If necessary, ask a friend to help. Don't be judgmental until you have the longest list you can think of. Then, decide which choices are good and, among these, which is best. The choices you select represent your first course of action, and alternative courses of action. After a while, you may find that identifying the choices you have in your life becomes a habit.

Good outcomes can result from bad beginnings. For now, remember to accept challenges as they arise. What you do when confronted by a stressor determines how difficult the stressful event or situation turns out to be.

Be Aware

Stressors often generate emotional responses. Sometimes it just can't be helped. We are all human, and our brains have powerful limbic systems that govern our emotions. However, it can help to know what's making you feel emotional. Many people project their feelings by lashing out at others when something else altogether is bothering them. Knowing what is making you emotional is the first step in dealing with the situation correctly. Box 12-7 lists unhelpful responses to stress.

Plan, Organize, Prioritize

As we have seen, change is inevitable. The good thing about something that's inevitable is that we can anticipate and plan for it. In many cases, we can control the change before it even occurs.

The first step in planning for change is usually to impose order and structure by either adopting or recommitting to a time management system while you adjust to the change, or by breaking a new project down into tangible subtasks. As you plan, decide what you will do first. Compare one task or appointment with another. Sometimes the priority is intuitively clear, or your supervisor has set the priority for you. Your job, once the priority is set, is to follow through, always pursuing the next most important task. The exercise in Box 12-8 offers a methodology for comparing similar items on a list to determine which has a higher priority.

Be Optimistic

Optimism is an attitude that helps people succeed and bounce back in the face of adversity. Optimistic people believe that good things happen to them because that is the normal course of things. They believe that they personally deserve good things, that goodness is pervasive and permanent. When bad things happen, they ascribe them to temporary, specific causes that are exceptions to the general rule and order of life. On the other hand, pessimists expect bad things to happen and explain good things by seeing them as accidental, temporary, or out of the ordinary. Fortunately, leaders of the Positive Psychology Movement, like Martin Seligman, have shown that you are not condemned to pessimism. You can *learn* optimism! Optimism and pessimism will be covered in greater detail in Chapter 13.

Laugh

Few things help you bounce back and regain your resiliency like humor. If you are blessed with a great sense of humor and the ability to laugh at yourself and your circumstances, you possess a powerful tool in your quest for resilience.

Humor is just another defense against the universe.

—Mel Brooks

Practice

Finally, remember that life pitches all kinds of crises at us, large and small; it's normal and constant. Practice building your resilience when small crises crop up. Return the unpleasant phone call. Schedule that dental appointment. Apologize to your co-worker. Get over your team's big loss. Decline the invitation.

BOX 12-7

Unhelpful Responses to Stress

- Personalizing
- Catastrophizing
- Isolation
- Worry
- Blame
- Victimization
- Self-pity
- Immobilization

BOX 12-8

Paired Task Comparisons for Setting Priorities

No.	Task	Checks	Rank	Compare
1	Pour medications	√√√	2	1-2; 1-3; 1-4; 1-5
2	Change Mr. Ott's bandage	√√√√	1	2-3; 2-4; 2-5
3	Write shift notes		5	3-4; 3-5
4	Set up search committee	√	4	4-5
5	Coach Lou	√√	3	

- Write down your tasks in no particular order.
- Compare each task with the others. Put the "√" in the box with the highest priority. Always decide, even if the difference is slight.
- Count up the checks.
- Re-rank based on checks. In case of a tie, compare the two tied tasks and decide which is more important.

Resilient people figure out the appropriate response to a problem and carry it out immediately rather than allowing problems to pile up. In fact, resilient people feel pretty good when they have solved their problems and put them safely in the past. Box 12-9 suggests resources to strengthen your resilience.

WHAT IF?

What if you oversleep and are late to work? How will you manage this minor crisis and stressor?

BOX 12-9

Sources of Resilience

- Love
- The truth
- Humor
- Forgiveness
- Exercise and recreation
- Vacation and breaks
- Sleep and rest
- Music
- Friends
- Deep breathing and meditation
- Reframing perceptions

CASE STUDY 12-4
Spark

The explosion was so loud they could hear it at the fire station on Grand Avenue, and the crew headed toward the blast even before they had an address to work with. They were the first on the scene, just as dazed neighbors were beginning to gather. It was dinner time, and most of the commuters were home by now.

Randy and Bob ran to the wreckage, while Debi called in the initial reports. There was nothing left of the home but tinder and smoke. Debi told the police dispatcher it looked like a natural gas explosion. Randy and Bob found four bodies in a quick systematic search of the rubble, three adults and a boy about twelve years of age. The bodies of the three adults were shredded, but the body of the boy was intact, although there were no clinical signs of life.

"He must have been protected by something," said Randy as he and Bob carried the body to the front lawn and began CPR. Debi came running up with the defibrillator. They shocked him twice, with no results, and continued CPR. Squad cars were converging on the scene, and several police officers helped carry the stretcher to the ambulance. Debi stowed the equipment and drove to the medical center while Randy and Bob continued CPR in the back.

At the medical center, Debi and some of the ER workers ran the gurney while Randy and Bob continued CPR until the doctors took over, rushing the boy into an operating room. Exhausted, Randy and Bob sprawled on chairs while Debi handled the reporting. After 20 minutes, Dr. Almano came out, and Randy and Bob rose to their feet. "He didn't make it," he said.

Debi came over, and the four of them huddled. Dr. Almano said, "He was dead at the scene. If there had been one spark of life left in that kid, you would have found it. Thank you."

QUESTIONS FOR THOUGHT AND REFLECTION

1. Did the EMTs do everything they could do?
2. Why did they keep working on the boy, even though there wasn't much hope?
3. Despite the outcome, do you think the EMTs felt positive about the effort they made?
4. Will they have the same resilience next time?

Down a Dark Road

At her supervisor's insistence, Jody took a long weekend to unwind, but now it was Tuesday and she didn't feel any better.

Jody was certified as an Occupational Therapy Assistant (COTA), but had also been filling in for the administrative assistant who was on maternity leave. Although everyone was pitching in, she was tired of tasks such as submitting insurance claims, writing up treatment plans, and recording progress reports.

Lydia, her supervisor, appeared in Jody's office almost as soon as Jody arrived. "I hope the long weekend helped."

Jody just looked at her.

"Jody, you have to speak to me when I speak to you."

Lydia's hovering reminded her of her mother. "Yes, thank you," she said, forcing a smile. "It was a big help."

"Why don't you tidy up your office a bit?" said Lydia. "I don't know how you find anything."

"I don't think that would work," said Jody. "I just need to keep focused." Lydia said nothing. "Don't worry," Jody said. "I'll get organized." She pretended to turn to the work on her desk.

Jody didn't make much progress. She really didn't know where to start. She made a few piles, then went in search of her friend, Thomasina, who was one of the nurses. She found her lounging in the break room. "I can't stand this paperwork," Jody started. "Did you see Lydia in that hideous dress?" Jody went on. "She acts like she's 20."

"No," Thomasina said. "She's a phony, though. I'm just glad I can wear these scrubs."

"When is she going to retire? I feel like she's watching me constantly. I could get a lot more done without her breathing down my neck every minute."

"She's got you in her sights, all right," said Thomasina.

"Yeah, OK," Jody said. "Well, I have an appointment with Calvin. He's getting worse."

When Calvin arrived at Jody's office in his wheelchair, he seemed to be in a good mood, smiling and calling her "Miss Jody." He had a miniature basketball clutched in one hand. He had cerebral palsy, and his arms were writhing more than usual today.

"Don't tell me you want to play catch," Jody said.

Calvin grinned and tried to throw the ball, but it went awry, bounced off the wall, and landed at Jody's feet with a thud.

"This ball's flat," said Jody, picking it up and tossing it in her wastebasket. Jody was in no mood for smiling.

She started with the usual assessments. In a few minutes, Lydia was at her door.

"Did you see Calvin's ball?" she asked brightly, winking at Calvin. "It's such a beautiful day, Jody. Why don't you take him outside and play catch with him?" Lydia looked around. "Where's the ball?"

Sheepishly, Jody pulled it out of her wastebasket. "It's flat," she said weakly.

At the end of the day, as Jody was leaving, Lydia suddenly appeared out of nowhere again. "You seem to be everywhere," said Jody.

"You've been here a long time, Jody," said Lydia, ignoring Jody's comment. "We could go through a long and painful process, but I don't want to go down that road. I hope you will come to the same conclusion that I have: it's time for you to look for a new job."

As Jody drove out of the parking lot, she honked her horn at some kids kicking a soccer ball. "Get away from the parking lot!" she yelled. She pulled out in traffic and was almost hit by a car she didn't see. "Everybody's crazy!" she said to no one. As she pulled onto the Interstate, she felt more miserable than ever. Great, she thought to herself. Who's going to hire me?

QUESTIONS FOR THOUGHT AND REFLECTION

1. In what ways did Lydia try to help Jody?
2. If you were Jody's supervisor, what else could you have done to help her?
3. Did Jody get any support from her friend Thomasina?
4. How is Jody's attitude affecting her job performance?
5. Where is Jody placing her anger and irritation?
6. Do you agree with Lydia's judgment and approach?

1. Make a playlist of motivational songs that you can listen to when you need to be resilient.
2. Take vitamins to improve your immune system.
3. Help a friend brainstorm possible solutions to a crisis.
4. Who do you call when you experience a crisis?
5. Take a problem you have to bed with you. Think about it before you drift off to sleep. Do any solutions emerge in the morning?

MANAGING STRESS: Resilience is the opposite of stressed. (pp. 203-210)

DEALING WITH DIFFICULT PEOPLE: So often, difficult people require us to be resilient. (pp. 231-238)

TAKING ACCOUNTABILITY: You are resilient when you take control of your life. (pp. 333-336)

EXUDING OPTIMISM, ENTHUSIASM, AND POSITIVITY: A recipe for resilience! (pp. 380-384)

CHAPTER 13

Managing Your Emotions

THEMES TO CONSIDER

- Recognize when your work and personal problems overlap.
- Describe the emotional problems that personal problems can cause at work.
- Describe the components of an anger management program.
- List the advantages of being optimistic.
- List the dangers of being pessimistic.

Separating Your Work and Personal Problems

LEARNING OBJECTIVE 1: SEPARATING YOUR WORK AND PERSONAL PROBLEMS

- Recognize when a personal problem is affecting you, your behavior, and your emotions at work.
- Articulate the work–life balance challenges facing health care professionals.
- Be aware of triggers that can spread personal problems to your workplace.
- Understand the consequences of being a problem employee.

Have you ever left for work in a huff, your temper as hot as your coffee? Sure you have. We all have. If your personal problems spill over into work, however, they will prevent your mood from improving. If you are unhappy at work, people will walk on eggshells around you. Worse, your unhappiness could create conflicts with your co-workers. In the end, you become your own problem, which only adds to your frustration.

Let's face it. Life is full of problems. No one is happy all the time. So how do you cope, when you have personal problems—as everyone does—and you have to go to work every day?

Contemporary Issues in Work–Life Balance

Health care presents unique challenges to its workers, who, like all workers, seek to balance work life with family and personal life and try to keep problems in one area from spreading to the other area. The health care industry places added demands on its workers because of the nature of the work. Patients cannot go without care, so mandatory overtime is required of some workers, and hours extend beyond the scheduled time as urgent issues demand attention. This state of emergency is absent from many other industries. Moreover, both single parents and young parents dominate most health care professions, and with the need for urgent and constant care for patients, it is easy to see why problems at work can spill over into the home, and problems at home become stressors at work.

Work as a Refuge from Your Personal Problems

Separating your personal problems from work can be relatively easy if you are successfully navigating both parts of your life and satisfied in both areas. In fact, many people find that work is therapeutic, or at least an escape from their personal problems. After all, you have friends at work who you look forward to seeing because they care about you and support you. However, maintaining such relationships does not mean that you should constantly burden your work friends with your problems. Recognize that if you can't do anything while you are at work to fix or improve your personal problems, you can use work as a chance to get away from your problems for a while.

Recognizing when You Have a Personal Problem at Work

Sometimes, however, your personal problems can spill over into work, leaving you at a significant disadvantage.

The first step in addressing such a problem is to recognize when it is affecting your mood. We all bring a long, deeply ingrained history of behavior patterns to work. Being able to assess your own mood takes work, commitment, and insight. You might not be able to help it, but you should at least recognize when your feelings about your personal problems are leaking over into your work.

Look for Patterns in Your Family History

One way to gain insight into your longstanding behavior patterns is to examine your family history. Specifically, what "invisible" role do you play in your family? What did your family think of you when you were growing up? Were you the responsible one? Were you the angry, resentful one? Were you the perfect child? Were you the rebel? If you can answer this question honestly, you have come a long way toward gaining insight into your behavior patterns. Box 13-1 offers some deeply ingrained patterns related

---

BOX 13-1

Behavioral Patterns in the Workplace

- *Super-achiever:* This person is talented but pursues success at the expense of relationships.
- *Rebel:* This person enjoys provoking others.
- *Procrastinator:* Everyone procrastinates to some extent, but this person easily makes promises but never delivers on deadlines.
- *Clown:* This person uses humor to defuse tension, but often may not be taken seriously.
- *Persecutors:* We know these people as bullies who intimidate and harass others.
- *Victim:* This person fears risk and scrutiny, and responds to negativity by complaining.
- *Rescuer:* This person can be helpful as long as other people's problems don't divert them from their own problems or work.

- *Drama Kings and Queens:* These people go to great lengths to receive any kind of attention, even if it is negative. They may elevate an event to a crisis to display their behavior patterns.
- *Martyr:* This person rarely refuses more work or a chance to be helpful, while secretly feeling underappreciated.
- *Pleaser:* Fearful of conflict and disapproval, this person appreciates clear direction and avoids controversy.
- *Avoider:* This person avoids dealing with problems or addresses problems passive-aggressively.
- *Denier:* Concerned with how things appear to outsiders, this person ignores problems.
- *Splitter:* This person quietly plays one person against another and then observes the conflict.

Modified from LaFair S: *Don't bring it to work,* San Francisco, 2009, Jossey Bass.

to families. Do you recognize one or more of these in yourself?

You might think especially about your relationship with your parents. Did you try to please them? Did you lack respect for them? Were you always disagreeing or fighting with them? Was one of them absent? For many people, their boss is a psychological surrogate for their parents. Do you see parallels between the way you treated your parents and the way you treat your supervisor?

These lifelong family patterns and roles can be so deeply ingrained in people that they automatically retreat to them in times of stress. It can be difficult to escape lifelong patterns while under the pressures of work.

 JOURNALING 13-1

What role did you play in your family? Explore how you demonstrate this role at work and in the rest of your life.

Triggers that Cause Personal Problems to Spill Over at Work

Work conditions and circumstances can resonate with your personal problems or remind you of them in ways that make you feel emotional. Perhaps a difficult person at work reminds you of a difficult person at home, and work seems like a continuation of your complicated personal life. In caring for a sick child, you might be reminded of the emotional attachments you have with your own child. If a co-worker treats you in a demeaning manner, or a patient is hostile toward you, it may take all your effort to avoid reacting as you would if you were confronted with the same behavior at home. Conversely, in today's economy, it is natural for these issues to trigger anxieties or arguments you are experiencing at home.

When Work Problems Cause Personal Problems

Just as work can be a therapeutic refuge from your personal problems, you can see home as a refuge from work problems. Usually, you cannot address work problems when you are not at work. You can only *worry* about work problems when you are not there. If you can, learn to use your commute as an effective transition period. Try to wrap up the problems of the work day and put them in the back of your mind.

Look forward to your home environment, even if it has its own problems.

Many people think the problems of work–life balance are caused by having too little time at home. However, it is usually an issue of attention. When you are home, give your personal life your complete and undivided attention. You will be more effective psychologically as an agent of change and progress in your personal life if you can simply be fully and mentally present by the time you arrive home. If you have children, they can tell if you are psychologically present. Whatever relationships you have at home, whether partners, roommates, or family members, they will benefit from your total attention. Ironically, when you can be totally engaged, whether you are at work or at home, you will have fewer problems in either place.

Finally, what if your boss demands your total commitment to work, and ignores the demands placed on you outside of work? You have two options. You can set limits on your work demands and educate your supervisor about the importance of work–life balance. If that proves unrealistic, you can find another employer who will see you as a person serving many roles in life. Fortunately, most health care employees understand the importance of balancing work and personal life. Trying to address the needs of your boss and the demands of your personal life simultaneously can lead to burnout.

When Personal Problems Become Serious Matters at Work

When personal problems become unresolved problems at work, negative behavior patterns can settle in. Such employees often become argumentative, sullen, rude, incommunicative, angry, uncooperative, and difficult to work with. They become known as "problem employees." Workplaces have definite response patterns in place to deal with problem employees.

Performance Improvement Plans

Usually, problem employees will have an opportunity to rectify their behavior to avoid termination. They will be presented with a "performance improvement plan," often called a "PIP." Usually crafted in a collaboration between the employee's manager and the Human Resources Department (if there is one),

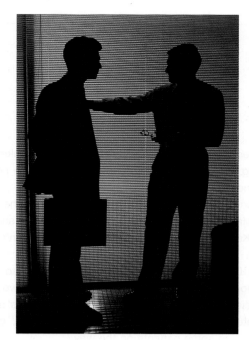

FIGURE 13-1 Employee receiving a performance improvement program (PIP). (From Proctor DB, Adams AP: *Kinn's the medical assistant: an applied learning approach*, ed 12, St Louis, 2014, Elsevier.)

the PIP will identify the problem behavior, prescribe expected behavioral improvements, and establish a deadline for progress, usually 30 or 60 days. Figure 13-1 shows a confidential discussion in which a manager places an employee on a PIP.

Performance improvement plans are confidential and serve as serious warnings. Employers do not want to spend their time micromanaging problem employees. They would rather inspire and motivate positive employees.

For some employees, a PIP serves as a wake-up call. They may be astounded that their behavior has gotten so out of control that it has come to this, and deeply search within themselves to address the issue.

? WHAT IF?

What if you were placed on a performance improvement plan? How would respond to that?

FIGURE 13-2 Balancing personal and work life.

Terminations

Employees in the vast majority of the United States are considered by the law to be "employees at will." That means as long as employers don't discriminate against you or treat you unfairly, they reserve the right to terminate you at any time. In most cases, people who lose their jobs are eligible for a certain amount of unemployment compensation. However, a person fired for reckless behavior cannot receive unemployment compensation.

A Final Word

In an ideal world, you will achieve a work–life balance that works just for you, because we are all unique. Ideally, you are a skilled, valued, and happy employee deriving enough satisfaction and income from your job that it allows you to pursue your personal and family goals with a clear mind and adequate resources. Work–life balance is always fluctuating and we all must work hard to restore this healthy equilibrium as seen in Figure 13-2. Our work–life balance is like our health, always seeking the homeostasis that will keep us healthy and achieve maximum results in the many roles we serve in our lives.

← JOURNALING 13-2

Describe the work–life balance you would like to achieve.

CASE STUDY 13-1
Holiday Spirit

It had been years since Paula had to work Christmas Eve, but this year it was unavoidable. There had been a big argument about working the holidays in the staff meeting, and somebody mentioned in a fit of anger that Paula hadn't worked the Christmas holidays in more than five years. "Who keeps track of that?" she had said, looking around the room to silent faces and averted eyes. "My daughter just turned two. Christmas is a big deal for a two-year-old." Still, no one spoke up.

"Don't fret," said her husband, Terry. "I'll bring Rosie over to the hospital before I put her to bed. You can take her down to the gift shop, and we'll all be together Christmas morning."

That made sense to Paula. She felt a little selfish objecting to the shift at the staff meeting. Everybody has to pitch in.

But by the time she arrived for her 3:00pm shift, the snow was coming down hard. Terry called to say he didn't think it would be a good idea to venture out with Rosie. Paula was disappointed, but she had to agree.

The snow kept coming as the evening wore on and the Director of Nursing asked the nurses to stay for the night shift. None of the night nurses could get their cars out of their garages, and the streets were mostly impassable. They would try to get them relief in the morning as soon as possible.

By 2:00 a.m., Paula and all the nurses were feeling fatigued. Paula was the most senior among the nurses, so she called a meeting. She thanked everyone for staying and providing such professional care. There were four of them,

and plenty of empty beds. She proposed they take turns working two hours, sleeping two hours. If anyone needed help, they could wake the sleepers.

Kenny volunteered to take the first shift. The other three let Paula sleep until 6:00. "You shouldn't have," she said when Kitty woke her up, but Kitty said the patients were all fine.

The Director called at 7:00 a.m. with more bad news. They hoped to get some relief by noon, but that would be the earliest. Paula felt like crying. She left the nurses' station and returned to the room where she had slept, quickly checking on some patients on the way.

In a few minutes, Kitty arrived with a surprise. Terry and Rosie had been up for about an hour and Kitty had called Terry to coordinate a mini–video conference with their cell phones.

Rosie showed her mother all the things that Santa had brought. When they hung up, Paula gave Kitty a big hug. "It's still early, Kitty, but you made my day!"

QUESTIONS FOR THOUGHT AND REFLECTION

1. Did Paula let her personal problems get the better of her at work?
2. How did the co-workers' kindness toward one another help them all get through the long shift together?
3. List examples of Paula's professionalism.
4. If you were Paula, would this be a Christmas to remember?

Down a Dark Road

Dr. Williamson got an earlier flight home from the medical convention and decided to drop by the office to catch up after his three-day absence. The receptionist greeted him nervously and glanced down the hall toward his office. Dr. Williamson checked to see that his office was locked, and opened it with a turn of a key. He was surprised to see that his medical assistant, Marianne Kolodny, was sitting in his chair and talking on his phone.

"I gotta go," she said, alarmed, and hung up. She stood up, as if at attention. "I...I...I was just talking to, um, my son's day care. It was private. I didn't think you would mind."

"I do mind, Marianne. This is completely inappropriate." He stood aside as Marianne rushed past him and out of the office.

"Thanks for the warning, Jill," she said to the receptionist.

Everybody knew that Marianne's marriage was disintegrating. Marianne talked endlessly about how difficult her husband, Marco, was. She was hoping she would not see the doctor before she could leave in a half-hour. She looked around the waiting room. Only one elderly gentleman was there, apparently waiting for someone.

"Do you know a good divorce lawyer?" she asked him.

He was so startled he could hardly mumble that he did not.

"Because I'm going to need one," she went on. "I have reason to suspect my husband is unfaithful, and even my three-year-old son seems afraid of him. He never talks to me," she said. "That's why I talk to strangers."

Just then, Dr. Williamson entered the room with a broad smile. "Carl, I didn't know you were here."

"I'm just waiting for Alice. She's getting some blood drawn."

"Do you know my medical assistant, Marianne?" he asked in his courtly manner.

"She works here?" said Carl.

Dr. Williamson quickly recovered. "Now that you've retired from your law practice, Carl, you'll have more time for golf," he said with a smile. "Come on back. I just returned from Houston."

In a few minutes, the men returned to the lobby, along with Alice. When he came back in from walking them to their car, Dr. Williamson asked to speak with Marianne in his office.

The next morning, everyone was surprised to see that Dr. Williamson was already there. He usually came in at 9:00 on the dot. When everyone had arrived, he asked the staff to join him in the conference room. "I just wanted to let you all know, before you heard it elsewhere, that I've decided to let Marianne go. I'm sure we all appreciated her service, but I felt that it was time for her to move on."

QUESTIONS FOR THOUGHT AND REFLECTION

1. What kind of mood did Marianne create in the office when she talked about her personal problems?
2. Did Dr. Williamson seem to value professionalism? Why or why not?
3. Why was Carl surprised to learn that Marianne worked in the office?
4. Was it upsetting for the staff to learn that Marianne no longer worked there?
5. Did Dr. Williamson handle the news of her termination appropriately? Why or why not?

⭐ EXPERIENTIAL EXERCISES

1. Identify a colleague at work who will be candid with you. Ask your colleague to give you honest feedback on your mood, attitude, and body language.
2. During your commute, practice making the transition from home to work and from work to home.
3. Have you encountered a patient who reminded you of a difficult family member? Did your treatment of the patient reflect your opinion of your family member?
4. Think of times when you had to overcome emotions associated with personal problems while you were at work. Is work therapeutic for you?

♻ CROSS CURRENTS WITH OTHER SOFT SKILLS

READING AND SPEAKING BODY LANGUAGE: Pay close attention to how your emotions are reflected in your body language. (pp. 277-284)

DEALING WITH DIFFICULT PEOPLE: Make sure you are not the difficult person your co-workers have to deal with. (pp. 231-238)

CONTROLLING ANXIETY: Anxiety can take over your emotions and lead to negative outcomes. (pp. 356-361)

Managing Anger and Strong Emotions

Anger is a short madness.

—Horace

LEARNING OBJECTIVE 2: MANAGING ANGER AND STRONG EMOTIONS

- Gain insight into why people become angry.
- Learn how to control your anger.
- Learn how to respond to angry patients and co-workers.
- Respond effectively to an angry supervisor.

Anger is the lynchpin of strong emotions at work. Everybody gets angry from time to time. Most of the time, however, we regret becoming angry because it can damage relationships and take its toll on us physically and mentally. Plus, anger rarely leads to any improvement.

Anger is only one letter short of danger.

—Anonymous

Why People Become Angry

Most of the time, people become angry because they are hurt or frustrated. They may feel they have been treated unfairly or thoughtlessly, ignored, disappointed, or taken for granted. Anger, then, substitutes for a deeper hurt. Sometimes anger is justified. Someone didn't empty the sharps container, and now it is full again. Sometimes problems arise that don't have immediate or obvious solutions, and they cause a great deal of frustration.

◀── JOURNALING 13-3

Describe an occasion when you became angry at work. Were you justified, or did you overreact? Are you glad you got angry, or do you regret it? Would you handle the incident differently if you could do it over again?

Controlling Your Anger

Everybody gets angry sometimes, but nobody likes to feel out of control. Anger rarely solves problems or makes you feel better. As soon as you feel your anger rising, try to stop it with one or more of the following strategies.

* *Try your favorite relaxation technique.* Breathe deeply and visualize a peaceful image. Do some isometric exercises or stretches if possible.
* *Try reframing the situation.* Try not to jump to conclusions or use extreme language. It probably isn't the *worst* day of your life. Your friend is not *always* late. Instead, state the problem accurately. For example, "I'm upset because this is the third weekend I've had to work in a row."
* *Refocus with problem-solving techniques.* Complicated problems can be frustrating, especially if you're in a hurry. For example, a pediatric medication dosage may not always be easy to calculate. You don't know how to spell the word you are looking for, so it's taking you a long time to find. Combine deep breathing with a step-by-step approach, talking yourself through a complicated calculation or seeing if you can break the tricky term down into known word parts from your medical terminology courses.
* *Adopt positive communication strategies.* When we are angry, being heard and understood often helps. Likewise, it is important to be a good listener. By listening, we are less likely to say something that escalates the conflict. Don't forget to listen to yourself, too. Angry people often jump to unwarranted conclusions. Despite what you might be thinking, expressing your thoughts might make things worse. Try to convey understanding when having a difficult conversation.
* *Combine humor with insight to defuse anger.* Sometimes, self-deprecating humor can defuse your anger by helping you to gain a new perspective. Humor must be used delicately, however. Never use sarcasm or cynicism in an angry situation.
* *Change your environment.* Often, a change of scene can defuse anger. Try leaving the area where you became angry to reflect and regain your perspective.

When You Are Confronted with Someone Else's Anger

Angry people can be very intimidating. That is part of the often destructive power of anger. How you respond when confronted by an intimidating angry person can determine whether the situation gets better or worse.

What Doesn't Work

Some people "take the bait" of an angry person and respond with anger. Suddenly, it becomes a competition of who is the angriest or the most intimidating. Although strong emotions can be contagious, it is a mistake to meet anger with anger. Such a response escalates anger, rather than defusing it. Now *two* people are likely to say something they will soon regret. Confrontation, no matter how well intentioned, is rarely a constructive approach to an angry person.

> *Speak when you are angry and you will make the best speech you will ever regret.*
>
> —Ambrose Bierce

Dealing with Angry Patients

With most people, and particularly in response to angry patients, it is best to be empathetic and comforting (Figure 13-3). Try to listen and ask nonconfrontational questions or objective questions. "When did this happen?" "What did she tell you then?" If someone is really angry because they have been hurt, disappointed, or disrespected, they want to be understood and validated. If possible, agree with the person to validate that they have a right to their emotions. As

FIGURE 13-3 A receptionist listens to a complaining patient (Copyright © istock.com).

a health professional, you want to defuse the anger so constructive problem solving can occur.

You never understand a person until you consider things from his point of view.

—Harper Lee

JOURNALING 13-4

Recount a time when you dealt effectively with an angry patient or co-worker. What happened? How did you deal with it?

Dealing with Angry Co-Workers

Co-workers who exhibit proper business etiquette and learn to separate their work problems from their personal problems rarely display anger at work, unless anger is truly a justified and limited response to a specific intentional or thoughtless provocation. Unfortunately, not all of your co-workers will be so mature and professional.

An effective technique for dealing with difficult or emotional co-workers is to give them honest feedback. Some of the statements in Box 13-2 offer strategies for initiating productive conversations with co-workers under stress.

Very often, the co-worker's emotional state doesn't have anything to do with you. Asking a direct question about the source of the anger will often be all that is needed to help your co-worker refocus on his or her work. If your co-worker is upset with you for some reason, your question will get the matter on the table, so it can be addressed effectively.

Dealing with an Angry Supervisor

Sometimes supervisors think it is their right as the boss to express anger toward their team. Some

BOX 13-2

Questions to Elicit Honest Feedback From Emotional Co-Workers

- You seem angry. What are you angry about?
- Is there anything I can do to help you?
- Can you communicate with me to solve this problem?
- I feel bad that you are so upset. Have I made you upset?
- Can I have your engagement with this problem?
- Are you having a difficult day?
- Has something happened you want to tell me about?
- Are you angry at me, or just angry?

ineffective supervisors think anger is an appropriate management strategy or a motivational tool. If you are a supervisor, parent, or anyone in charge of someone else, you should seriously consider removing anger from your array of management tools.

It is tempting, if the only tool you have is a hammer, to treat everything as if it were a nail.

—Abraham Maslow

Nevertheless, as workers, we are sometimes confronted by an angry supervisor. You hope that the supervisor's angry behavior is highly unusual. You recognize that managers get angry sometimes just like everybody else. If your manager is rarely angry, you want to be empathetic and helpful, so listen and respond in the same way you would respond to an angry patient.

If your supervisor is angry frequently or seems especially angry toward you, select a strategy that puts an end to your boss's outbursts. As always, confrontation is not the way to go, particularly in a public place.

WHAT IF?

What if your supervisor embarrassed you in public? How would you respond?

If you have an ongoing concern about the way your supervisor treats you, make a private appointment with her and give her the same direct feedback you would offer to an emotional co-worker. This tactic may be enough to end the abuse. At the very least, it will lead to a mature discussion of the issues your supervisor may have with you.

Forgiveness and Letting Go

Many people misunderstand what forgiveness means. They refuse to forgive someone for their actions or mistakes. It is liberating when you can truly get past what someone did to you, and forgive them without holding a grudge. Everyone makes mistakes, and you will be perceived as an understanding member of your team if you are able to treat your co-workers compassionately through your forgiveness.

For every minute you are angry, you lose sixty seconds of happiness.

—Ralph Waldo Emerson

CASE STUDY 13-2
Lifetime Achievement

Molly Griffin was a speech therapist and was having a difficult time communicating with the administrative medical assistant, Lou. He had received a poor performance evaluation from the office manager, Kenosha Cooper, and still seemed mad about it. Although his cubicle was directly across the hall from Molly's office, he sent her a series of emails instead of speaking to her in person as he had done before his evaluation.

She walked over to his cubicle. "Lou, could you please share these kinds of messages with me in person, as you always have?"

"Soooo, that would be one way I could improve my communications with the staff?"

"Sure," Molly said.

In her 9:00 meeting with the business manager, Walter Everts, Molly discussed the following year's budget.

"We've got a huge problem, here," said Walter, passing out a spreadsheet. "Our budget will be $600,000 less next year."

Molly scrutinized the spreadsheet. "It says here that the cut is $60,000, Walter," she said.

"You're right, Molly. Who constructs a spreadsheet in increments of hundreds?"

"It's just a mistake," said Molly.

"Well, they're cutting us by $60,000, and that's a huge problem."

Molly smiled. "Well, Walter, it's one-tenth the problem it was a few minutes ago."

"What, you think we can cut $60,000 in paper clips?"

"Let's look elsewhere."

The meeting ended on an upbeat note and Walter agreed that they might be able to eliminate the problem with minor cuts and some revenue increases.

Molly used the time freed up by her 11:00 cancellation to catch up on her paperwork. She also wrote a note to Walter thanking him for his ideas at the meeting. She was early for her lunch with her supervisor, Margaret Ong.

"I can't believe you're actually early," said Margaret.

Molly had never been late, but she made a mental note to erase that perception by making an extra effort to be on time, especially around Margaret.

"Molly, I have some bad news. I nominated you for the Frank R. Kleffner Award, and you didn't get it."

"That's it? You nominated me for an ASHA award, and I didn't get it?"

"I'm sorry, Molly. You deserved it."

"Margaret, if you nominated me, then I'm already a winner. Thank you."

Margaret was relieved that Molly took the news so well.

The last appointment in Molly's schedule that day was for a new patient, Mr. Kaulawi, who had suffered a stroke the previous week and was experiencing aphasia. Molly introduced herself.

Mr. Kaulawi said something that most people wouldn't have been able to understand.

"You can't talk?" asked Molly.

Mr. Kaulawi was surprised that she could understand him, but she had heard the phrase many times before.

"That's not a problem," Molly said, "Let's get started."

Before she left that afternoon, Molly checked out the Frank R. Kleffner Award on the ASHA web site. It was an award for lifetime achievement in the communications disorders professions. Molly smiled to herself. She was barely 30.

QUESTIONS FOR THOUGHT AND REFLECTION

1. In what ways does Molly demonstrate resilience?
2. What provocations does Molly choose to ignore?
3. How did Molly make Mr. Kaulawi feel welcome?
4. How did Molly's optimism help get her through her day?

Down a Dark Road

Management at the assisted living facility brought in a new director to cut costs and streamline operations. Peter Harmon was put in charge of both of the facilities and reported to the owner, Dr. Houdek. "Everybody's job is on the line," he announced in his first meeting with the staff.

He flashed a notebook and a red pen. "Now, I want to get everyone's views on what we can do to reduce costs and increase services. Say what's on your mind." No one spoke.

Pretty soon, however, a voice came over the speakerphone. It was Jeff, the Recreational Therapist at the Greene Street facility. He was advocating for combined field trips because there was plenty of room on the bus and it would be a good social opportunity for the two facilities. Pretty soon, Peter was rolling his eyes. Finally, he jammed the mute button on the phone as Jeff continued outlining his ideas. "I really can't make out what that guy is saying," said Peter, "but he's clearly clueless." He interrupted Jeff. "Field trips cost money. We're not doing that. Any other ideas?"

"I didn't think that was such a bad idea," said Eve.

"Oh, you don't, Miss?" said Peter.

"Deming," she said. "Eve Deming."

"So what's *your* big idea?" said Peter.

"I don't have an idea. I just thought Jeff—"

"Miss Deming. No ideas. Anyone else?"

"I don't think I like your attitude," Eve pressed on.

"Oh, you don't have any ideas, but you don't like my attitude," he said. "Well, here's the deal, Miss Deming. We're going to make some big changes around here."

QUESTIONS FOR THOUGHT AND REFLECTION

1. How would you describe Peter?
2. What efforts did Peter make to intimidate his new staff?
3. Do you think that, in being this provocative, Peter was hoping that someone would challenge him?
4. Should Eve have taken the bait?
5. In your opinion, what should Eve have done? What were her options?

⭐ EXPERIENTIAL EXERCISES

1. Keep track of the number of negative thoughts, inaccurate assessments, unkind evaluations, and mental insults you make about other people during the course of an entire day. If you can, write them down so you can look at them and reevaluate them the next day.
2. What kind of anger would you tolerate from someone else? Does it matter who the person is? At what point would you walk away from the person, refusing to subject yourself to further abuse? Where do you draw the line, personally?
3. For an idea of how destructive anger can be, watch the film *The War of the Roses* with Michael Douglas and Kathleen Turner.
4. Pretend to get angry and shout at yourself in a mirror. What do you see? Would you be intimidating to others? Unpleasant? Ugly? Scary?
5. Avoid challenging an angry person by locking eye contact with him, by focusing at a spot low on his forehead just between his eyes. Try this out with a friend. Tell each other what it felt like.

🔄 CROSS CURRENTS WITH OTHER SOFT SKILLS

MODELING BUSINESS ETIQUETTE: A well-mannered employee can command respect in the workplace without ever being angry or difficult. (pp. 170-178)

SHOWING EMPATHY, SENSITIVITY, AND CARING: Empathy is the best way to disarm an angry patient or co-worker. (pp. 218-222)

DEALING WITH DIFFICULT PEOPLE: Emotional people can be difficult. (pp. 231-238)

PRACTICING PATIENCE: A thoughtful, patient, considered response defuses many emotional situations. (pp. 361-364)

Exuding Optimism, Enthusiasm, and Positivity

I wish I could show you, when you are lonely or in darkness, the astonishing light of your own being.

—Hafiz of Shiraz

LEARNING OBJECTIVE 3:
EXUDING OPTIMISM, ENTHUSIASM, AND POSITIVITY

- State the benefits of optimism.
- Understand the limitations and strengths of pessimism.
- Connect optimism with good health.
- Relate goal achievement to optimism.

We can view optimism and pessimism as ways to explain life. We are either optimists who believe that the world is good at its core, and good things await us. Or we are pessimists who believe that the world is a hostile place with danger lurking everywhere. These pervasive explanations have been part of us since we were small, driven into us by the attitudes of our parents and teachers.

If something bad happens to an optimist, that person sees the incident as a product of specific circumstances and a learning opportunity. Optimists expect things to go well for them, and with astounding consistency, they do.

If something good happens to a pessimist, that person sees that as a lucky break in a bleak world and the product of circumstances not likely to reoccur. Pessimists expect things to go wrong, so they usually do.

← JOURNALING 13-5

Write about two instances in your life, one when you gave up more easily than you should have, and one when you were resilient in the face of a challenge. Which characteristics did you display in each of these instances? Would you choose one of your "selves" over the other?

Both optimism and pessimism are more than self-fulfilling prophesies. These attitudes actually influence the small and large outcomes in your life. As psychologist Martin Seligman announced in the title of his best-known book, *Learned Optimism*, optimism can be learned. Review 25 benefits of optimism in Box 13-3. Why wouldn't everyone want to be an optimist, especially now that we know you can learn to be one?

BOX 13-3

Benefits of Optimism

- It enables you to generate an alternative, more hopeful explanation for difficulties experienced.
- It reduces your level of stress.
- It increases longevity.
- It promotes happiness.
- It forges persistence, which is an essential trait required for achieving success.
- It creates a sense of fulfillment and satisfaction.
- It promotes healthy living.
- It creates a positive anticipation of the future.
- It allows you to deal with failure and mistakes constructively.
- It makes you proactive.
- It enables you to deal with the constant negative thoughts that arise.
- It increases the likelihood of effective problem solving.

- It creates a positive attitude.
- It increases your level of motivation.
- It promotes laughter.
- It welcomes any form of constructive change.
- It creates positive expectations.
- It sets your mood for the day.
- It promotes positive relationships.
- It builds resilience in the face of adversity.
- It promotes self-confidence and boosts self-esteem.
- It improves your social life.
- It increases your spiritual development and awakening.
- It increases your mental flexibility.
- It is therapeutic.

Why Some People Are Pessimists

Many people were raised as pessimists. Their parents and teachers indicated that the world is a hostile place full of negative experiences. They take their bad luck personally, which attracts more bad luck. In their world, the deck is stacked against them, and they are helpless to do anything about it.

If it wasn't for bad luck, I wouldn't have no luck at all.
—William Bell

The Benefits of Pessimism

Studies show that pessimists tend to be more realistic in their assessment of a situation than optimists. This means that optimists sometimes overlook obstacles when making and pursuing plans. Optimists can learn from their pessimistic counterparts by analyzing all sides of a situation carefully, listening with an open mind to opposing views, and being skeptical when appropriate. A balanced view of what optimists can learn from pessimists is suggested in Box 13-4. Still, even if pessimists and optimists fully agree on their analysis of a situation, optimists are much more likely to succeed because they don't view the obstacles as major setbacks. They see themselves as innovators searching for hidden angles and insights.

The Downside of Pessimism

Martin Seligman, a prolific optimism researcher from the University of Pennsylvania, a past president of the American Psychological Association, and a founder of the Positive Psychology movement, has discovered some rather startling facts about the dangers of being pessimistic. His research has shown that pessimistic people are eight times more likely to suffer from depression than optimistic people.

In addition, pessimists lead shorter lives than optimists and suffer from more illnesses. The cause of this gap is still being explored, but it is clear that depression lowers immune function. Some studies suggest that people who feel helpless are more susceptible to cancer and fare much more poorly in fighting disease and infection. Pessimists are also less likely to seek medical help early or social support later.

Pessimists have essentially accepted that fate is working against them, and that the best they can do is avoid uncertainty by playing it safe. As a result, they set goals that are easily attainable.

> **? WHAT IF?**
>
> *What if you accomplished something great, and you overheard someone say you didn't deserve it? What would your self-talk sound like?*

Benefits of Optimism

Optimists advance quicker than pessimists and lead richer lives with more experiences, friends, and opportunities. They are resilient in the face of adversity.

Resilience and Perseverance

Optimists don't take failures personally, and they don't view setbacks as permanent. They try to learn from their experiences, confident that with renewed energy and strategies, they can overcome even big obstacles. Optimists are more likely to succeed simply because success requires the perseverance and resilience that an optimistic explanation of events provides. As illustrated in Figure 13-4, the way you view an event influences the outcome.

Health

Evidence shows that an optimistic outlook strengthens the immune system. Optimistic people believe their fate is in their own hands and pursue healthier lifestyles. They eat a balanced diet and exercise regularly. They seek help from health care professionals when they have health concerns, and they seek support from friends when they are dealing with problems. By being proactive about their health, optimists possess physical resiliency and positive health outcomes.

BOX 13-4

What Optimists Can Learn from Pessimists

- Analyze situations to uncover risks and obstacles.
- Evaluate risks realistically.
- Know when to cut your losses and move on.
- Pay attention to safety-related issues.
- Be open-minded.
- Be flexible rather than blind.
- Sympathize with those going through hard times.

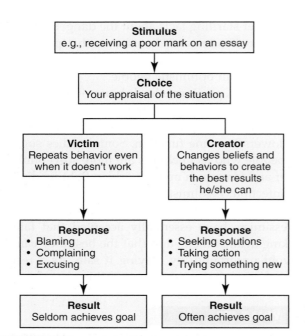

FIGURE 13-4 How two responses to an event can influence the outcome.

Accomplishment, Happiness, and Meaning

Optimistic people, as captains of their own fates, place few limits on themselves. They set high goals and believe in their ability to achieve them. Achieving your goals adds happiness and meaning to your life. Optimism is virtually synonymous with happiness.

You can either be an actor in your own life, or a reactor in somebody else's.

—Hillary Rodham Clinton

How to Be an Optimist

Some people are hesitant to be optimistic. They are not quite sold on it. They may feel that optimistic people are naïve or foolishly hopeful. Living enthusiastically and optimistically will yield success in every area of your life, from work to family.

The hardest challenge is to be yourself in a world where everyone is trying to make you be somebody else.

—E. E. Cummings

Self-talk

Self-talk can be either your best asset or your worst critic. Being optimistic involves *choosing* optimism and adjusting your attitudes and self-talk accordingly. What you say when you talk to yourself matters tremendously. You don't blame yourself for making a mistake, you learn from it. You don't call it a failure if something doesn't work. It just means you have to try another approach. You keep telling yourself that, if you take command of your circumstances, set goals, and make plans, things will improve.

Enthusiasm

Enthusiasm gives you the energy to do things well. Enthusiasm is based on the belief that effort, energy, and engagement lead to results. Much like optimism, enthusiasm is a choice. To be enthusiastic, *act* enthusiastic. Energy drives its own rewards.

Positivity

Positivity keeps your focus on the future you want to achieve. Positive expectations lead to positive results. This is not just because positivity is a self-fulfilling philosophy. Instead, it is also because anything you undertake with a positive attitude will move you toward your goal. People like positive people, and they want to help them. Just think about your own workplace. Isn't it more rewarding to be part of the enthusiastic, high-energy, and positive crowd?

Whether you think you can, or whether you think you can't, you're right.

—Henry Ford

CASE STUDY 13-3
Health Care for Science and Humanity

Lucinda studied anthropology because it interested her, but even she had to admit that there were not a lot of obvious employment opportunities for someone with an anthropology degree. Lucinda decided to enroll in a medical assisting certificate program, which she could complete in one year.

Lucinda got a job as soon as she graduated. Within three years, Lucinda had been promoted to operations management in the Emergency Department. She was frequently asked to join task forces and committees, support new initiatives, and participate in community outreach programs. As far as her own department was concerned, she was a presence on all three shifts, and she knew every single team member. In order to make others aware of all of the great opportunities in health care, Lucinda developed a plan to reach out to high school students.

First, she did a lot of research. She interviewed guidance counselors and principals at the nine major high schools in the city, to share her ideas and solicit theirs. She reviewed all the statistics she was given about graduation rates, employment, college attendance, and a full array of other postsecondary options ranging from trade schools to union apprenticeships to the military.

She also researched the resources available at the hospital and drafted a proposal, which she presented in a quarterly meeting. The VP for Administration, Bob Lake, suggested she get someone from the business office to examine the costs. Lucinda also recruited the support of Kim Delancey, the Director of Public Relations.

Initially, her colleagues raised many objections. The business office in particular opposed her ideas because they would be costly. But Lucinda worked with Kim to show how much money could be saved in recruiting, labor, and volunteer costs with the program. Kim was willing to co-sponsor the program as a project of her Public Relations Office. Eventually, many were on board, and others dropped their objections. In the fall, Lucinda and Kim rolled out the new program, branded "Health Care for Science and Humanity," with an internal promotion program. Representatives of all 42 health professions signed on as volunteers.

Lucinda set up Health Care Career Fairs at local high schools. The volunteers staffed booths labeled with each profession or group of professions, and talked to students about careers and opportunities and passed out literature. The program was a big success at the schools, and there was a lot of positive press about the hospital and the program.

For the second year of the program, Lucinda sent surveys to over 400 stakeholders, including the volunteers, key stakeholders at the hospital, high school officials, and students. She recruited area career colleges and also some vendors who worked closely with the hospital, to expand the number of careers included and also connect students with educational opportunities. She also invited medical equipment reps to demonstrate the latest technology, including software applications.

It never occurred to Lucinda that this was the kind of initiative that the Employee-of-the-Year Committee had been looking for over the past few years. The award usually went to prominent clinicians, so Lucinda was surprised to receive the honor for her Health Care for Science and Humanity initiative.

QUESTIONS FOR THOUGHT AND REFLECTION

1. What did Lucinda do that was more than required of her in her position at the hospital?
2. What did Lucinda do in the face of opposition?
3. What benefits did the Health Care for Science and Humanity create?
4. Why did Lucinda work to make a good program even better?

Down a Dark Road

Fairmont Hospital was very fortunate to find a health information management professional like Connie Derderian. She had a background in software development and computer programming and thought that all health care facilities would have to move to electronic health records (EHR) eventually. Fairmont was about to install an EHR system, but their main concern was the lack of expertise to test, install, and maintain the system. It was as if Connie was a feature that came with the software.

In fact, Connie's hiring was a real positive for Don Kendall, the CIO and Chief Privacy Officer, because he could easily imagine all the nightmares that a poorly implemented EHR system could cause in terms of functionality, security, and the internal reputation of his department. He made Connie a good offer and gave her a generous budget.

After three weeks, when Don saw that Connie's office was just about as bare as the day she moved in, he broached the topic with her. "Not planning to stay long?" he asked her in a half-joking way.

She just looked at him.

"Your office," he said, waving his hand. "It doesn't look like anyone works here."

"Oh," she said. "I'm pretty moved in."

"No calendars, art, pictures of the family?"

"All of that stuff is electronic these days, Don. I'm pretty moved in."

Don found it difficult to connect with Connie. One day he offered to put her on the committee that planned the holiday activities at the hospital. He thought she might meet and connect with some people if she got out and about in a more social setting.

"I don't think so, Don. We're at a critical stage in the implementation. I don't think we want to screw this up."

Don was at a loss. The job wasn't just technical. It required some leadership skills. So he decided to appoint her as the manager for three of the programmers.

"These guys aren't working on EHR, Don."

"I know that, Connie. They work on all different kinds of software projects all over the hospital. Wouldn't it be interesting to learn more about the environment here?"

"Yes. I would like to learn more about the other systems, because we'll have to integrate the EHR eventually. Maybe I could go to a class, though, or maybe the guys could just make a presentation for me."

"Well, I need a manager for them, and you are the logical choice."

"I don't think I could do it. I never managed anyone before, and I think I should stick to the EHR, don't you think?"

A week later, Don told her she was going to the AHIMA convention with him.

"I don't know if I can take the time, Don."

"Yes, you can," he said. "You're definitely going."

At the convention, Connie went to the functions Don planned for her but otherwise stayed in her room. When she didn't arrive at the exhibit hall on the third day, Don called her room. She said she was sick and needed to return home right away. She wasn't even sure she could fly. She said it was her stomach. Maybe it was her gallbladder or appendix. Don called an ambulance for her right away.

QUESTIONS FOR THOUGHT AND REFLECTION

1. What kinds of risks was Connie willing to assume?
2. What is it about Connie that Don couldn't understand?
3. Why wouldn't Connie assume any extra responsibilities?
4. Were you surprised when Connie became ill?

⭐ EXPERIENTIAL EXERCISES

1. See a health care professional, whether a dentist, a massage therapist, or a pharmacist, as soon as possible about a health concern you have been putting off.
2. Volunteer somewhere that interests you.
3. Dispute a pessimistic belief that you have.
4. Draw a line on a piece of paper and label the left end "pessimistic" and the right end "optimistic." Put the names of your friends, family members, and co-workers at the place on the continuum where you think they fit.

CROSS CURRENTS WITH OTHER SOFT SKILLS

ADOPTING A POSITIVE MENTAL ATTITUDE: Optimism is the best attitude to adopt. (pp. 2-11)

THINKING CRITICALLY: Critical thinking suggests that the many benefits of optimism make it the obvious attitude choice. (pp. 320-325)

SETTING GOALS AND PLANNING ACTIONS: Optimism makes significant goal achievement possible. (pp. 286-291)

STRENGTHENING RESILIENCE: Any attitude that strengthens your immune system strengthens your resilience. (pp. 364-368)

UNIT VI

GO FORTH AND PROSPER

CHAPTER 14

Go Forth and Prosper

THEMES TO CONSIDER	■ Expect acceptance for yourself and accept all others without hesitation.
	■ Plan for success.
	■ Project confidence from deep down inside of yourself.
	■ Respect yourself.

Expect Acceptance

I long to accomplish a great and noble task, but it is my chief duty to accomplish small tasks as if they were great and noble.

—Helen Keller

LEARNING OBJECTIVE 1: EXPECT ACCEPTANCE

■ Understand, give, and expect acceptance.
■ Learn how to plan for success.
■ Recall skills taught in this text.

If you live to be 70 years old, you have been given a few more than 25,500 days. How you live them is up to you. A good place to start is to expect acceptance from everyone and to give your acceptance to others.

? WHAT IF?

What if you lived to be 100 years old? What can you do today and in the coming days to make that 100th birthday party the incredible experience you deserve?

Your success at work depends as much on who you are as a person as it does on your credentials and or your skills. No matter how well educated you are, you still have to be someone who treats patients, clients, and customers respectfully and empathetically. No matter how skillful you are in performing the most difficult procedures in your profession, you still have to be someone your co-workers want to spend eight hours a day with, day after day. No matter how high your grades were in school, or how high you scored on your licensing or certification exam, your supervisor wants you to be someone who is respectful, open to learning and coaching, and an example for your co-workers.

Be the best person you can be and expect acceptance for it. As executive coach D.A. Benton put it, "Forget your blushing, sweating, trembling, and shaking as you expect and give acceptance. Ignore the heart palpitations from dealing with intimidating people, the embarrassment in talking to strangers, the fear of authority, or the possibility that someone may criticize you."

Relate to the people in your life as if you are in traffic, assuming you are a courteous driver. As Figure 14-1 demonstrates, you don't know who is driving the car in front of you, whether it is a police officer, your boss, your neighbor, your friend's grandmother, or a celebrity. You should treat them all with courtesy as you all follow the rules of the road. Apply this philosophy to your workplace. Why wouldn't you give acceptance to everyone?

FIGURE 14-1 Interact with others as if you were all in traffic together, without knowing who is in each car (Copyright © istock.com).

You were hired based on your credentials, abilities, and soft skills. Live up to this acceptance every single day on the job.

You experience your world from the inside out. Everyone else experiences your world from the outside in. Just because someone else looks confident from the outside doesn't mean they are without any insecurities. Make sure the "outside" you, the "you" that others see, projects confidence and assurance. If you feel nervous, don't announce it. If you are intimidated, demonstrate courage. Expect acceptance.

Whatever we expect with confidence becomes our own self-fulfilling prophecy.

—Brian Tracy

Plan for Success

You are embarking on a brand new phase of life. This is no time for coasting. Instead, start the rest of your life right now by using what you have learned in this book to set goals for yourself, make a concrete plan to achieve them, and become the best person you can be. Commit now to setting high standards for yourself at work and in your life. With a solid plan in place, you will meet your targets as seen in Figure 14-2. Your success and happiness depend on this plan and your efforts to stick to it.

FIGURE 14-2 Looking toward your goals by following a plan will help you hit your targets.

Rules of Thumb

We revisit some of the main insights in this book, listed in Box 14-1. If you integrate these and other positive practices into your work life, and you have good clinical and work skills, you will be a highly valued employee and enjoy work. You will be appreciated by your patients and your supervisor, and you will make friends among your co-workers.

Not knowing when the dawn will come, I open every door.

—Emily Dickinson

You are a very special person who has chosen a career in health care. Congratulations, and thank you. You can be incredible.

CASE STUDY 14-1

Big Rocks

Charlie was only 25, but he had just earned a promotion at work. He was glad he decided to get a bachelor's degree as a laboratory technologist with a minor in management. Later, he planned to go to graduate school to study cell biology, pharmacology, or pathology.

In his new position, he would be managing fifteen lab techs in the pathology lab. Although Charlie was a whiz in clinical chemistry, he was most proud of his people skills because he thought that managing people would end up being more important to his success than anything else.

When he learned that he would be promoted, the first thing Charlie did was set up a dinner with his grandfather. Charlie's grandfather was retired from a long career as an engineer and an inventor, and Charlie admired him greatly.

Charlie's grandfather, whose name was also Charles, accepted Charlie's invitation and told Charlie to pick him up at 6:00.

When Charlie arrived, his grandfather was working at the carpenter's bench in his garage. Charlie had spent many happy hours in this place with his grandfather when he was growing up.

"Wha'cha doin', Grandpa?" asked Charlie.

"Oh, just thinking about you, and your career, and all the success you're going to have. The 21st century is a wonderful time to be young, Charlie."

"Wha'cha got there?" asked Charlie.

"This is a five-gallon jar with a big wide mouth," he said, answering Charlie's question literally.

"What are you going to use it for?"

"To find out something."

"An experiment?"

"Yup." His grandfather had an assortment of big rocks, and he proceeded to fill up the jar with the rocks. "Now, Charlie," he said. "Is this jar full?"

"Yes," said Charlie, puzzled at the obvious.

His grandfather took a big galvanized scooper, went out to the driveway, and scooped up a large amount of gravel. Charlie followed him back into the garage, and his grandfather emptied the scoop into the jar, shaking the jar to get the gravel to the bottom and all around the bigger rocks. "Full now?" said his grandfather.

"Yup," said Charlie.

His grandfather went to a corner of the garage and hefted a large sack of sand he used for winter traction. He started pouring the sand into the jar, again shaking it down to fill the jar completely. "Full now?

Charlie laughed. "I guess it is now!"

His grandfather took a bucket, went over to the zinc sink, and filled it with water. Carefully, he poured the water into the jar all the way up to the top. He looked at Charlie.

"What do you make of that?"

Charlie thought for a moment. "Well, I guess it means that there's always room for more in your schedule and in your life."

"Hmmm. Let's go to dinner. I'm getting hungry."

They got the same booth they had when Charlie's grandfather took him there shortly after Charlie's twenty-first birthday.

Charlie answered his grandfather's questions about his new job, and said how he hoped to be like his grandfather, inventing new biomaterials and new manufacturing processes, but for now, he wanted to learn more about the end users, and how to manage people successfully.

"Managing people successfully, Charlie. That's a high goal," said his grandfather. His grandfather gave Charlie lots of tips and advice about how to handle his new job. "Expect acceptance," his grandfather told him, "and treat everybody as an equal, including the higher-ups."

When the check came, Charlie grabbed it, and his grandfather let him. On the way home, Charlie said, "So that wasn't the right answer, about the jar. You can always fill your life with more stuff."

"Well, that wasn't bad," said his grandfather, "but that's not the lesson."

"So …?"

"Put the big rocks in first."

QUESTIONS FOR THOUGHT AND REFLECTION

1. What are the big rocks you want to be sure and put in your jar of life?
2. When is the best time to choose the big goals you want to achieve in life and start working on them?
3. Do you agree with Charlie that people skills are the most important?
4. In your opinion, will Charlie achieve his aspirations?

Down a Dark Road

It was Jessica's third week on the job at the pharmacy, and she didn't like it. She had been late a couple of times in the second week, and her boss yelled at her. She was fed up with this guy, and she decided to let her Facebook friends know. On Monday after work, she wrote this message:

"OMG. Almost late again!! No time for shower. Ick!!! Bossman says time 2 learn new program for med pharm. Boring!!! Then it CRASHED. ☺ He acted like I did it! Another great day on the job!"

By Tuesday, a lot of her friends had responded to her post, so she wrote another one:

"YIKES!!! Pulling my hair out today. Bossman gave me 80 scripts 2 fill. Customers all ancient fossils, kept alive on DRUGS!!! LOL."

On Wednesday, Jessica awoke to more comments on her Facebook page, so she wrote another post:

"New rules today. No tongue rings allowed??? Ugh!"

Thursday was really a bad day for Jessica. She was late again, and the pharmacist said it was her last chance. He would let her go if she was late once more. Jessica stewed all day. She was so tired by the end of the day that she decided to take a nap before going out with her friends. But before she lay down, she wrote her Facebook post for the day:

"I hate my job. Bossman is an IDIOT!! Need 411 on NEW JOB!! He wants 2 fire me!!! Keyed his car on way out!!! ☺"

When she was getting ready to party, she decided to check her Facebook page once more and found this surprising post: "Did you forget you friended me? Since you have apparently already resigned, there is no need for you to come in tomorrow. Your things will be in a box at the front desk. BOSSMAN."

QUESTIONS FOR THOUGHT AND REFLECTION

1. Why didn't Jessica like her job as a pharm tech?
2. Were her online posts about work inappropriate, or should she be allowed to say whatever she thinks?
3. What is Jessica's opinion on rules?
4. Based on her posts, name at least three reasons that could be used to justify Jessica's termination.

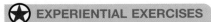 **EXPERIENTIAL EXERCISES**

1. If you ever talk to a person in a wheelchair, kneel down so they can look you straight in the eye. The next time you talk to someone who is higher up than you, think how grateful you are to be able to look them straight in the eye.
2. Talk to somebody you respect about the aspirations you have for your career and your life.

 CROSS CURRENTS WITH OTHER SOFT SKILLS

ADOPTING A POSITIVIE MENTAL ATTITUDE: Adopting a positive attitude will take you far. (pp. 2-11)

Bibliography

Benton DA. *Executive charisma*, New York, 2003, McGraw-Hill, p. 22.

INDEX